MR Imaging of the Shoulder

Editors

NAVEEN SUBHAS
SOTERIOS GYFTOPOULOS

MAGNETIC RESONANCE IMAGING CLINICS OF NORTH AMERICA

www.mri.theclinics.com

Consulting Editors
SURESH K. MUKHERJI
LYNNE S. STEINBACH

May 2020 • Volume 28 • Number 2

ELSEVIER

1600 John F. Kennedy Boulevard • Suite 1800 • Philadelphia, Pennsylvania, 19103-2899

http://www.mri.theclinics.com

MRI CLINICS OF NORTH AMERICA Volume 28, Number 2
May 2020 ISSN 1064-9689, ISBN 13: 978-0-323-79088-8

Editor: John Vassallo (j.vassallo@elsevier.com)
Developmental Editor: Kristen Helm

Magnetic Resonance Imaging Clinics of North America (ISSN 1064-9689) is published quarterly by Elsevier Inc., 360 Park Avenue South, New York, NY 10010-1710. Months of issue are February, May, August, and November. Business and Editorial Offices: 1600 John F. Kennedy Blvd., Ste. 1800, Philadelphia, PA 19103-2899. Customer Service Office: 3251 Riverport Lane, Maryland Heights, MO 63043. Periodicals postage paid at New York, NY and additional mailing offices. Subscription prices are $404.00 per year (domestic individuals), $773.00 per year (domestic institutions), $100.00 per year (domestic students/residents), $437.00 per year (Canadian individuals), $1007.00 per year (Canadian institutions), $550.00 per year (international individuals), $1007.00 per year (international institutions), $100.00 per year (Canadian students/residents), and $275.00 per year (international students/residents). International air speed delivery is included in all *Clinics* subscription prices. All prices are subject to change without notice. **POSTMASTER:** Send address changes to *Magnetic Resonance Imaging Clinics*, Elsevier Health Sciences Division, Subscription Customer Service, 3251 Riverport Lane, Maryland Heights, MO 63043. Customer Service (orders, claims, online, change of address): Elsevier Health Sciences Division, Subscription **Customer Service, 3251 Riverport Lane, Maryland Heights, MO 63043. Tel:1-800-654-2452 (U.S. and Canada); 314-447-8871 (outside U.S. and Canada). Fax: 314-447-8029. E-mail: journalscustomerservice-usa@elsevier.com (for print support); journalsonlinesupport-usa@elsevier.com (for online support).**

Reprints. For copies of 100 or more of articles in this publication, please contact the Commercial Reprints Department, Elsevier Inc., 360 Park Avenue South, New York, NY 10010-1710. Tel.: 212-633-3874; Fax: 212-633-3820; E-mail: reprints@elsevier.com.

Magnetic Resonance Imaging Clinics of North America is covered in the *RSNA Index of Imaging Literature, MEDLINE/PubMed (Index Medicus),* and *EMBASE/Excerpta Medica.*

Contributors

CONSULTING EDITORS

SURESH K. MUKHERJI, MD, MBA, FACR
Clinical Professor, Marian University, Director,
Head and Neck Radiology, ProScan Imaging,
Regional Medical Director, Envision Physician
Services, Carmel, Indiana, USA

LYNNE S. STEINBACH, MD, FACR
Emeritus Professor of Radiology on Full Recall,
Department of Radiology and Biomedical
Imaging, University of California, San
Francisco, San Francisco, California, USA

EDITORS

NAVEEN SUBHAS, MD, MPH
Associate Professor, Department of Diagnostic
Radiology, Musculoskeletal Division, Imaging
Institute, Cleveland Clinic, Cleveland, Ohio, USA

SOTERIOS GYFTOPOULOS, MD, MSc
Associate Professor, Radiology and
Orthopedic Surgery, NYU Langone Health,
New York, New York, USA

AUTHORS

ERIN F. ALAIA, MD
Assistant Professor, Department of Radiology,
Musculoskeletal Division, NYU Langone
Health, NYU Langone Orthopedic Hospital,
New York, New York, USA

DOMENICO ALBANO, MD
IRCCS Istituto Ortopedico Galeazzi, Milano,
Italy; Sezione di Scienze Radiologiche,
Dipartimento di Biomedicina, Neuroscienze e
Diagnostica Avanzata, Università degli Studi di
Palermo, Palermo, Italy

FAYSAL ALTAHAWI, MD
Staff Musculoskeletal Radiologist, Cleveland
Clinic Foundation, Cleveland, Ohio, USA

LUIS BELTRAN, MD
Department of Radiology, Brigham and Women's
Hospital, Boston, Massachusetts, USA

SAMY BOUAICHA, MD
Faculty of Medicine, University of Zurich,
Department of Orthopaedic Surgery, Balgrist
University Hospital, Zurich, Switzerland

CHRISTOPHER J. BURKE, MBChB
Department of Radiology, NYU Langone
Health, NYU Langone Orthopedic Center,
New York, New York, USA

CONNIE Y. CHANG, MD
Division of Musculoskeletal Imaging and
Intervention, Department of Radiology,
Massachusetts General Hospital, Boston,
Massachusetts, USA

FILIPPO DEL GRANDE, MD
Department of Radiology, Ospedale
Regionale di Lugano, Lugano,
Switzerland

**TERENCE PATRICK FARRELL, MB BCh,
BAO, MRCPI, FFRRCSI, FRCRUK**
Clinical Musculoskeletal Radiology
Fellow, Department of Radiology,
Thomas Jefferson University Hospitals,
Radiology Admin, Philadelphia,
Pennsylvania, USA

DAVID C. GIMARC, MD
Assistant Professor, Department of Radiology,
University of Colorado School of Medicine,
Aurora, Colorado, USA

SOTERIOS GYFTOPOULOS, MD, MSc
Associate Professor, Radiology
and Orthopedic Surgery, NYU
Langone Health, New York,
New York, USA

JAMES THOMAS PATRICK DECOURCY HALLINAN, MBChB
Department of Diagnostic Imaging, National University Health System, Yong Loo Lin School of Medicine, National University of Singapore, Singapore, Singapore

BRADY K. HUANG, MD
Department of Radiology, University of California, San Diego School of Medicine, UCSD Teleradiology and Education Center, San Diego, California, USA

JAD S. HUSSEINI, MD
Division of Musculoskeletal Imaging and Intervention, Department of Radiology, Massachusetts General Hospital, Boston, Massachusetts, USA

KENNETH S. LEE, MD
Professor, Department of Radiology, University of Wisconsin-Madison School of Medicine and Public Health, Madison, Wisconsin, USA

MARC LEVIN, MD
Department of Radiology, Mt. Auburn Hospital, Cambridge, Massachusetts, USA

ERIN McCRUM, MD
Division of Musculoskeletal Imaging, Clinical Instructor, Department of Radiology, Duke University Medical Center, Duke University, Durham, North Carolina, USA

CARMELO MESSINA, MD
IRCCS Istituto Ortopedico Galeazzi, Dipartimento di Scienze Biomediche per la Salute, Università degli Studi di Milano, Milano, Italy

JOSHUA M. POLSTER, MD
Associate Professor, Cleveland Clinic Lerner College of Medicine, Cleveland Clinic Foundation, Cleveland, Ohio, USA

TATIANE CANTARELLI RODRIGUES, MD
Department of Radiology, NYU Langone Health, NYU Langone Orthopedic Center, New York, New York, USA

DAVID A. RUBIN, MD, FACR
All Pro Orthopedic Imaging Consultants, LLC, St Louis, Missouri, USA; Radsource, Brentwood, Tennessee, USA; NYU Langone Medical Center, New York, New York, USA

MOHAMMAD SAMIM, MD, MRCS
Department of Radiology, NYU Langone Orthopedic Hospital, New York, New York, USA

LUCA MARIA SCONFIENZA, MD, PhD
IRCCS Istituto Ortopedico Galeazzi, Dipartimento di Scienze Biomediche per la Salute, Università degli Studi di Milano, Milano, Italy

CHRISTOPH STERN, MD
Radiology, Balgrist University Hospital, Faculty of Medicine, University of Zurich, Zurich, Switzerland

NAVEEN SUBHAS, MD, MPH
Associate Professor, Department of Diagnostic Radiology, Musculoskeletal Division, Imaging Institute, Cleveland Clinic, Cleveland, Ohio, USA

RETO SUTTER, MD
Radiology, Balgrist University Hospital, Faculty of Medicine, University of Zurich, Zurich, Switzerland

ADAM ZOGA, MD, MBA
Professor, Department of Radiology, Thomas Jefferson University Hospitals, Sidney Kimmel Medical Center, Vice Chair for Clinical Practice, Director of Musculoskeletal MRI, Philadelphia, Pennsylvania, USA

Contents

> MR imaging is the standard diagnostic modality that provides a comprehensive and accurate assessment for both osseous and soft-tissue pathologic conditions of the shoulder. This article discusses standard MR imaging and arthrography protocols used routinely in clinical practice, as well as more innovative sequences and reconstruction techniques, facilitated by the increasing availability of high-field-strength magnets and multichannel phased array surface coils and incorporation of artificial intelligence. These exciting innovations allow for a more detailed and diagnostic imaging assessment, improvements in image quality, and more rapid image acquisition.

> The cause of rotator cuff tears is multifactorial with both intrinsic and extrinsic contributing factors. Understanding the normal MR anatomy of the rotator cuff and using an appropriate search pattern can help readers identify common pathologic conditions. Accurate designation using classification systems for tear thickness, size, and degree of retraction and muscle fatty infiltration and atrophy are important in guiding surgical management. Knowledge of common disease locations for the rotator cuff tendons can help focus reader searches and increase sensitivity.

> MR imaging interpretation following rotator cuff repair can be challenging and requires familiarity with various types of rotator cuff tear, their surgical treatments, normal postoperative MR imaging appearance, and complications. This article reviews the common surgical procedures for the reparable and nonreparable massive rotator cuff tears, their expected postoperative MR imaging findings, and imaging appearance of a range of complications.

> Most first-time anterior glenohumeral dislocations occur as the result of trauma. Many patients suffer recurrent episodes of anterior shoulder instability (ASI). The

anatomy and biomechanics of ASI is addressed, as is the pathophysiology of capsulolabral injury. The roles of imaging modalities are described, including computed tomography (CT) and MR imaging with the additional value of arthrography and specialized imaging positions. Advances in 3D CT and MR imaging particularly with respect to the quantification of humeral and glenoid bone loss is discussed. The concepts of engaging and nonengaging lesions as well as on-track and off-track lesions are examined.

Posterior shoulder instability is often hard to diagnose with clinical examination. Patients generally present with vague pain, weakness, and/or joint clicking but less frequently complaining of frank sensation of instability. Imaging examinations, especially MR imaging and magnetic resonance arthrography, have a pivotal role in the identification and management of this condition. This review describes the pathologic micro/macrotraumatic magnetic resonance features of posterior shoulder instability as well as the underlying joint abnormalities predisposing to this condition, including developmental anomalies of the glenoid fossa, humeral head, posterior labrum, and capsular and ligamentous structures.

MR imaging of the postoperative shoulder after instability surgery is challenging. The radiologist must be familiar with surgical procedures, altered anatomy, and expected postoperative findings for correct interpretation of normal findings versus a true pathology. Artifacts from metallic hardware or abrasions further complicate MR image interpretation, but are reduced with metal artifact reduction techniques. This article focuses on capsulolabral surgery, bone block transfers, and humeral bone loss procedures in patients with shoulder instability and their postoperative imaging evaluation. Surgical procedures and common complications are explained, and normal and pathologic postoperative imaging findings are presented.

In this article, the authors aim to focus on the challenges of interpreting shoulder MR imaging in the throwing athlete with an approach formed by evidence-based literature and clinical experience, with a particular focus on superior labrum tears.

The capsular and ligamentous structures of the glenohumeral joint are important for stability of the shoulder. These structures are best evaluated by MR imaging. Familiarity with normal and abnormal appearance of the capsular structures of the shoulder is important to ensure that important pathology is not overlooked. Injury to the capsular structures can occur in the setting of trauma and most commonly involves the inferior glenohumeral ligament and axillary pouch. Adhesive capsulitis is a common inflammatory condition with characteristic imaging features that should be considered in the absence of alternative diagnoses.

Terence Patrick Farrell and Adam Zoga

Acromioclavicular joint (ACJ) pathology is a common source of shoulder girdle pain, frequently coexisting with and sharing overlapping clinical features of rotator cuff and glenohumeral articular lesions. ACJ trauma and osteoarthritis dominate clinical presentation; however, an array of pathologies can affect the joint. MR imaging of the ACJ is a powerful secondary diagnostic tool in early diagnosis of ACJ pathology and in accurate assessment of ACJ injuries, helping to resolve clinically challenging cases and allowing for individualized treatment planning. Knowledge of ACJ anatomy, biomechanics, and pathology is fundamental to interpreting and providing a clinically relevant ACJ MR imaging report.

David A. Rubin

Muscle atrophy in shoulders with rotator cuff tendon tears is a negative prognosticator, associated with decreased function, decreased reparability, increased retears after repair, and poorer outcomes after surgery. Muscle edema or atrophy within a neurologic distribution characterizes denervation. Because most nerve entrapments around the shoulder are not caused by mass lesions and show no nerve findings on routine MR imaging sequences, pattern of muscle denervation is often the best clue to predicting location of nerve dysfunction, which narrows the differential diagnosis and guides clinical management. The exception is suprascapular nerve compression in the spinoglenoid notch caused by a compressing cyst.

James Thomas Patrick Decourcy Hallinan and Brady K. Huang

This article discusses the most common tumor and tumor-like lesions arising at the shoulder. Osseous tumors of the shoulder rank second in incidence to those at the knee joint and include benign osteochondromas and myeloma or primary malignant lesions, such as osteosarcoma or chondrosarcomas. Soft tissue tumors are overwhelmingly benign, with lipomas predominating, although malignant lesions, such as liposarcomas, can occur. Numerous tumor-like lesions may arise from the joints or bursae, due to either underlying arthropathy and synovitis (eg, rheumatoid arthritis and amyloid) or related to conditions, including tenosynovial giant cell tumor and synovial osteochondromatosis.

David C. Gimarc and Kenneth S. Lee

Imaging evaluation of the shoulder is performed using multiple modalities, including ultrasound (US) and MR imaging. Clinicians often wonder which modality to use to work up their patients with shoulder pain. Although MR imaging has remained the workhorse of shoulder imaging, US has increased in popularity among academic and private institutions. Both modalities offer similar diagnostic information in regards to rotator cuff pathology and other soft tissues, although they differ in their technique, indications, and interpretation. A thorough understanding of these differences is imperative to appropriately use these modalities in clinical practice, including the unique interventional opportunities available with US.

MAGNETIC RESONANCE IMAGING CLINICS OF NORTH AMERICA

VISIT THE CLINICS ONLINE!
Access your subscription at:
www.theclinics.com

PROGRAM OBJECTIVE
The goal of *Magnetic Resonance Imaging Clinics of North America* is to keep practicing physicians up to date with current clinical practice by providing timely articles reviewing the state of the art in patient care.

TARGET AUDIENCE
All practicing physicians and healthcare professionals who provide patient care utilizing findings from Magnetic Resonance Imaging.

LEARNING OBJECTIVES
Upon completion of this activity, participants will be able to:
1. Review the anatomy, pathology, and imaging findings seen in the most common conditions affecting the shoulder.
2. Discuss clinical applications of shoulder MRI and improve diagnostic accuracy and improve patient outcomes.
3. Recognize the clinical value of shoulder MRI as the imaging modality of choice for select shoulder pathologies.

ACCREDITATION
The Elsevier Office of Continuing Medical Education (EOCME) is accredited by the Accreditation Council for Continuing Medical Education (ACCME) to provide continuing medical education for physicians.

The EOCME designates this journal-based CME activity enduring material for a maximum of 12 *AMA PRA Category 1 Credit*(s)™. Physicians should claim only the credit commensurate with the extent of their participation in the activity.

All other healthcare professionals requesting continuing education credit for this enduring material will be issued a certificate of participation.

DISCLOSURE OF CONFLICTS OF INTEREST
The EOCME assesses conflict of interest with its instructors, faculty, planners, and other individuals who are in a position to control the content of CME activities. All relevant conflicts of interest that are identified are thoroughly vetted by EOCME for fair balance, scientific objectivity, and patient care recommendations. EOCME is committed to providing its learners with CME activities that promote improvements or quality in healthcare and not a specific proprietary business or a commercial interest.

The planning committee, staff, authors and editors listed below have identified no financial relationships or relationships to products or devices they or their spouse/life partner have with commercial interest related to the content of this CME activity:
Erin F. Alaia, MD; Domenico Albano, MD; Faysal Altahawi, MD; Luis Beltran, MD; Samy Bouaicha, MD; Christopher J. Burke, MBChB; Connie Y. Chang, MD; Filippo Del Grande, MD; Terence Patrick Farrell, MB BCh, BAO, MRCPI, FFRRCSI, FRCRUK; David C. Gimarc, MD; Soterios Gyftopoulos, MD, MSc; James Thomas Patrick Decourcy Hallinan, MBChB; Brady K. Huang, MD; Jad S. Husseini, MD; Marilu Kelly, MSN, RN, CNE, CHCP; Pradeep Kuttysankaran; Marc Levin, MD; Erin McCrum, MD; Carmelo Messina, MD; Suresh K. Mukherji, MD, MBA, FACR; Joshua M. Polster, MD; Tatiane Cantarelli Rodrigues, MD; David A. Rubin, MD, FACR; Mohammad Samim, MD, MRCS; Luca Maria Sconfienza, MD, PhD; Lynne S. Steinbach, MD, FACR; Christoph Stern, MD; Naveen Subhas, MD, MPH; Reto Sutter, MD; John Vassallo; Adam Zoga, MD, MBA.

The planning committee, staff, authors and editors listed below have identified financial relationships or relationships to products or devices they or their spouse/life partner have with commercial interest related to the content of this CME activity:
Kenneth S. Lee, MD: research support from General Electric Company, DePuy Mitek Inc., and Supersonic Imagine; royalties from Elsevier.

UNAPPROVED / OFF-LABEL USE DISCLOSURE
The EOCME requires CME faculty to disclose to the participants:
1. When products or procedures being discussed are off-label, unlabelled, experimental, and/or investigational (not US Food and Drug Administration [FDA] approved); and
2. Any limitations on the information presented, such as data that are preliminary or that represent ongoing research, interim analyses, and/or unsupported opinions. Faculty may discuss information about pharmaceutical agents that is outside of FDA-approved labelling. This information is intended solely for CME and is not intended to promote off-label use of these medications. If you have any questions, contact the medical affairs department of the manufacturer for the most recent prescribing information.

TO ENROLL
To enroll in the *Magnetic Resonance Imaging Clinics of North America* Continuing Medical Education program, call customer service at 1-800-654-2452 or sign up online at http://www.theclinics.com/home/cme. The CME program is available to subscribers for an additional annual fee of USD 260.00.

METHOD OF PARTICIPATION
In order to claim credit, participants must complete the following:

1. Complete enrolment as indicated above.
2. Read the activity.
3. Complete the CME Test and Evaluation. Participants must achieve a score of 70% on the test. All CME Tests and Evaluations must be completed online.

CME INQUIRIES/SPECIAL NEEDS

For all CME inquiries or special needs, please contact elsevierCME@elsevier.com.

Foreword
Shoulder Imaging

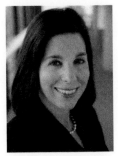

Lynne S. Steinbach, MD, FACR
Consulting Editor

I would like to thank editors, Naveen Subhas from Cleveland Clinic and Soterios Gyftopoulos from New York University, for spearheading this valuable state-of-the-art update on shoulder MR imaging. These leaders in musculoskeletal imaging are well known for their expertise in shoulder MR imaging, and they have chosen authors from around the globe who are at the top of their field for each section of the issue. The topics are timely and important for radiologists evaluating musculoskeletal shoulder imaging.

New advances in shoulder MR imaging and MR angiography techniques are an important subject in a review that includes innovative sequences and reconstruction techniques, issues with high-field-strength magnets and multichannel phased array surface coils as well as artificial intelligence. Assessment of the rotator cuff anatomy and pathologic condition by MR imaging is discussed along with a differential diagnosis and pitfalls. Imaging of anterior shoulder instability includes details about the challenging hot topic of engaging and nonengaging Hill-Sachs lesions that are on and off track. The less common posterior shoulder instability is

also comprehensively discussed in a separate article. The unique biomechanics of the thrower's shoulder leads to predictable pathologic condition that is succinctly reviewed. The postoperative shoulder reviews include new types of rotator cuff surgical treatment and repairs of the lesions of shoulder instability. More detailed evaluation of capsular and ligamentous trauma, the acromio-clavicular joint, nerve and muscle abnormalities, shoulder tumors, along with an important discussion of how to choose between shoulder MR imaging and ultrasound rounds out the issue.

This issue is a timely reference for shoulder imaging. Fantastic work, editors and authors!

Lynne S. Steinbach, MD, FACR
Department of Radiology and
Biomedical Imaging
University of California, San Francisco
505 Parnassus
San Francisco, CA 9413-0628, USA

E-mail address:
lynne.steinbach@ucsf.edu

Magn Reson Imaging Clin N Am 28 (2020) xi
https://doi.org/10.1016/j.mric.2020.02.002
1064-9689/20/© 2020 Published by Elsevier Inc.

Preface
MR Imaging of the Shoulder

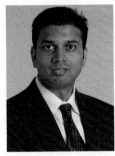

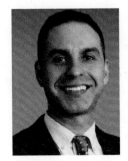

Naveen Subhas, MD, MPH   Soterios Gyftopoulos, MD, MSc
Editors

In this issue of *Magnetic Resonance Imaging Clinics of North America*, we are delighted to provide you with an update on shoulder MR imaging. The articles are written by experts in the field, and they not only review the current literature and latest advances in the field but also provide practical tips that are useful in daily clinical practice.

We begin with an update on the current state of shoulder MR and MR angiographic imaging. Drs Alaia and Subhas provide a comprehensive review of current MR imaging practices for the shoulder along with updates on recent technological advances and their clinical utility.

One of the most common indications for shoulder MR imaging is for the evaluation of rotator cuff pathologic condition. Dr McCrum discusses the pathophysiology of rotator cuff disease and highlights clinically relevant imaging features and pitfalls when evaluating the rotator cuff. In the next article, Drs Samim and Beltran discuss the normal postoperative appearance and complications after standard rotator cuff repair as well as postoperative imaging after newer techniques, such as patch graft augmentation and superior capsular reconstruction.

Evaluation of shoulder instability is another frequent indication for MR imaging. This broad and important topic is discussed over 3 articles in this issue. Drs Burke, Rodrigues, and Gyftopoulos discuss what to look for in the setting of anterior instability with a review of soft tissue injuries that can result in instability and the role and value of MR imaging for the evaluation of bone loss. In the next article, Drs Albano, Messina, and Sconfienza discuss what to look

for in the setting of posterior instability, a less common but increasingly recognized source of instability. In the last of these 3 articles, MR imaging after instability surgery is reviewed by Drs Stern, Bouaicha, Del Grande, and Sutter with helpful tips of the normal postoperative appearance and complications that may arise after soft tissue repairs and bone augmentation procedures.

Shoulder MR imaging is the imaging modality of choice in evaluating shoulder pain in throwing athletes. Drs Altahawi and Polster discuss how to recognize the normal adaptive changes and imaging abnormalities that are unique to this population.

A wide range of pathologic conditions outside of the rotator cuff and labrum can be causes of shoulder pain. Drs Husseini, Levin, and Chang provide a review on an increasingly important symptom generator in the shoulder, the joint capsule. This article provides a comprehensive overview of the anatomy, pathologic condition, and imaging findings seen in the most common conditions affecting the glenohumeral joint capsule along with pearls to improve your diagnostic accuracy.

Drs Farrell and Zoga discuss the most common ailments of the acromioclavicular joint and how MR imaging can provide useful information that impacts clinical care.

Nerve-related muscle pathologic conditions remain one of the most difficult conditions to diagnose, with MR imaging becoming an increasingly popular tool utilized by clinicians to help with these patients. Dr Rubin provides a comprehensive overview of how MR imaging can help you

Magn Reson Imaging Clin N Am 28 (2020) xiii–xiv
https://doi.org/10.1016/j.mric.2020.02.001
1064-9689/20/© 2020 Published by Elsevier Inc.

understand and more accurately characterize the nerve-related shoulder muscle pathologic conditions commonly seen in everyday practice.

Drs Hallinan and Huang provide a detailed review of how MR imaging can provide clinical value in the diagnosis of shoulder tumor and tumorlike conditions.

Although the focus of this issue is on shoulder MR imaging, shoulder ultrasound can be a useful complement to MR imaging. Drs Gimarc and Lee discuss how both MR imaging and ultrasound can be used to evaluate the patient with shoulder pain. This review includes the strengths and limitations of each modality as well as the appropriate indications for each imaging tool.

We would like to thank all of the authors for their contributions to this issue and hope that you enjoy reading this update on shoulder MR imaging.

Naveen Subhas, MD, MPH
Department of Diagnostic Radiology
Cleveland Clinic
9500 Euclid Avenue
Cleveland, OH 44195, USA

Soterios Gyftopoulos, MD, MSc
Radiology and Orthopedic Surgery
NYU Langone Health
333 East 38th Street
New York, NY 10016, USA

E-mail addresses:
subhasn@ccf.org (N. Subhas)
Soterios.Gyftopoulos@nyulangone.org
(S. Gyftopoulos)

Shoulder MR Imaging and MR Arthrography Techniques: New Advances

Erin F. Alaia, MD[a],*, Naveen Subhas, MD, MPH[b]

KEYWORDS

• Shoulder • MR imaging • MR arthrography • Techniques • Accelerated imaging • 3D imaging

KEY POINTS

- An accelerated shoulder MR imaging protocol, obtained with parallel imaging technique, is feasible, diagnostic performance comparable with that of a standard protocol.
- Artificial intelligence holds promise for improvement in image quality, speed of image acquisition, and tissue segmentation in shoulder MR imaging.
- ABER images increase diagnostic yield for Perthes lesions, but have the risk of engaging a Hill-Sachs lesion while in the scanner.
- Techniques such as SEMAC and MAVRIC have improved postoperative shoulder image quality, with ultrasonography being a good alternative modality.

CURRENT STATUS OF SHOULDER MR IMAGING AND MR ARTHROGRAPHY
Introduction

MR imaging is the standard diagnostic modality that provides a comprehensive and accurate assessment for both osseous and soft-tissue pathologic conditions of the shoulder. This article discusses standard MR imaging and arthrography protocols used routinely in clinical practice, as well as more innovative sequences and reconstruction techniques, facilitated by the increasing availability of high-field-strength magnets, multichannel phased array surface coils, and incorporation of artificial intelligence. These exciting innovations allow for a more detailed and diagnostic imaging assessment, improvements in image quality, and more rapid image acquisition.

Equipment

At the authors' institutions, most routine shoulder MR imaging examinations are performed on either a 1.5-T or 3-T system, using a multichannel phased array shoulder coil to obtain the best signal-to-noise ratio and to accelerate the acquisition through the use of parallel imaging.

Shoulder MR Imaging: Standard Institutional Protocol

For the routine shoulder MR imaging protocol, the patient is placed supine on the scan table, with the body shifted to the contralateral side so that shoulder to be imaged is as close to the isocenter as possible. The arm is placed to the side and the hand is positioned in supination with the thumb facing outward, achieving a position of external rotation, with a sandbag placed over the hand to maintain position. The elbow is supported and secured to immobilize the arm in a comfortable externally rotated position, and a pad is placed within the shoulder surface coil to maximize signal and improve fat saturation (**Fig. 1**). When a shoulder coil cannot be used, as is often the case with larger or obese patients, a large multichannel

a Department of Radiology, Musculoskeletal Division, NYU Langone Health, NYU Langone Orthopedic Hospital, 301 East 17th Street, 6th Floor, New York, NY 10003, USA; b Department of Radiology, Musculoskeletal Division, Imaging Institute, Cleveland Clinic, 9500 Euclid Avenue, A21, Cleveland, OH 44195, USA
* Corresponding author.
E-mail address: Erin.Fitzgerald@nyumc.org

Magn Reson Imaging Clin N Am 28 (2020) 153–163
https://doi.org/10.1016/j.mric.2019.12.001

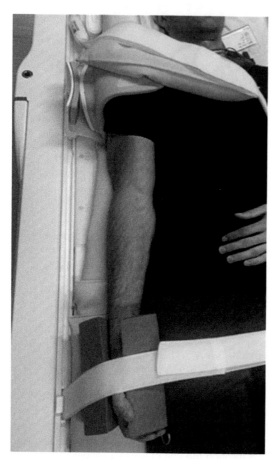

Fig. 1. Routine shoulder MR imaging setup, whereby the shoulder is placed within the dedicated shoulder coil in a position of external rotation, with the elbow supported and the hand in a supinated position.

phased array flexible coil is used, wrapped around the shoulder.

Axial images in mild obliquity are obtained with a reference line orthogonal to the articular surfaces of the glenohumeral joint on scout coronal images, scanning from just superior to the acromioclavicular joint to the inferior margin of the glenohumeral joint. Straight axial images are obtained for the Dixon 3-dimensional (3D) protocol, and occasionally used by some imaging centers in a routine shoulder protocol, covering a similar craniocaudal field of view in the axial plane, without a reference line orthogonal to the glenohumeral joint. Coronal plane images are obtained in mild obliquity, with the reference line orthogonal to the glenohumeral joint in the axial plane, scanning from the anterior margin of the subscapularis muscle to the posterior margin of the infraspinatus and teres minor muscles. Finally, sagittal images are obtained in mild obliquity, with the reference line aligned parallel to the glenohumeral joint on both coronal and axial images, scanning from the scapular body to the lateral margin of the humeral greater tuberosity, including the entirety of the rotator cuff insertion. This standard institutional protocol is presented in **Table 1**.

Accelerated Imaging: What Do We Compromise?

There are an increasing number of motivating factors for improving imaging speed, namely: operational efficiency (by increasing patient throughput), patient satisfaction (especially for claustrophobic and pediatric patients), and image quality (by reduction in motion artifact). Common techniques that have been used in musculoskeletal imaging for the purpose of improving imaging speed include isotropic 3D acquisition, parallel imaging, and, increasingly, machine learning.

Isotropic three-dimensional imaging

MR images obtained with 3D technique provide thin, contiguous slices, which have the potential to accelerate imaging speed, as a single acquisition with high-resolution (submillimeter) isotropic voxels may be reformatted in multiple planes. Isotropic 3D fast-spin echo (FSE) protocols of the knee have been developed in the hopes of improving imaging speed as well as diagnostic performance with reduction in partial volume averaging.[1] Diagnostic performance of an isotropic knee protocol, however, has been found to be inferior to a standard 2-dimensional (2D) FSE protocol with regard to diagnosis of meniscal tears,[2] has not surpassed standard 2D FSE sequences for the assessment of ligamentous disorder, and has increased sensitivity but lower specificity for articular cartilage defects,[3] limiting more widespread use in clinical practice. In addition, the long acquisition times required for obtaining a high-resolution 3D sequence makes them more susceptible to motion artifact than traditional 2D sequences.

Parallel imaging

Parallel imaging has become the mainstay of accelerated imaging, largely because of its increasing availability in modern MR systems, and the ability to use this technique with any MR imaging pulse sequence. Each phased array surface coil of a multichannel system samples local spatial information in parallel, affording time savings by decreasing the number of phase encoding steps.[4] Potential disadvantages of parallel imaging, including a reduction in signal-to-noise ratio (SNR) and acceleration artifact, are partially overcome by higher-field-strength magnets and multichannel surface coils available in clinical practice. Loss in signal, however, precludes acceptable

Table 1
Standard institutional parameters for routine shoulder MR imaging

Sequence	Plane	TR Range	TE Range	Slice Thickness (mm)	Field of View	Resolution	Acceleration Factor	Time (min:s)
PD FS	Axial oblique	3000	32	3	140	320 × 272	2	2:11
T2 FS	Coronal oblique	4000	54	3	140	320 × 256	1	3:02
T1	Sagittal oblique	747	12	3	140	320 × 240	2	2:22
PD TSE	Coronal oblique	3200	37	3	140	384 × 307	2	3:02
TSE T2 FS	Sagittal oblique	4600	53	3	140	320 × 240	1	3:01
Dixon	Straight axial	10	2.4/3.6 (TE^1/ TE^2)	1	200	192 × 100	2	3:28

Abbreviations: FS, fat saturation; PD, proton density; TE, echo time; TR, repetition time; TSE, turbo spin echo.

image quality at high acceleration factors.[3] For clinical use, acceleration with parallel imaging techniques is limited to a factor of 2.

Recently, the authors' institutions demonstrated that an accelerated shoulder protocol consisting of 4 2D multiplanar sequences using parallel imaging, completed at an average of 5 minutes 23 seconds at 3 T (62% reduction in image acquisition time) and 4 minutes 30 seconds at 1.5 T (71% reduction in image acquisition time), had comparable diagnostic performance with a standard nonaccelerated protocol.[2] At one author's institution, an accelerated protocol using parallel imaging consisting of 5 2D sequences requiring approximately 7 minutes is now used routinely in patients older than 50 years imaged on a 3-T magnet (**Fig. 2**). The other author's institution also uses an accelerated shoulder protocol, but not routinely, and only when a series needs to be repeated because of motion artifact, or if a patient has severe claustrophobia. Details of the institutional accelerated shoulder protocol are presented in **Table 2**.

Artificial intelligence and machine learning

Machine learning is increasingly coming to the forefront of musculoskeletal MR imaging, with potential to impact and improve everything from image acquisition, image interpretation, and quantitative image analysis.[5] For the purposes of increasing MR imaging speed, deep neural networks are trained through exposure to both fully sampled data with optimal image quality and accelerated images obtained with undersampled data and resultant poorer image quality. Deep neural networks learn how to best reconstruct highly undersampled data by comparing the image quality with that reconstructed from fully sampled data in an iterative fashion.[3] Machine learning acceleration techniques have the promise of allowing for much higher acceleration factors than with parallel imaging, with recent work presented by Subhas and colleagues[6] showing similar diagnostic performance in the knee with an acceleration factor of 6.

Shoulder MR Arthrography: Standard Institutional Protocol

Shoulder MR arthrography with direct intra-articular injection is performed most commonly in patients with a history of glenohumeral instability or other clinical suspicion for labral tear. First, the patient is taken to the interventional unit for direct glenohumeral joint intra-articular injection, which can be performed under ultrasound or fluoroscopic guidance. After intra-articular injection is completed, the patient is escorted to the MR imaging suite, with images acquired within 30 minutes following injection.

For a shoulder MR imaging arthrogram, the patient is placed in external rotation using the phase array surface coil, similar to the routine MR imaging protocol. Soft-tissue contrast is optimized on fat-suppressed T1-weighted images, not only between the contrast distended joint capsule and the subcutaneous fat but also between intra-articular gadolinium and cartilage.[7] Parameters for this standard institutional MR imaging arthrogram protocol are listed in **Table 3**.

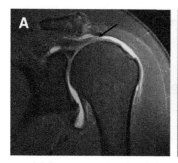 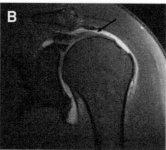

Fig. 2. Comparison of fast and routine shoulder MR imaging protocols. Coronal T2 fat-suppressed (FS) image obtained on a 3-T magnet, with routine shoulder protocol, in a 59-year-old man with shoulder pain after injury, demonstrating a full-thickness, retracted tear of the supraspinatus tendon (*arrow* in *A*). The full-thickness tendon tear (*arrow* in *B*) is also well demonstrated on a coronal T2 FS image obtained from the same patient using a fast protocol.

MR arthrography has been found to have high accuracy in the detection of most capsulolabral injuries[8] except for Perthes lesions, for which routine axial images are able to detect only 50% of tears.[8,9] In the abduction external rotation (ABER) position, however, the anterior band of the inferior glenohumeral ligament exerts traction on the anteroinferior capsulolabral complex.[10] This traction pulls the torn labrum away from the glenoid, displaying an otherwise potentially occult Perthes labral tear (**Fig. 3**). For the ABER series, the patient is taken out of the phased array surface coil and placed into a flex coil, with the arm positioned behind the head in abduction and external rotation (**Fig. 4**). Despite its clinical utility, ABER positioning has the potential for a Hill-Sachs lesion to engage while in the MR imaging scanner (**Fig. 5**), and as a result is not performed routinely at one of the authors' institutions.

Rarely an indirect shoulder arthrogram is performed, typically for patients unable to tolerate direct articular injection (ie, pediatric patients) or postoperative assessment, or in patients with inflammatory arthropathy. The robust vascularity intrinsic to the glenohumeral joint capsule permits indirect shoulder arthrography with the understanding that intravenous gadolinium will diffuse into the glenohumeral joint, which can be enhanced in patients with underlying pathologic synovitis, or after exercising the shoulder (**Fig. 6**).[11]

For the institutional protocol, the shoulder is exercised through repeated rotation, abduction, and adduction for approximately 10 to 15 minutes following the intravenous injection of 0.1 mL/kg of gadolinium contrast. Postcontrast images are acquired 15 to 20 minutes after injection. The major downside of indirect arthrography is the lack of substantial capsular distension when compared with direct injection. The pressure achieved by a distended joint capsule in the setting of direct arthrogram forces contrast into labral tears and increases diagnostic yield. For this reason, most of the referring providers prefer the direct technique, and indirect arthrography is not routinely performed at either of the authors' institutions.

CURRENT ADVANCED APPLICATIONS IN SHOULDER MR IMAGING AND MR ARTHROGRAPHY
Bone Modeling: Can MR Imaging Replace Computed Tomography?

2D and 3D MR imaging sequences can be used to evaluate bone anatomy, especially in the setting of

Table 2
Accelerated shoulder protocol

Sequence	Plane	TR Range	TE Range	Slice Thickness (mm)	Field of View	Resolution	Acceleration Factor	Time (min:s)
PD FS	Axial	2800	41	3	120	256 × 179	2	1:14
T2 FS	Coronal oblique	3580	51	3	120	256 × 179	2	1:06
T1	Sagittal oblique	600	8.5	3	120	256 × 166	2	1:05
PD TSE	Coronal oblique	2800	41	3	120	320 × 240	2	1:12
TSE T2 FS	Sagittal oblique	4100	57	3	120	256 × 166	2	1:11

Table 3
Standard institutional parameters for direct shoulder MR arthrogram

Sequence	Plane	TR Range	TE Range	Slice Thickness (mm)	Field of View	Resolution	Acceleration Factor	Time (min:s)
T1 FS	Axial	825	24	3	140	320 × 320	2	4:09
T1 FS	Coronal oblique	825	24	3	140	320 × 320	2	4:09
T1	Sagittal oblique	689	12	3	140	448 × 358	2	2:11
TSE T2 FS	Coronal oblique	4000	75	3	140	320 × 320	1	3:46
ABER	Axial oblique	825	24	4	140	320 × 320	2	4:09

shoulder instability and preoperative planning for shoulder arthroplasty, negating the need to obtain a concomitant computed tomography (CT) scan.

Isotropic high-resolution (submillimeter) 3D sequences, similar to thin-section CT, can be reformatted in different 2D planes to evaluate bone anatomy and can be postprocessed to produce images with "CT-like" contrast that can be used to generate 3D bone models. A 3D dual echo time T1-weighted FLASH sequence, with separation of water and fat using the technique originally described by Dixon,[12] can be used for evaluation of bone anatomy. In this technique, the water-only source images can be postprocessed to produce inverted subtraction images with signal-avid osseous structures and signal-void soft-tissue structures simulating CT contrast. The "CT-like" images can then be manually segmented using standard CT volume-rendering tools to generate 3D models of the proximal humerus and scapula (Fig. 7).[13] In a similar fashion, an isotropic high-resolution 3D fat-suppressed VIBE (volumetric interpolated breath-hold) sequence can also be used to produce "CT-like" 2D images and 3D bone models.[14,15] These 3D sequences are used in clinical practice at the request of the referring clinician, with Dixon image parameters outlined in **Table 1**.

With traditional MR sequences, osseous structures, in particular cortical bone, have little to no signal because of an inherent short T2 relaxation time. Ultrashort echo time and zero echo time (ZTE) imaging, however, can be used to acquire signal from bone and other short T2 structures by acquiring signal almost immediately after application of the radiofrequency pulse.[16] This results in an image with positive bone contrast similar to that in CT. An advantage of this technique is that postprocessing to create "CT-like" images easier than with the previously mentioned conventional MR imaging sequences because the acquired signal is only from short T2 structures such as bone. The major limitation is that it is still experimental and not currently available for routine clinical use.

Utility in Anterior Shoulder Instability

In patients with anterior shoulder instability, preoperative assessment includes standard MR imaging for the identification capsulolabral injury, articular cartilage defect, rotator cuff tear, and presence

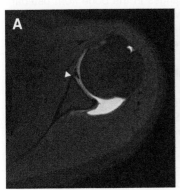
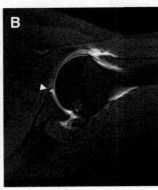

Fig. 3. Shoulder arthrogram demonstrating utility of abduction external rotation (ABER) view for Perthes lesion. (*A*) Axial T1 FS image of a 36-year-old woman, demonstrating no evidence of anteroinferior labral tear (*arrowhead*). (*B*) T1 FS ABER view of the same patient, demonstrating contrast imbibition of an otherwise occult anteroinferior labral tear (*arrowhead*).

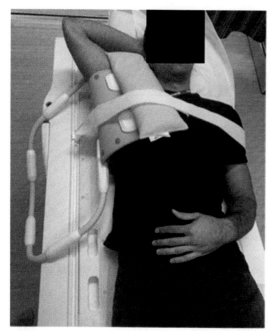

Fig. 4. ABER setup. The patient is positioned into a flex coil, with elbow flexed and hand placed behind the head.

of osseous injury, including Hill-Sachs lesion and glenoid fracture or bone loss. Patients with glenoid bone loss commonly undergo CT with 3D reconstruction, which is the current gold standard in preoperative assessment of glenoid bone loss,[17,18] and increasingly is being used for the assessment of bipolar bone loss, the combination of bone loss from both the anterior-inferior glenoid and the Hill-Sachs lesion. CT, however, is not ideal, requiring a separate appointment and radiation exposure. For these reasons, 3D reconstructions with MR imaging have been increasingly used for the assessment of glenoid bone loss and have been found to have similar diagnostic performance.[13,14,19]

Preoperative Planning for Shoulder Arthroplasty

Both MR imaging and CT of the shoulder are often obtained as part of the standard preoperative shoulder arthroplasty assessment. MR imaging is obtained to evaluate rotator cuff integrity and rotator cuff muscle atrophy, whereas CT is obtained to evaluate the degree of glenoid erosion and retroversion. As glenohumeral osteoarthritis evolves, biomechanical forces eccentrically increase contact pressure along the posterior glenoid rim, leading to posterior glenoid erosion, retroversion, and subsequent posterior translation of the humeral head. If not addressed at the time of arthroplasty, either with posterior glenoid augmentation or anterior glenoid reaming, the glenoid component is more predisposed to failure.[20] The criteria originally described by Walch and colleagues[21] are used clinically in the classification of glenoid morphology, with the most advanced B2 (biconcave glenoid) or C (dysplastic, severely retroverted) subgroups the most prone to failure if not adequately addressed. Although standard clinical assessment is with axial 2D CT images, Scalise and colleagues[22,23] have found 3D modeling to effectively demonstrate complex anatomy of the glenoid vault, serving as a reliable and accurate measure of glenoid erosion and retroversion. Axial 2D MR imaging for the assessment of glenoid retroversion has been found to be inferior to standard 2D CT in the more advanced Walch glenoid types B2 and C; thus, CT remains the diagnostic modality of choice.[24] Preliminary results using ZTE imaging for Walch classification and evaluation of cystic changes in the bone from osteoarthritis has, however, shown high and nearly identical inter-reader agreement with CT.[16] It is hoped that future studies will show similar diagnostic accuracy with 3D MR imaging to negate the need to obtain a preoperative CT.

POSTOPERATIVE IMAGING: CAN MR IMAGING BE USEFUL?
Role of MR Imaging in the Postoperative Shoulder

The role of MR imaging following shoulder arthroplasty has been previously limited, largely because

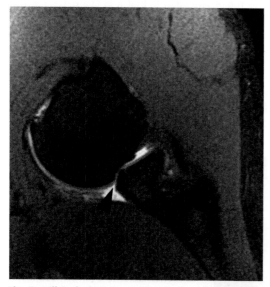

Fig. 5. Hill-Sachs lesion engaging in the ABER position. T1 FS ABER image of a 23-year-old man with recurrent dislocations, demonstrating engagement of a Hill-Sachs lesion along the anteroinferior glenoid (*arrowhead*).

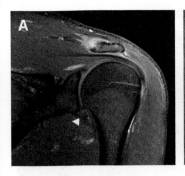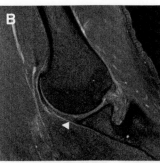

Fig. 6. Indirect shoulder arthrogram of a 23-year-old man for evaluation of labral tear. (*A*) Coronal T1 FS indirect arthrogram image demonstrates mild, likely physiologic enhancement of the glenohumeral joint capsule (*arrowhead*). Note lack of capsular distension with indirect technique. (*B*) T1FS ABER image of the same patient, demonstrating no evidence of anteroinferior labral tear (*arrowhead*).

of the susceptibility artifact produced by the prosthesis, degrading the regional osseous and soft-tissue structures, often precluding diagnostic evaluation of rotator cuff integrity. Because rotator cuff tear is a common complication following shoulder arthroplasty, diagnostic shoulder ultrasonography has been used as an alternative modality, useful not only for the diagnosis of rotator cuff tear but also for rotator cuff muscle atrophy, biceps disorder, and periarticular fluid collections.[25]

However, with the continual development and improvement of metal artifact reduction sequences and protocols, the role of MR imaging in the postoperative shoulder has recently expanded.

Standard Metal Artifact Reduction Techniques

In MR imaging of patients with orthopedic hardware, several standard techniques are used to minimize susceptibility artifact. Examinations are scheduled on the 1.5-T, not a 3-T magnet, to reduce image degradation and artifact inherent to imaging most hardware at higher field strengths. Pulse sequence selection is also important because certain sequences, namely gradient echo and frequency-selective fat-saturation pulse sequences, inherently magnify artifact generated from orthopedic hardware. When imaging patients with metal hardware, fat saturation instead is achieved with the short-tau inversion recovery (STIR) technique, which is less sensitive to field inhomogeneity. The frequency-encoding gradient is routinely oriented parallel to the long axis of hardware.[26]

At the authors' institutions, standard approaches for optimizing image quality in patients with metallic hardware include an increase in both turbo factor and bandwidth, an increase in number of excitations (to improve SNR), decreasing slice thickness, and switching from frequency-selective fat saturation to STIR.

Advanced Metal Artifact Reduction Techniques

The standard techniques to reduce metal artifact discussed earlier primarily focus on reducing in-plane artifact but do not reduce out-of-plane or through-plane artifact. Advanced metal artifact reduction (MAR) techniques, however, such as multiacquisition variable-resonance imaging combination (MAVRIC) and slice encoding for metal artifact correction (SEMAC), which are now available commercially, can, reduce both in-plane and through-plane resolution, thereby achieving a much greater degree of artifact reduction compared with conventional methods.[27] The MAVRIC technique acquires and combines multiple 3D FSE data sets at various frequency bands offset from the resonance frequency to minimize signal voids and signal pile-ups generated by orthopedic hardware.[28,29] Similarly, SEMAC acquires and combines multiple 2D FSE data sets above and below the excited slice with a slice-encoding gradient and view-angle tilting at readout to minimize through-plane and in-plane distortion from metallic hardware[30] (**Fig. 8**).

EMERGING TECHNIQUES: THE NEXT FRONTIER BEYOND MORPHOLOGY
Automated Tissue Segmentation

Tissue segmentation, which is used primarily in musculoskeletal imaging for the assessment of articular surfaces, is extremely time consuming when performed manually, requiring the user to scroll through an examination and manually segment each slice.[31] This time requirement, and the potential for poor reproducibility, has triggered interest in developing fully automated segmentation programs, which have been recently developed using deep convolutional neural networks (DCNNs). Fully automated tissue segmentation of knee osseous and articular surfaces with DCNNs has been shown to be both quick and accurate.[32,33] More recently, Gyftopoulos and colleagues[25]

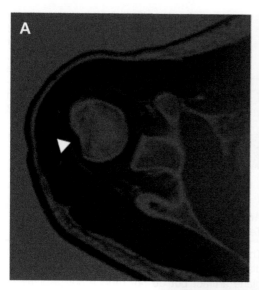
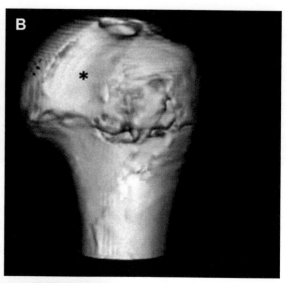
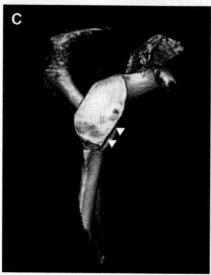

Fig. 7. Dixon technique for 3D shoulder MR imaging. (*A*) Axial subtracted Dixon image obtained from a 17-year-old man with shoulder instability, demonstrating signal-avid osseous structures, with Hill-Sachs lesion along the superior posterolateral humeral head (*arrowhead*). Manually 3D reconstructed images, obtained from Dixon source images, better demonstrate the Hill-Sachs lesion (*asterisk* in *B*) and anteroinferior glenoid bone loss (*arrowheads* in *C*).

demonstrated DCNNs to have high accuracy in automatic segmentation of shoulder MR imaging when compared with manual segmentation, for the purpose of creating 3D models used to quantify both Hill-Sachs lesions and glenoid bone loss used for preoperative planning, and assessment of on-track and off-track lesion status (**Fig. 9**).

Quantitative Assessment of Tendon Abnormality

MR imaging is the standard diagnostic modality in the diagnosis of rotator cuff tear. However, diagnostic accuracy for qualitative assessment of rotator cuff disorder is variable for partial-thickness rotator cuff tears and tendinopathy, and even more so in the postoperative rotator cuff. Biochemical composition of the rotator cuff tendons, formed from highly organized collagen fibrils, allow for a more quantitative assessment of rotator cuff disorder with T2 mapping, permitting a microscopic assessment of tissue integrity.[34] Early studies have found T2 mapping of the supraspinatus to reliably differentiate partial-thickness and full-thickness rotator cuff tears from normal tendons and tendinosis.[35,36] Future studies are

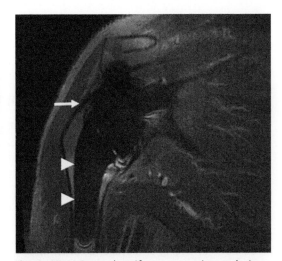

Fig. 8. SEMAC metal artifact suppression technique. Coronal STIR SEMAC image obtained on a 1.5-T magnet from a 65-year-old man with shoulder weakness following reverse shoulder arthroplasty, permitting visualization of the rotator cuff (*arrow*) and the humeral arthroplasty-bone interface (*arrowheads*).

needed to determine whether biochemical imaging can predict tendon functionality, longitudinally assess tendon degeneration, predict the outcome of rotator cuff repair surgery, and assess the quality of repaired tissue. T2 mapping is not currently performed in routine clinical practice at either of the authors' institutions.

Quantitative Assessment of Rotator Cuff Fatty Atrophy

Fatty degeneration of rotator cuff musculature is a morphologic characteristic observed in rotator

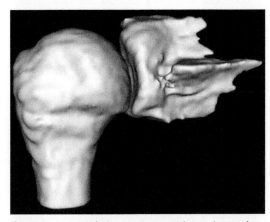

Fig. 9. Automated tissue segmentation using a deep convolutional neural network. Fully automated 3D image of the glenohumeral joint of a 28-year-old man, obtained using a deep convolutional neural network. (*Courtesy of* S. Gyftopoulos, MD, New York, NY.)

cuff tears, and is positively correlated with both tear chronicity and extent.[37] Fatty degeneration of the rotator cuff muscles has been found to be associated with overall poor postoperative outcomes, in both quantitative and qualitative assessments.[37,38] The qualitative scoring system first described by Goutallier on CT, and later modified by Fuchs on parasagittal MR images,[37,39] is used routinely in clinical practice, subdividing fatty atrophy into 5 separate stages: stage 0, normal skeletal muscle, with absence of fatty infiltration; stage 1, muscle containing fatty streaks; stage 2, fatty infiltration with overall more muscle than fat; stage 3, fatty infiltration with equal fat and muscle; and stage 4, fatty infiltration with more fat than muscle.

The degree of fatty atrophy is an important element in the decision tree on whether to proceed with rotator cuff repair, with many advocating advanced fatty degeneration as an absolute or relative contraindication to attempted rotator cuff repair.[40] Despite its ubiquitous use in clinical decision making, the qualitative Goutallier scoring system has been found to have poor reproducibility.[41] Moreover, assessment of fatty atrophy on the most lateral sagittal image where the scapular spine touches the remainder of the scapula, as recommended by Fuchs and colleagues,[39] may give a false estimation in patients with substantially retracted tears.[42]

The limitations of the qualitative Goutallier scoring system have led many to push for a validated quantitative assessment of fatty atrophy. More recently, the two-point Dixon sequence[12] has been used to quantify rotator cuff fat fraction. Nozaki and colleagues[43] found a significantly higher preoperative fat fraction in rotator cuff muscles with failed repair, and also found patients with failed repair to have progressed fatty degeneration on follow-up MR imaging. Although quantitative assessment of muscle atrophy is not currently performed in routine clinical practice at either of the authors' institutions, this may be a better predictor of outcomes than the qualitative Goutallier assessment that is currently being carried out.

SUMMARY

This article reviewed MR imaging and MR arthrography protocols used routinely in the authors' clinical practice as well as newer techniques that are increasingly being used in clinical practice, such as accelerated imaging facilitated by high-field-strength magnets and multichannel phased array surface coils, bone imaging with "CT-like" post-processed images, and standard and advanced MAR techniques. Also reviewed were some emerging techniques that are not currently used in clinical practice but show promise for future applications, such as automated tissue segmentation using artificial intelligence and quantitative assessment of rotator cuff tendon and muscle abnormality using novel sequences such as T2 mapping. These exciting innovations allow for more rapid image acquisition, improvements in image quality, and imaging assessment beyond morphology.

DISCLOSURE

Nothing to disclose (E.F. Alaia, N. Subhas).

REFERENCES

1. Kijowski R, Davis KW, Blankenbaker DG, et al. Evaluation of the menisci of the knee joint using three-dimensional isotropic resolution fast spin-echo imaging: diagnostic performance in 250 patients with surgical correlation. Skeletal Radiol 2012; 41(2):169–78.
2. Subhas N, Kao A, Freire M, et al. MRI of the knee ligaments and menisci: comparison of isotropic-resolution 3D and conventional 2D fast spin-echo sequences at 3 T. AJR Am J Roentgenol 2011; 197(2):442–50.
3. Garwood ER, Recht MP, White LM. Advanced imaging techniques in the knee: benefits and limitations of new rapid acquisition strategies for routine knee MRI. AJR Am J Roentgenol 2017;209(3):552–60.
4. Glockner JF, Hu HH, Stanley DW, et al. Parallel MR imaging: a user's guide. Radiographics 2005;25(5): 1279–97.
5. Gyftopoulos S, Lin D, Knoll F, et al. Artificial intelligence in musculoskeletal imaging: current status and future directions. AJR Am J Roentgenol 2019; 213(3):506–13.
6. Subhas N, Li H, Polster JM, et al. Highly accelerated knee MRI using a novel deep convoluted neural network algorithm: a multi-reader comparison study. Society of Skeletal Radiology Annual Meeting. Scottsdale (AZ), March 10-13, 2019.
7. Vahlensieck M, Peterfy CG, Wischer T, et al. Indirect MR arthrography: optimization and clinical applications. Radiology 1996;200(1):249–54.
8. Waldt S, Burkart A, Imhoff AB, et al. Anterior shoulder instability: accuracy of MR arthrography in the classification of anteroinferior labroligamentous injuries. Radiology 2005;237(2):578–83.
9. Wischer TK, Bredella MA, Genant HK, et al. Perthes lesion (a variant of the Bankart lesion): MR imaging and MR arthrographic findings with surgical correlation. AJR Am J Roentgenol 2002;178(1):233–7.
10. Tirman PF, Bost FW, Steinbach LS, et al. MR arthrographic depiction of tears of the rotator cuff: benefit of abduction and external rotation of the arm. Radiology 1994;192(3):851–6.
11. Bergin D, Schweitzer ME. Indirect magnetic resonance arthrography. Skeletal Radiol 2003;32(10): 551–8.
12. Dixon WT. Simple proton spectroscopic imaging. Radiology 1984;153(1):189–94.
13. Gyftopoulos S, Yemin A, Mulholland T, et al. 3DMR osseous reconstructions of the shoulder using a gradient-echo based two-point Dixon reconstruction: a feasibility study. Skeletal Radiol 2013;42(3): 347–52.
14. Tian CY, Shang Y, Zheng ZZ. Glenoid bone lesions: comparison between 3D VIBE images in MR arthrography and nonarthrographic MSCT. J Magn Reson Imaging 2012;36(1):231–6.
15. Stillwater L, Koenig J, Maycher B, et al. 3D-MR vs. 3D-CT of the shoulder in patients with glenohumeral instability. Skeletal Radiol 2017;46(3): 325–31.
16. Breighner RE, Endo Y, Konin GP, et al. Technical developments: zero echo time imaging of the shoulder: enhanced osseous detail by using MR imaging. Radiology 2018;286(3):960–6.
17. Bishop JY, Jones GL, Rerko MA, et al. 3-D CT is the most reliable imaging modality when quantifying glenoid bone loss. Clin Orthop Relat Res 2013; 471(4):1251–6.
18. Rerko MA, Pan X, Donaldson C, et al. Comparison of various imaging techniques to quantify glenoid bone loss in shoulder instability. J Shoulder Elbow Surg 2013;22(4):528–34.
19. Gyftopoulos S, Beltran LS, Yemin A, et al. Use of 3D MR reconstructions in the evaluation of glenoid bone loss: a clinical study. Skeletal Radiol 2014;43(2): 213–8.
20. Sears BW, Johnston PS, Ramsey ML, et al. Glenoid bone loss in primary total shoulder arthroplasty: evaluation and management. J Am Acad Orthop Surg 2012;20(9):604–13.
21. Walch G, Badet R, Boulahia A, et al. Morphologic study of the glenoid in primary glenohumeral osteoarthritis. J Arthroplasty 1999;14(6):756–60.
22. Scalise JJ, Bryan J, Polster J, et al. Quantitative analysis of glenoid bone loss in osteoarthritis using three-dimensional computed tomography scans. J Shoulder Elbow Surg 2008;17(2):328–35.
23. Scalise JJ, Codsi MJ, Bryan J, et al. The three-dimensional glenoid vault model can estimate normal glenoid version in osteoarthritis. J Shoulder Elbow Surg 2008;17(3):487–91.
24. Lowe JT, Testa EJ, Li X, et al. Magnetic resonance imaging is comparable to computed tomography for determination of glenoid version but does not accurately distinguish between Walch B2 and C classifications. J Shoulder Elbow Surg 2017;26(4): 669–73.

25. Annual Meeting Abstracts of the Society of Skeletal Radiology (SSR) 2019, Scottsdale, Arizona, USA. Skeletal Radiol 2019;48(3):479–98.

26. Harris CA, White LM. Metal artifact reduction in musculoskeletal magnetic resonance imaging. Orthop Clin North Am 2006;37(3):349–59, vi.

27. Gupta A, Subhas N, Primak AN, et al. Metal artifact reduction: standard and advanced magnetic resonance and computed tomography techniques. Radiol Clin North Am 2015;53(3):531–47.

28. Koch KM, Lorbiecki JE, Hinks RS, et al. A multispectral three-dimensional acquisition technique for imaging near metal implants. Magn Reson Med 2009;61(2):381–90.

29. Hayter CL, Koff MF, Shah P, et al. MRI after arthroplasty: comparison of MAVRIC and conventional fast spin-echo techniques. AJR Am J Roentgenol 2011;197(3):W405–11.

30. Lu W, Pauly KB, Gold GE, et al. SEMAC: slice encoding for metal artifact correction in MRI. Magn Reson Med 2009;62(1):66–76.

31. McWalter EJ, Wirth W, Siebert M, et al. Use of novel interactive input devices for segmentation of articular cartilage from magnetic resonance images. Osteoarthritis Cartilage 2005;13(1):48–53.

32. Liu F, Zhou Z, Jang H, et al. Deep convolutional neural network and 3D deformable approach for tissue segmentation in musculoskeletal magnetic resonance imaging. Magn Reson Med 2018;79(4): 2379–91.

33. Liu F, Zhou Z, Samsonov A, et al. Deep learning approach for evaluating knee MR images: achieving high diagnostic performance for cartilage lesion detection. Radiology 2018;289(1):160–9.

34. Anz AW, Lucas EP, Fitzcharles EK, et al. MRI T2 mapping of the asymptomatic supraspinatus tendon by age and imaging plane using clinically relevant subregions. Eur J Radiol 2014;83(5):801–5.

35. Ganal E, Ho CP, Wilson KJ, et al. Quantitative MRI characterization of arthroscopically verified supraspinatus pathology: comparison of tendon tears, tendinosis and asymptomatic supraspinatus tendons with T2 mapping. Knee Surg Sports Traumatol Arthrosc 2016; 24(7):2216–24.

36. Krepkin K, Bruno M, Raya JG, et al. Quantitative assessment of the supraspinatus tendon on MRI using T2/T2* mapping and shear-wave ultrasound elastography: a pilot study. Skeletal Radiol 2017; 46(2):191–9.

37. Goutallier D, Postel JM, Bernageau J, et al. Fatty muscle degeneration in cuff ruptures. Pre- and postoperative evaluation by CT scan. Clin Orthop Relat Res 1994;304:78–83.

38. Thomazeau H, Rolland Y, Lucas C, et al. Atrophy of the supraspinatus belly. Assessment by MRI in 55 patients with rotator cuff pathology. Acta Orthop Scand 1996;67(3):264–8.

39. Fuchs B, Weishaupt D, Zanetti M, et al. Fatty degeneration of the muscles of the rotator cuff: assessment by computed tomography versus magnetic resonance imaging. J Shoulder Elbow Surg 1999;8(6): 599–605.

40. Burkhart SS, Barth JR, Richards DP, et al. Arthroscopic repair of massive rotator cuff tears with stage 3 and 4 fatty degeneration. Arthroscopy 2007;23(4): 347–54.

41. Slabaugh MA, Friel NA, Karas V, et al. Interobserver and intraobserver reliability of the Goutallier classification using magnetic resonance imaging: proposal of a simplified classification system to increase reliability. Am J Sports Med 2012;40(8):1728–34.

42. Chitkara M, Albert M, Wong T, et al. Rotator cuff fatty infiltration are coronal images more helpful for characterization than sagittal images? Bull Hosp Jt Dis (2013) 2016;74(2):130–4.

43. Nozaki T, Tasaki A, Horiuchi S, et al. Quantification of fatty degeneration within the supraspinatus muscle by using a 2-point Dixon method on 3-T MRI. AJR Am J Roentgenol 2015;205(1):116–22.

MR Imaging of the Rotator Cuff

Erin McCrum, MD

KEYWORDS

• Rotator cuff tear • Classification • Shoulder MR imaging

KEY POINTS

- The cause of rotator cuff disease is multifactorial, but the most important risk factor is patient age.
- Use of an appropriate search pattern and knowledge of common disease locations can increase reader sensitivity for pathologic condition.
- Accurate reporting of tear thickness, AP tear size, degree of tear retraction, and fatty infiltration and fatty atrophy helps guide surgical management.

INTRODUCTION

Shoulder pain is a pervasive problem. Estimated lifetime prevalence varies but is reported to be as high as 70%.[1] Shoulder pain attributed to rotator cuff tears is responsible for 4.5 million annual patient visits and 250,000 operative interventions in the United States.[2] Because many rotator cuff tears are asymptomatic, true prevalence is unknown. Cadaver studies yield a wide range of reported tendon defects ranging from 5% to 40%.[3] Similarly, patient studies with MR imaging and ultrasound (US) also yield variable results. Sher and colleagues[4] found the overall prevalence of tears to be 34% by MR imaging. Templehof and colleagues[5] used US to evaluate asymptomatic patients and found a prevalence of 23% of rotator cuff tears, which increased to 51% in subjects older than the age of 80. Yamaguchi and colleagues[6] evaluated patients presenting with shoulder pain and, consistent with studies by Sher and Templehof, determined that prevalence increased with increasing age. They also determined that if a patient had a symptomatic rotator cuff tear, there was a 35% chance of a rotator cuff tear in the asymptomatic shoulder, which increased to 50% at age 66 and older.

Several risk factors have also been shown to be associated with rotator cuff tears. Prevalence data suggest that the most important of these is advancing patient age.[5,6] Trauma, such as repetitive macrotrauma or microtrauma, also contributes to rotator cuff tearing. Interestingly, smoking, high cholesterol, and genetics have also recently been implicated as risk factors. Smoking has been shown to increase the risk for rotator cuff tearing, to increase the tear size, and to impede healing after repair and is associated with worsened outcomes after surgical intervention.[7] In a study of 160 patients, Abboud and Kim[8] found elevated serum cholesterol in 64% of patients with a tear compared with 24% in a control group with shoulder pain but normal shoulder MR. Tashjian and colleagues[4] demonstrated increased incidence of rotator cuff tearing in second- and third-degree relatives of patients less than 40 years old with rotator cuff tears (in whom rotator cuff tears are reportedly uncommon), suggesting that genetics also predispose an individual toward tearing.[3]

Understanding of the pathogenesis of rotator cuff disease is continually evolving. The "intrinsic" theory was put forth in 1934 and espouses that age-related tendon wear compounded by chronic microtrauma results in partial-thickness tearing, which then progresses to full-thickness tearing. The "extrinsic" theory was formulated in 1972 and holds that extrinsic causes, namely

Division of Musculoskeletal Imaging, Department of Radiology, Duke University Medical Center, Duke University, Box 3808, Durham, NC 27707, USA
E-mail address: erin.mccrum@duke.edu

Magn Reson Imaging Clin N Am 28 (2020) 165–179
https://doi.org/10.1016/j.mric.2019.12.002
1064-9689/20/© 2020 Elsevier Inc. All rights reserved.

subacromial impingement, underlie rotator cuff tears.[9] Today, the cause of rotator cuff disease is thought to be multifactorial with both intrinsic and extrinsic factors contributing to tendon breakdown.

The differential diagnosis for a patient presenting with pain and/or functional limitations of the glenohumeral joint is broad and not limited to rotator cuff disease. Clinical examinations can offer high sensitivity or specificity and are confounded by subjective interpretation, which makes definitive diagnosis based on physical examination difficult.[10] Radiologists aid their surgical colleagues through accurate reporting of cuff status and identification of factors that are associated with poor outcomes. Although US has been validated in the evaluation of rotator cuff tears with reported sensitivities and specificities that rival that of conventional MR,[11] MR provides more comprehensive evaluation of the glenohumeral joint, including more accurate evaluation of articular cartilage and labroligamentous structures, factors that dictate conservative treatment, guide surgical management, and help set patient expectations.

NORMAL ROTATOR CUFF ANATOMY

The rotator cuff is a laminated structure comprising 4 naked tendons and their respective muscles: the supraspinatus, infraspinatus, subscapularis, and teres minor. The supraspinatus originates from the posterior aspect of the scapula and inserts on the superior facet of the greater tuberosity and, together with the deltoid, contributes to shoulder abduction. The infraspinatus arises along the posterior scapula in the infraspinatus fossa just below the scapular spine, inserts at the middle facet on the greater tuberosity, and provides external rotation force at the glenohumeral joint. The subscapularis is a multipennate structure arising from the subscapular fossa usually consisting of 4 to 6 tendon slips, which insert on the inferior facet of the lesser tuberosity of the humerus, and has fibers that blend with the transverse humeral ligament to form the floor of the bicipital groove. The subscapularis is innervated by both the upper and the lower subscapular nerve and internally rotates and adducts the shoulder. Teres minor arises from the lateral border of the scapula and inserts on the most inferior facet of the greater tuberosity after blending with the posterior capsule. Teres minor is innervated by the axillary nerve and provides 20% to 45% of the external rotation power of the shoulder.[12]

The rotator cuff fibers blend together: the anterior fibers of the supraspinatus and subscapularis blend together to envelop the biceps tendon, the posterior supraspinatus and anterior infraspinatus interleave at their junction, and the inferior infraspinatus and teres minor merge at the posterior aspect of the capsule. The blending of fibers allows the tendons to work in concert to center the humeral head on the glenoid and enables a wide range of dynamic motion at the glenohumeral joint.[10,13]

IMAGING TECHNIQUE

Accurate interpretation of shoulder MR imaging relies on proper technique. For further discussion of noncontrast and MR arthrography technique, refer to Drs Erin F. Alaia and Naveen Subhas' article, "Shoulder MR Imaging and MR Arthrography Techniques: New Advances," in this issue.

MR arthrography offers increased sensitivity for both labral tears and rotator cuff pathologic condition. In 2009, Magee[14] evaluated 150 patients who underwent conventional MR and shoulder MR arthrography and compared them with the results of arthroscopy. They found that sensitivity and specificity for full-thickness tears of 92% and 100% and partial-thickness articular-sided tears of 68% and 100% on conventional MR. MR arthrography improved sensitivities with sensitivities and specificities for full-thickness tears of 100% and 100% and for partial-thickness articular-sided tears of 97% and 100%, respectively. Although institutional practices vary, it is reasonable to reserve MR arthrography for surgical candidates in whom labral pathologic condition is suspected or whose cuff tears are not well delineated on conventional MR.

ROTATOR CUFF TENDINOSIS

Normal rotator cuff tendons are composed of type I collagen molecules, which form dense highly ordered fiber bundles, which aggregate parallel to the long axis of the tendon.[15] The regular structure of the fibers alters the rotational motion of the water molecules, which results in a uniform reduction of signal in all MR sequences.[15] As a result, normal tendons appear uniformly hypointense on MR sequences.[16] As tendons begin to undergo histopathologic changes of mucoid degeneration and scarring, increased signal is evident on proton density images without changes on T2-weighted imaging. As tendon disease and degeneration progress, disruption of the highly ordered tendinous structure becomes evident as increased

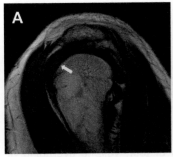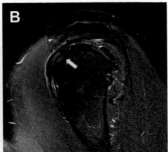

Fig. 1. Supraspinatus tendinosis seen on sagittal oblique images, indicated by the arrows. Tendinosis appears as intermediate signal on (A) T1-weighted imaging. (B) Increased signal that does not approach that of fluid on fat-saturated T2-weighted imaging.

signal on T1- and T2-weighted imaging, which does not reach the signal intensity of fluid (Fig. 1).[17] The morphology of tendons with tendinosis is variable, and they can appear thickened (Fig. 2) or normal in caliber (Fig. 3), with focal or diffuse alterations in normal signal intensity. In a study of 52 athletes, Sein and colleagues[18] showed high intraobserver reliability classifying tendinosis as mild if there was mild focally increased tendon signal on PD and T2 fat-saturated imaging, moderate if there was moderate focally increased tendon signal on PD and T2 fat-saturated imaging, or marked if there was diffusely increased signal on PD and T2 fat-saturated imaging, which did not yet reach fluid signal intensity. Interobserver agreement was less reliable, reinforcing the adage that as radiologists, we may be "often wrong, but never in doubt." Although a strict criterion for grading tendinosis has not been widely adopted, the author's group typically categorizes tendinosis into mild, moderate, and severe categories based on their own internal metric.

ROTATOR CUFF TEARS

A partial-thickness tear is a noncommunicating tear involving either the substance or the articular or bursal side of the tendon. Ellman classified tear depth based on the expected tendon thickness of 10 to 12 mm. Small and medium tears are those that are less than 3 mm deep and 3- to 6 mm deep, respectively, and involve less than 50% of tendon thickness. Large partial-thickness tears are those that are greater than 6 mm deep and thus involve greater than 50% of tendon thickness.[19] However, this grading system does not account for the natural variation in tendon thickness and in daily practice, and reporting follows surgical management; partial-thickness tears are denoted as "low grade" if they occupy less than 50% of the tendon thickness (Fig. 4) or high grade if fluid signal intensity spans greater than 50% of the expected tendon thickness (Fig. 5). Although treatment is not standardized, accurate designation of low- versus high-grade tearing is important because surgical repair is often reserved for high-grade tendon tears,

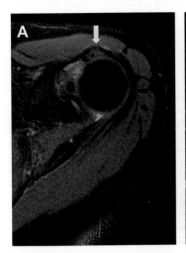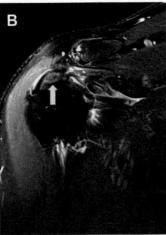

Fig. 2. (A) Thickening and intermediate signal in the supraspinatus on axial fat-saturated proton density images consistent with tendinosis as indicated by the arrow. Note that the shoulder is markedly internally rotated. (B) Corresponding coronal fat-saturated T2-weighted imaging demonstrating increased signal within the thickened supraspinatus as indicated by the arrow.

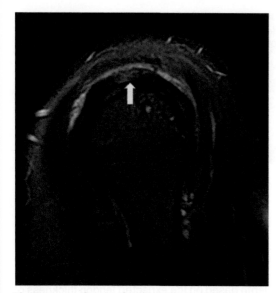

Fig. 3. Arrow denotes focal tendinosis at the junction of the supraspinatus and infraspinatus with preserved tendon morphology in T2 fat-saturated sagittal oblique plane.

whereas low-grade tendon tears are frequently conservatively treated or debrided.[20,21] Bursal-sided tears (**Fig. 6**) are far less frequent than articular-sided tears with a reported incidence of 2.9%.[22]

Partial-thickness tears within the substance of a tendon likely arise because of shear stresses on degenerated tendon tissue and may represent up to 33% of partial-thickness tears (**Fig. 7**). Although also known as intrasubstance tears, delaminating tears, or interstitial clefts, the author refers to a tear that is contained entirely within the substance of a tendon with or without communication with articular- or bursal-sided tears[22] as an interstitial tear. Interstitial tears are important to note because of difficult visualization at arthroscopy.

Tears are said to be full thickness if there is communication between the bursal and articular side of the cuff. Although up to 87% of full-thickness tears demonstrate the classic appearance with fluid or gadolinium (**Fig. 8**) signal attenuation filling the communicating gap between articular and bursal surfaces, a smaller percentage demonstrate heterogenous T2 signal, likely because of inflammation with subsequent scar and granulation tissue formation within the region of tear, volume averaging of focal tears, or coaptation of torn tendon edges (**Fig. 9**).[10,14] Identification of these nonclassic tears remains problematic and, in these situations, secondary findings, such as muscular edema and atrophy, intramuscular cysts, subacromial-subdeltoid bursal fluid, and cyst formation in the humeral head, can be supportive, but are not diagnostic of rotator cuff tears.[23] Arthrography can be used as a problem-solving technique.

TENDONS
Supraspinatus

When evaluating for supraspinatus tendon tear, the T2 fat-saturated sagittal oblique and coronal oblique images are the most useful. In a well-positioned shoulder MR imaging, the supraspinatus spans the 10 to 11 o'clock position and blends with the anterior infraspinatus at approximately the 12 o' clock position. The footprint of the supraspinatus on the superior facet of the greater tuberosity is the most commonly torn portion of the supraspinatus.[22] A partial articular-sided supraspinatus tendon avulsion (PASTA), a type of rim rent tear,[24] is the mostly commonly seen partial-thickness rotator cuff tear and may comprise up to 91% of all partial-thickness tears (**Fig. 10**).[19,25] These tears are frequently missed because of their far anterior position and suboptimal visualization on the sagittal oblique images on an incorrectly

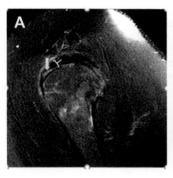
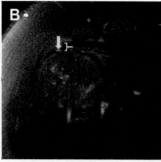

Fig. 4. Low-grade partial-thickness articular-sided tear involving less than 50% of thickness of the tendon. (*A*) Fat-saturated sagittal oblique T2-weighted image demonstrating fluid signal intensity tear (*arrow*) along the articular side of the tendon involving less than 50% of the tendon thickness. (*B*) Corresponding T2 fat-saturated coronal oblique image with low-grade partial-thickness articular-sided tear (*arrow*). Normal tendon thickness is indicated by the yellow calipers in both figures.

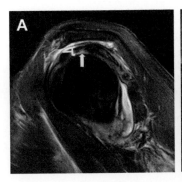
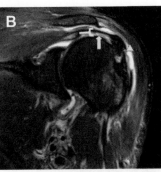

Fig. 5. High-grade partial-thickness articular-sided tearing of the supraspinatus. (*A*) Fat-saturated sagittal oblique T2-weighted image demonstrating a fluid signal intensity tendon tear (*arrow*) spanning greater than 50% of the expected tendon thickness (*caliper*) along the articular side of the tendon. (*B*) Corresponding T2 fat-saturated coronal oblique image demonstrating high-grade articular-sided tear (*arrow*) involving more than half of the expected tendon thickness (*calipers*). The patient also had a greater tuberosity fracture (*arrowhead*). The supraspinatus remains attached to the displaced tuberosity fracture fragment.

positioned internally rotated shoulder MR imaging. As such, interrogation of the coronal oblique images and axial images is critical. The most anterior fibers of the supraspinatus are located just posterior to the extraarticular biceps tendon on the coronal oblique images and just peripheral to the bicipital groove on axial imaging.

Infraspinatus

In a well-positioned shoulder MR, the infraspinatus tendon spans the 1 to 2 o' clock position with anterior fibers that blend with the posterior fibers of the supraspinatus. Tears of the infraspinatus generally occur in conjunction with tears of the supraspinatus with an extent similar to that of supraspinatus tear.[20] Similar to the supraspinatus, evaluation of the T2 fat-saturated coronal oblique and sagittal oblique images is most useful. Isolated tears of the infraspinatus are reportedly rare.[26] The "novel lesion" of the infraspinatus is an isolated atraumatic rupture of the interstitial infraspinatus (**Fig. 11**). Although unusual, these tears are important to note because of difficult visualization at arthroscopy and progression to severe fatty atrophy, which may occur despite surgical intervention.[27,28]

Subscapularis

Previously regarded as the "forgotten tendon" because of difficulty assessing the tendon

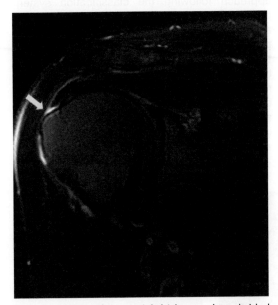

Fig. 6. High-grade partial-thickness bursal-sided tearing. Fat-saturated coronal oblique T2-weighted images demonstrating fluid signal intensity tear (*arrow*) along the bursal side of the tendon with intact articular-sided fibers.

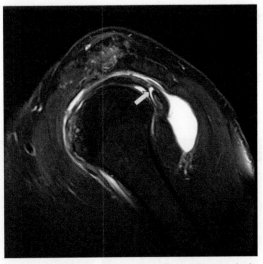

Fig. 7. Interstitial tearing. Fat-saturated sagittal oblique T2-weighted image demonstrating fluid signal at the myotendinous junction of the infraspinatus (*arrow*).

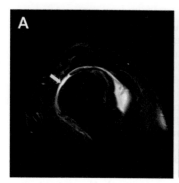
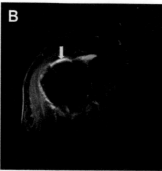

Fig. 8. Full-thickness supraspinatus tear. (*A*) Fat-saturated sagittal oblique T2-weighted image demonstrating a bare humeral head and full-thickness tendon defect (*arrow*) in the expected location of the supraspinatus tendon. (*B*) Corresponding T2 fat-saturated coronal oblique image with arrow indicating the full thickness supraspinatus tear.

during rotator cuff repair, the subscapularis is an important stabilizer of the shoulder girdle because newer arthroscopic techniques permit improved visualization, and new repair techniques have expanded therapeutic options.[29] The arthroscopic incidence of subscapularis tears is reported as 31.4% with only 6.4% of patients having an isolated subscapularis tear.[30] MR arthrography offers both great sensitivity and specificity for subscapularis tears, reportedly 91%/91% and 86%/79%, respectively, for 2 readers in a study by Pfirrmann and colleagues.[31]

Routine MR does not fare as well with sensitivity and specificity of 36% and 100%, respectively, with some evidence that sensitivity and specificity may be related to the size of the tear.[32] Improved sensitivities and specificities of 73% and 94% were reported by Adams and colleagues[33] with a 4-step approach to subscapularis evaluation:

1. Subscapularis is evaluated for tear on axial T2-weighted images,
2. The biceps tendon is evaluated for evidence of subluxation,
3. The presence of subscapularis fatty infiltration and atrophy is assessed on T1-weighted images,
4. Presence of tear is assessed on T2-weighted fat saturated sagittal oblique images.[33]

Shi and colleagues[34] reported a positive predictive value of only 35% for subscapularis tears in the presence of biceps tendon subluxation, which challenges the belief that subscapularis must be torn for the biceps to exit the bicipital groove. In the author's experience, T2-weighted fat-saturated sagittal oblique sequences are also helpful to characterize the thickness of tears, and T2-weighted fat-saturated sagittal oblique and coronal oblique images are helpful to confirm the cranial caudal extent of subscapularis tears (**Fig. 12**).

Although consensus regarding reporting of subscapularis tears is lacking, a descriptive approach following the classification system proposed by Fox in which tears are described as follows: (1) partial thickness; (2) complete tears of the upper 25%; (3) complete tears of the upper 50%; or (4) complete tears of the tendon with retraction, helps guide management.[29,31] As in other tendon tears, the degree of fatty infiltration correlates with the severity and chronicity of tear, and more advanced fatty infiltration is associated with negative outcomes after arthroscopy.

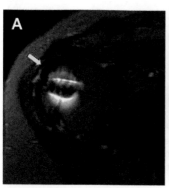
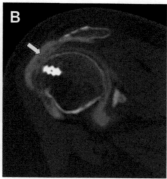

Fig. 9. (*A*) Hypointense tissue approximating a suture anchor in the humeral head was thought to represent intact supraspinatus (*arrow*) status after rotator cuff tear. (*B*) Subsequent evaluation with CT arthrography demonstrated a full-thickness recurrent tear (*arrow*) with a paucity of normal tendon tissue.

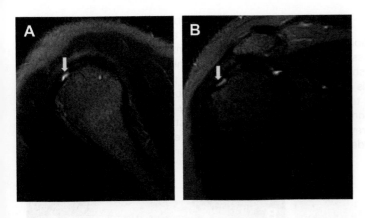

Fig. 10. PASTA. High-grade partial-thickness articular-sided tearing at the footplate. (A) T2 fat-saturated sagittal oblique image demonstrating fluid signal intensity involving greater than 50% of tendon thickness (arrow). (B) Corresponding T2 fat-saturated coronal oblique image demonstrating the same PASTA tear (arrow).

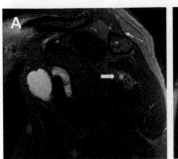
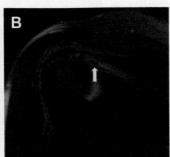

Fig. 11. A "novel lesion" of the infraspinatus. (A) Sagittal oblique T2 fat-saturated image demonstrating an isolated interstitial tear of the infraspinatus (arrow) with surrounding muscular edema. (B) Coronal oblique T2 fat-saturated images demonstrate torn and retracted infraspinatus fibers (arrow).

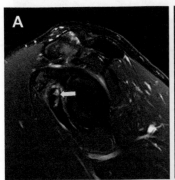
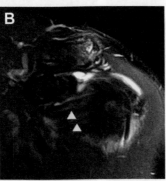
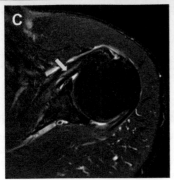

Fig. 12. Three-plane evaluation of the subscapularis. The cranial-caudal extent of a subscapularis interstitial tear is assessed in (A) the sagittal oblique T2 fat-saturated plane where the arrow denotes the interstitial tear and (B) the coronal oblique planes where the arrowheads denote the interstitial tearing. (C) Preservation of the articular and bursal surfaces in the axial plane confirms the interstitial nature of the tear. The interstitial tear is denoted by the yellow arrow. The axial plane is also used to evaluate the position of the biceps tendon in the bicipital groove.

TERES MINOR

Teres minor becomes an important stabilizer of the glenohumeral joint in the setting of massive irreparable rotator cuff tears and counters shear forces induced by unopposed subscapularis or deltoid muscles.[35,36] In fact, preservation of teres minor function and muscle bulk is an important prognostic factor in patients undergoing reverse total shoulder arthroplasties and shoulder tendon transfers.[35] The reported incidence of teres minor tears is only 0.9% and is usually seen in association with supraspinatus and infraspinatus tears.[36] Reported mechanisms of teres injury include both anterior and posterior dislocations and are seen in association with multitendon injury or concomitant injury of the infraspinatus, posterior capsule, and posterior inferior glenoid labrum, respectively. Isolated teres minor tears are notably rare.[37] Teres minor integrity is best evaluated on

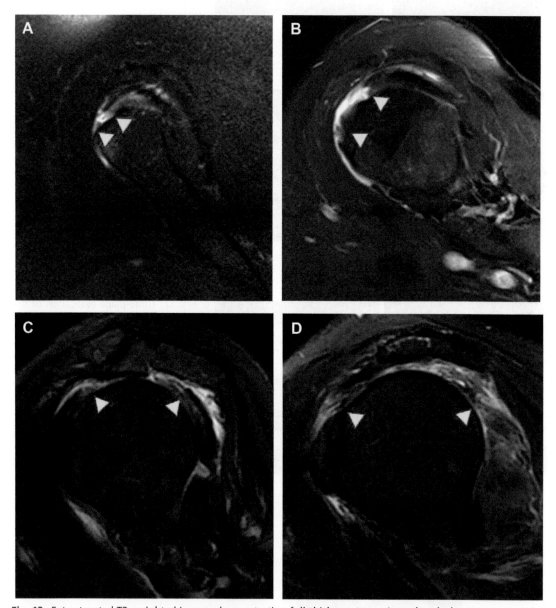

Fig. 13. Fat-saturated T2-weighted images demonstrating full-thickness tears. Arrowheads denote tear margins. (*A*) Small full-thickness tear measuring less than 1 cm in the AP dimension. (*B*) Medium tear measuring 1 to 3 cm in AP dimension. (*C*) Large full-thickness tear measuring 3 to 5 cm. (*D*) Massive tear spanning greater than 5 cm and involving both the supraspinatus and the infraspinatus.

T2 fat-saturated sagittal oblique, and assessment for injuries to the capsule and posterior inferior glenoid labrum is most evident on the axial T2 fat-saturated sequences and confirmed on sagittal oblique T2 fat-saturated and coronal T2 fat-saturated sequences.

Denervation change in the teres minor is far more frequent with a reported incidence of 3% to 5%.[10] In addition to the quadrilateral space, axillary nerve is also susceptible to injury as it courses around the glenoid and posterior capsule and can be injured by repetitive micro-trauma associated with humeral head instability.[37] Teres minor volume is reported using the Walch classification. Teres minor is reported as hypertrophic if it is the same width as the same slice glenoid, normal if the half the width of the glenoid, atrophic if thinner than half the width, and absent if absent.[35] Interestingly, although normal in approximately 90.8% of shoulders, Melis and colleagues[36] report that teres minor hypertrophy has been associated with anterior tears and teres minor atrophy with posterior superior tears.

ADDITIONAL TEAR DESCRIPTORS

Radiologic findings of AP tear size, degree of tendon retraction, degree of fatty infiltration of the musculature, and degree of muscle atrophy are important full-thickness tear descriptors, which help guide surgical management.

Tear size descriptors are placed into 4 categories: Small tears of less than 1 cm, medium tears of 1 to 3 cm, large tears of 3 to 5 cm, and massive tears, which are tears larger than 5 cm (**Fig. 13**).[38] Although tear management is surgeon and institution specific, small tears are usually treated conservatively.

Reporting the degree of tendon retraction can help guide surgical approach and is designated in 1 of 3 locations: near the humeral insertion, at the humeral apex, or at the level of the glenoid (**Fig. 14**).[10] Primary repair is often performed if the tendon remains near the humeral insertion, which keeps tension on the repair low and aids healing. Tears medial to the level of the glenoid are often regarded as irreparable.[13]

The degree of fatty atrophy and infiltration of the musculature are described using Warner's and modifications to Goutallier's classification schemes, which are discussed further in later discussion.

FATTY INFILTRATION AND ATROPHY OF ROTATOR CUFF MUSCULATURE

Although both fatty infiltration and volume atrophy are likely part of the same process, they have been found to be independent predictors of surgical outcomes.[39] In assessing muscle quality and quantity, T1 and T2 signal characteristics should be assessed on sagittal oblique series. High T2-weighted signal, although nonspecific, suggests

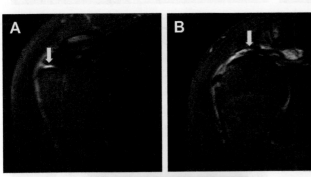

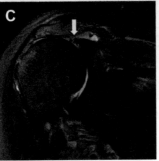

Fig. 14. (*A*) Coronal oblique T2-weighted fat-saturated images demonstrate full-thickness supraspinatus tear, which remains near the humeral insertion, (*arrow*) (*B*) with tendon retraction to the level of the humeral apex, (*arrow*) (*C*) with retraction to the level of the glenoid (*arrow*).

recent trauma or denervation change, whereas increased T1-weighted signal suggests a more chronic process.[40]

Goutallier and colleagues developed a staging system to grade fatty infiltration of the rotator cuff muscles after noting the association of rotator cuff tear with fatty infiltration. This grading system was based on axial computed tomography (CT) images and was subsequently modified for MR by Fuchs, which allowed grading of muscles based on the most lateral sagittal image in which the scapular spine is in contact with the scapular body. However, these grading systems are complicated by variability in interobserver interpretation and spatial variation of fatty infiltration within a muscle. In practice, the Fuchs staging system has been further qualified, and muscle is evaluated on T1 sagittal oblique images, and the degree of fatty infiltration is reported as normal if there are no fatty streaks, minimal if there are a few fatty streaks, mild if there is less fat than muscle in the fossa, moderate if the volume of fat and muscle is roughly equivalent in the fossa, and advanced if there is more fat than muscle (**Fig. 15**).[39]

Fatty infiltration is associated with higher rates of retear and poor surgical outcomes.[41] Although the cause of fatty infiltration is not definitive, it is

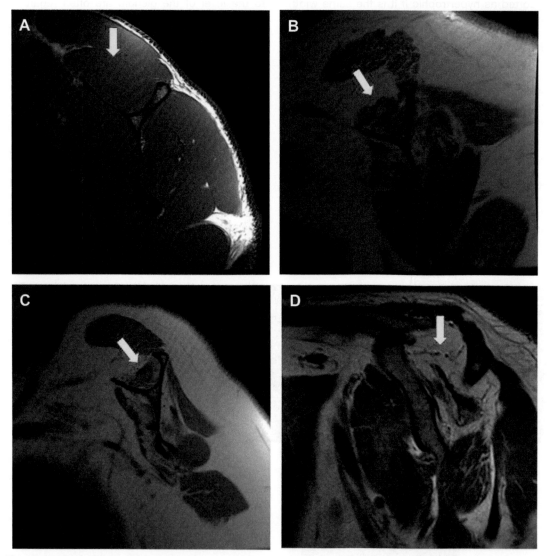

Fig. 15. Sagittal oblique T1-weighted images demonstrating supraspinatus fatty infiltration as indicated by the arrows in each of the images. (*A*) Normal cuff musculature. (*B*) Mild supraspinatus fatty infiltration with more muscle than fat. (*C*) Moderate supraspinatus fatty infiltration with muscle roughly equal to the amount of fat. (*D*) Severe supraspinatus fatty infiltration with paucity of normal muscle identified.

likely the consequence of decreased mechanical load and denervation. Fat deposition within muscles and tendons decreases their elastic potential, making mobilization for repair more difficult and decreases the quality of tissue.[42] Factors that have been associated with progression of fatty infiltration include size and location of tear, degree of retraction, age, and time of onset of symptoms to diagnosis. Infraspinatus fatty infiltration also predicts a poor surgical outcome. As Kuzel and colleagues[39] elegantly note, the natural history of fatty infiltration is one of progression. Current interventions may halt or slow the process of fatty infiltration but have not consistently been shown to reverse the process. Furthermore, in patients with failed repairs, the process of fatty infiltration is accelerated.[39,41,43] Melis and colleagues[42] recommend attempting rotator cuff repair before the development of Goutallier stage 2 fatty infiltration, which is associated with a definitive loss of muscular function and moderate atrophy.

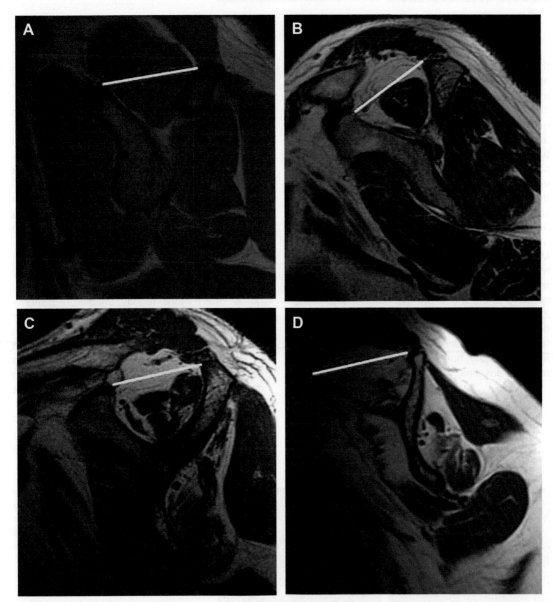

Fig. 16. Sagittal oblique T1-weighted images used to assess supraspinatus volume atrophy relative to a tangent line between the coracoid and scapular spine. (*A*) Normal volume with muscle above the line, (*B*) mild atrophy with superior margin of the muscle touching the line, (*C*) moderate atrophy with concavity of the superior muscle margin, and (*D*) severe atrophy with little to no muscle present.

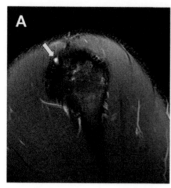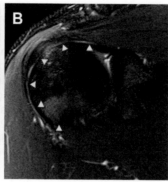

Fig. 17. (A) T2-weighted fat-saturated sagittal oblique image demonstrates a small fluid signal intensity cleft in the anterior fibers of supraspinatus suspicious for tear (arrow). (B) Correlation with coronal T2-weighted fat-saturated image demonstrates a curvilinear vessel (arrowheads) confirming the vascular cause of this tear mimic.

Like fatty infiltration, muscle atrophy is also likely the consequence of decreased mechanical load and denervation changes, which results in proliferation of adipocytes. Also, like fatty infiltration, atrophy leads to decreased tissue elasticity and quality, which demonstrate impaired healing. The author describes atrophy using the grading system proposed by Warner, which modified the classification developed by Zanetti to include evaluation of the subscapularis. In this system, the cuff muscle is evaluated on T1-weighted sagittal oblique images relative to a series of lines between the coracoid process and scapular spine and the scapular spine and tip of the scapula. Muscles are reported as normal if they are convex relative to the tangent line, mildly atrophied if they touch the line, moderately atrophied if they are concave to the line (a positive tangent sign in the Zanetti classification), and severely atrophied if little normal muscle is identified (Fig. 16).[39] Unlike fatty infiltration, successful rotator cuff repair can reverse atrophy; however, muscle volume will not return to baseline.[44]

ROTATOR CUFF PITFALLS

Rotator cuff disease mimics can confound MR interpretation. Prominent blood vessels may course through muscles and tendons but often appear serpiginous and should not be mistaken for tears (Fig. 17).[45] Magic angle can contribute to a hyperintense appearance of tendon at short echo time (TE), which can be misinterpreted as tendinosis or partial tearing; however, this finding will not persist on T2 sequences with longer TE.[46,47] The rotator cable is an inconsistently seen band of fibrous tissue that courses obliquely along the articular surface of infraspinatus and supraspinatus approximately 1.3 cm medial to the greater tuberosity. The dark fibers of the rotator cable can be mistaken for torn and retracted undersurface fibers of the supraspinatus or infraspinatus if the reader is not aware of this structure. However, the rotator cable may hypertrophy in response to tendinous laxity and is often more readily visible in patients with a partial-thickness rotator cuff tear (Fig. 18); thus, identification of this structure can often lead to the correct diagnosis.[48–51] In the setting of trauma, a rotator cuff contusion can cause focal high signal of the cuff, which can be mistaken for tear.[52] Hydroxyapatite deposition within the substance of a tendon, also known as calcific tendinosis, can incite a striking inflammatory response in the surrounding tissue. The edematous tendon tissue can

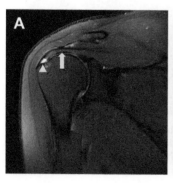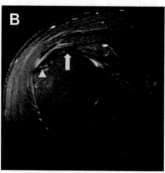

Fig. 18. (A, B) The rotator cable is visible as a band of hypointense tissue perpendicular to the articular surface supraspinatus (arrows). A high-grade (arrowhead in A) and low-grade (arrowhead in B) partial-thickness rotator cuff tear was also present.

be mistaken for tearing if the reader does not identify the foci of calcification, which will be hypointense on both T1- and T2-weighted imaging.

SUMMARY

Management of rotator cuff disease is continually evolving as knowledge of the natural history and pathogenesis of tendon pathologic condition advances. Appropriate treatment depends on accurate interpretation of MR images, aided by knowledge of rotator cuff anatomy and understanding of typical disease patterns. Factors that are currently thought to affect surgical outcomes, such as tear size and depth, degree of retraction, muscle status, and tendon quality, should be reported to help guide optimal management (**Boxes 1–3**).

DISCLOSURE

Neither I nor my immediate family members have a financial relationship with a commercial organization that may have a material interest in the content of this article.

REFERENCES

1. Cadogan A, Laslett M, Hing WA, et al. A prospective study of shoulder pain in primary care: prevalence of imaged pathology and response to guided diagnostic blocks. BMC Musculoskelet Disord 2011;12:119.
2. Rahman H, Currier E, Johnson M, et al. Primary and secondary consequences of rotator cuff injury on joint stabilizing tissues in the shoulder. J Biomech Eng 2017;139(11).
3. Tashjian RZ. Epidemiology, natural history, and indications for treatment of rotator cuff tears. Clin Sports Med 2012;31(4):589–604.
4. Sher JS, Uribe JW, Posada A, et al. Abnormal findings on magnetic resonance images of asymptomatic shoulders. J Bone Joint Surg Am 1995;77(1):10–5.
5. Tempelhof S, Rupp S, Seil R. Age-related prevalence of rotator cuff tears in asymptomatic shoulders. J Shoulder Elbow Surg 1999;8(4):296–9.
6. Yamaguchi K, Ditsios K, Middleton W, et al. The demographic and morphological features of rotator cuff disease: a comparison of asymptomatic and symptomatic shoulders. J Bone Joint Surg Am 2006;88(8):1699–704.
7. Carbone S, Gumina S, Arceri V, et al. The impact of preoperative smoking habit on rotator cuff tear: cigarette smoking influences rotator cuff tear sizes. J Shoulder Elbow Surg 2012;21(1):56–60.
8. Abboud JA, Kim JS. The effect of hypercholesterolemia on rotator cuff disease. Clin Orthop 2010;468(6):1493–7.
9. Spargoli G. Supraspinatus tendon pathomechanics: a current concepts review. Int J Sports Phys Ther 2018;13(6):1083–94.
10. MRI of the shoulder: rotator cuff. Available at: https://www.appliedradiology.com/articles/mri-of-the-shoulder-rotator-cuff. Accessed July 31, 2019.

11. de Jesus JO, Parker L, Frangos AJ, et al. Accuracy of MRI, MR arthrography, and ultrasound in the diagnosis of rotator cuff tears: a meta-analysis. Am J Roentgenol 2009;192(6):1701–7.

12. DePalma AF. The classic. Surgical anatomy of the rotator cuff and the natural history of degenerative periarthritis. Surg Clin North Am. 1963;43:1507-1520. Clin Orthop 2008;466(3):543–51.

13. Morag Y, Jacobson JA, Miller B, et al. MR imaging of rotator cuff injury: what the clinician needs to know. Radiographics 2006;26(4):1045–65.

14. Magee T. 3-T MRI of the shoulder: is MR arthrography necessary? Am J Roentgenol 2009;192(1):86–92.

15. Franchi M, Trirè A, Quaranta M, et al. Collagen structure of tendon relates to function. ScientificWorldJournal 2007;7:404–20.

16. Chang A, Miller TT. Imaging of tendons. Sports Health 2009;1(4):293–300.

17. Kjellin I, Ho CP, Cervilla V, et al. Alterations in the supraspinatus tendon at MR imaging: correlation with histopathologic findings in cadavers. Radiology 1991. https://doi.org/10.1148/radiology.181.3.1947107.

18. Sein ML, Walton J, Linklater J, et al. Reliability of MRI assessment of supraspinatus tendinopathy. Br J Sports Med 2007;41(8):e1–4.

19. Spargoli G. Partial articular supraspinatus tendon avulsion (PASTA) lesion. Current concepts in rehabilitation. Int J Sports Phys Ther 2016;11(3):462–81.

20. Wolff A, Sethi P, Sutton K, et al. Partial-thickness rotator cuff tears. J Am Acad Orthop Surg 2006;14(13):715–25.

21. Strauss EJ, Salata MJ, Kercher J, et al. The arthroscopic management of partial-thickness rotator cuff tears: a systematic review of the literature. Arthroscopy 2011;27(4):568–80.

22. Vinson EN, Helms CA, Higgins LD. Rim-rent tear of the rotator cuff: a common and easily overlooked partial tear. Am J Roentgenol 2007;189(4):943–6.

23. Hodgson RJ, O'Connor PJ, Grainger AJ. Tendon and ligament imaging. Br J Radiol 2012;85(1016):1157–72.

24. Smith CD, Corner T, Morgan D, et al. Partial thickness rotator cuff tears: what do we know? Shoulder Elb 2010;2(2):77–82.

25. Gartsman GM, Milne JC. Articular surface partial-thickness rotator cuff tears. J Shoulder Elbow Surg 1995;4(6):409–15.

26. Yeol Lee K, Hoon Kim S, Han Oh J. Isolated ruptures of the infraspinatus: clinical characteristics and outcomes. Clin Shoulder Elb 2017;20:30–6.

27. Walch G, Nové-Josserand L, Liotard J-P, et al. Musculotendinous infraspinatus ruptures: an overview. 2009. Available at: https://www.em-consulte.com/en/article/231060/Data/revues/18770568/v95i7/S1877056809001273/. Accessed July 29, 2019.

28. Lunn JV, Castellanos-Rosas J, Tavernier T, et al. A novel lesion of the infraspinatus characterized by musculotendinous disruption, edema, and late fatty infiltration. J Shoulder Elbow Surg 2008;17(4):546–53.

29. Lee J, Shukla DR, Sánchez-Sotelo J. Subscapularis tears: hidden and forgotten no more. JSES Open Access 2018;2(1):74–83.

30. Narasimhan R, Shamse K, Nash C, et al. Prevalence of subscapularis tears and accuracy of shoulder ultrasound in pre-operative diagnosis. Int Orthop 2016;40(5):975–9.

31. Pfirrmann CW, Zanetti M, Weishaupt D, et al. Subscapularis tendon tears: detection and grading at MR arthrography. Radiology 1999;213(3):709–14.

32. Adams CR, Schoolfield JD, Burkhart SS. Accuracy of preoperative magnetic resonance imaging in predicting a subscapularis tendon tear based on arthroscopy. Arthroscopy 2010;26(11):1427–33.

33. Adams CR, Brady PC, Koo SS, et al. A systematic approach for diagnosing subscapularis tendon tears with preoperative magnetic resonance imaging scans. Arthroscopy 2012;28(11):1592–600.

34. Shi LL, Mullen MG, Freehill MT, et al. Accuracy of long head of the biceps subluxation as a predictor for subscapularis tears. Arthroscopy 2015;31(4):615–9.

35. Williams MD, Edwards TB, Walch G. Understanding the importance of the teres minor for shoulder function: functional anatomy and pathology. J Am Acad Orthop Surg 2018;26(5):150–61.

36. Melis B, DeFranco MJ, Lädermann A, et al. The teres minor muscle in rotator cuff tendon tears. Skeletal Radiol 2011;40(10):1335–44.

37. Pathology of the teres minor. Radsource. 2018. Available at: http://radsource.us/pathology-teres-minor/. Accessed August 1, 2019.

38. Patte D. Classification of rotator cuff lesions. Clin Orthop 1990;(254):81–6.

39. Kuzel BR, Grindel S, Papandrea R, et al. Fatty infiltration and rotator cuff atrophy. J Am Acad Orthop Surg 2013;21(10):613–23.

40. Kamath S, Venkatanarasimha N, Walsh MA, et al. MRI appearance of muscle denervation. Skeletal Radiol 2008;37(5):397–404.

41. Chaudhury S, Dines JS, Delos D, et al. Role of fatty infiltration in the pathophysiology and outcomes of rotator cuff tears. Arthritis Care & Research. 2012. Available at: https://onlinelibrary.wiley.com/doi/abs/10.1002/acr.20552. Accessed July 27, 2019.

42. Melis B, DeFranco MJ, Chuinard C, et al. Natural history of fatty infiltration and atrophy of the supraspinatus muscle in rotator cuff tears. Clin Orthop 2010;468(6):1498–505.

43. Deniz G, Kose O, Tugay A, et al. Fatty degeneration and atrophy of the rotator cuff muscles after

arthroscopic repair: does it improve, halt or deterio-rate? Arch Orthop Trauma Surg 2014;134(7): 985–90.

44. Chung SW, Kim SH, Tae S-K, et al. Is the supraspi-natus muscle atrophy truly irreversible after surgical repair of rotator cuff tears? Clin Orthop Surg 2013; 5(1):55–65.

45. Motamedi D, Everist BM, Mahanty SR, et al. Pitfalls in shoulder MRI: part 1–normal anatomy and anatomic variants. AJR Am J Roentgenol 2014; 203(3):501–7.

46. Carroll K, Helms C. Magnetic resonance imaging of the shoulder: a review of potential sources of diag-nostic errors. Skeletal Radiol 2002;31(7):373–83.

47. Marcon GF, Macedo TAA. Artifacts and pitfalls in shoulder magnetic resonance imaging. Radiol Bras 2015;48(4):242–8.

48. Rotator cuff pitfalls. Radsource. 2013. Available at: http://radsource.us/rotator-cuff-pitfalls/. Accessed August 1, 2019.

49. Sheah K, Bredella MA, Warner JJP, et al. Transverse thickening along the articular surface of the rotator cuff consistent with the rotator cable: identification with MR arthrography and relevance in rotator cuff evaluation. AJR Am J Roentgenol 2009;193(3): 679–86.

50. Gyftopoulos S, Bencardino J, Nevsky G, et al. Rota-tor cable: MRI study of its appearance in the intact rotator cuff with anatomic and histologic correlation. Am J Roentgenol 2013;200(5):1101–5.

51. Podgórski MT, Olewnik Ł, Grzelak P, et al. Rotator cable in pathological shoulders: comparison with normal anatomy in a cadaveric study. Anat Sci Int 2019;94(1):53–7.

52. Cohen SB, Towers JD, Bradley JP. Rotator cuff contusions of the shoulder in professional football players: epidemiology and magnetic resonance imaging findings. Am J Sports Med 2007;35(3): 442–7.

The Postoperative Rotator Cuff

Mohammad Samim, MD, MRCS[a],*, Luis Beltran, MD[b]

KEYWORDS

- Rotator cuff tear • Irreparable massive rotator cuff tear • Postoperative imaging • MR imaging

KEY POINTS

- The expected appearance of the postoperative rotator cuff tendon is variable and depends on the stage and duration of the underlying disease process and the time interval between MR imaging and surgery.
- The greatest predictive factor for re-tear is the size of the original tear.
- Knowledge of surgical techniques for irreparable massive rotator cuff tears, including patch graft augmentation/bridging, superior capsular reconstruction, and muscle tendon transfer, and their postoperative MR imaging appearance, is critical for correct interpretation of MR imaging.

INTRODUCTION

Treatment options for rotator cuff tears (RCTs) include conservative and surgical treatments, with various techniques. Surgical treatment for RCT has substantially increased in recent years. From 1996 to 2006, open repairs increased by 34% while arthroscopic repairs increased by 600%,[1] with 250,000 to 300,000 rotator cuff repairs now being performed annually in the United States.[1,2]

Despite recent improvements in surgical techniques, including newer advanced arthroscopic techniques for treating RCTs, re-tear remains a major concern after arthroscopic treatment[3] for both reparable and irreparable RCTs. Hence, MR imaging is often requested for patients who had surgical intervention for their RCT and continue to have symptoms. MR imaging evaluation of postoperative patients remain challenging due to altered normal anatomy, postoperative metallic artifacts, and irregular and heterogenous appearance of repaired tissue especially at least within the first 3 months.[4] Given increasing number of shoulder rotator cuff repairs performed in the United States[5,6] it is, therefore, crucial for radiologist to understand the more commonly performed surgical or arthroscopic procedures and their impact on the appearance of the relevant anatomic structures.

This article reviews the common surgical procedures performed for rotator cuff repairs for the reparable tears and surgical procedures, including augmentation and reconstruction techniques for nonreparable massive RCTs. The expected postoperative MR imaging findings are discussed as well as the imaging appearance of a range of complications, predominantly focusing on re-tears or failures of the repaired tissue that may be identified with the use of MR imaging and MR arthrography (MRA).

TECHNICAL CONSIDERATIONS IN MR IMAGING

One of the challenges of postoperative MR imaging following rotator cuff repair is the metal artifact from screws, anchors, and metal shavings related

---

IRB: No IRB approval was required.
[a] Department of Radiology, NYU Langone Orthopedic Hospital, 301 East 17th Street, Room 600, New York, NY 10003, USA; [b] Department of Radiology, Brigham and Women's Hospital, RA3, 75 Francis Street, Boston, MA 02115, USA
* Corresponding author.
E-mail address: mohammad.samim@nyulangone.org

Magn Reson Imaging Clin N Am 28 (2020) 181–194
https://doi.org/10.1016/j.mric.2019.12.003
1064-9689/20/© 2019 Elsevier Inc. All rights reserved.

to burring by surgical instruments. Metal artifact can be reduced by modifying MR imaging protocols,[7] including using a lower magnetic field strength (1.5T rather than 3T), using fast spin-echo sequences with long echo trains, avoiding gradient-echo sequences, using short tau inversion recovery rather than frequency-selective fat suppression sequences, increasing the bandwidth and echo train length, using a larger matrix size, thinner slices, lower time-to-echo, switching the phase and frequency-encoding directions, and reducing the voxel size (**Fig. 1**).[8] Please refer to the Erin F. Alaia and Naveen Subhas' article, "Shoulder MRI and MRA Techniques: New Advances," in this issue for more specific information on optimizing shoulder MR imaging protocols. Direct MRA can improve diagnostic accuracy in postoperative shoulder due to the joint distension from intraarticular injection of gadolinium and increase in signal-to-noise ratio.[7]

REPARABLE ROTATOR CUFF TEARS

The RCT is considered reparable if size of tear, number of tendons involved, quality of the tendon and muscle allow surgeons to perform primary repair of the tear. These tears should be able to be reduced to the greater tuberosity footprint and do not meet the criteria for irreparable massive RCT that are discussed in detail below. Although there is considerable variations among orthopedic surgeons in management of patients with RCT,[9] the decision to perform a repair of RCT generally depends on the size of the tear, duration of symptoms, duration or failure of nonoperative treatment, nocturnal pain, history of trauma, and limitations of daily living activities.[10,11] Repair is usually not indicated when there is a fixed humeral head elevation, nonfunctioning deltoid muscle, and advanced rotator cuff muscle atrophy and fatty infiltration.[12] Arthroscopic repair is currently the most popular initial approach versus open surgery. Detachment or splitting of the deltoid muscle is required for the open and mini-open approach, adding to comorbidity and recovery time compared with an arthroscopic approach. In addition, there is no differences in clinical outcomes or complication rates between arthroscopy and open surgery.[13,14]

The morphology, thickness, and orientation of the RCT can determine the type of repair.[6] Smaller partial-thickness tears are typically treated with debridement, longitudinal tears oriented in the long axis of the tendon are treated with tendon-to-tendon suturing, while higher-grade partial-thickness (50% tendon thickness or greater) or full-thickness tears are treated by attaching the torn tendon to the greater tuberosity osseous footprint.[6,15] These high-grade partial-thickness tears may be converted to full-thickness tear during surgery and then being treated as such.[6] The tendon attachment to the osseous footprint is performed using a single or a double row of sutures placed in the tendon and along the medial and lateral margin of the footprint. Double-row repairs have a significantly higher rate of intact tendon healing compared with single-row repair.[16,17]

Normal Postoperative Imaging Findings

The expected appearance of the postoperative rotator cuff tendon is variable and depends on the stage and duration of the underlying disease process and the time interval between MR imaging and surgery. A major challenge of evaluating repaired rotator cuff tendons is that intermediate signal or disorganized appearance of tendon fibers can be an expected finding and does not necessarily indicate recurrent or residual disease, such as tendinosis or partial tear, nor does it correlate

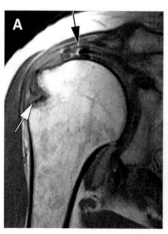
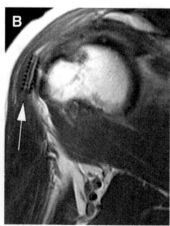

Fig. 1. 64-year-old man with prior primary rotator cuff repair (RCR) with re-tear of the repaired supraspinatus tendon. (*A, B*) Coronal proton density (PD) MR images following surgery show full-thickness re-tear of repaired supraspinatus tendon with retraction and susceptibility artifact related to surgical sutures (*black arrow*). The empty screw tract in the supraspinatus tendon footprint (*white arrow* in *A*) with screw displaced into the deltoid muscle (*white arrow* in *B*).

with clinical outcome following surgery.[18,19] Intact repaired tendons are usually thinner (earlier) or thicker (later) than normal tendons[18,19] and contain increased T2 signal intensity due to granulation tissue, fibrosis, suture material, or metal artifacts (**Fig. 2**).[18,20] This signal change involves almost 90% of the repaired tendons[18] and starts improving between 3 and 12 months following surgery,[19] although it can persist for several months to years.[21] This appearance is part of the normal spectrum of the postoperative repaired tendon. Therefore, it is prudent not to consider tendon re-tear following repair especially within the first year from surgery based on tendon irregularity, thinning, or signal hyperintensity.[19] On the other hand, parts of an abnormal tendon may not have been debrided or repaired during surgery due to poor tendon tissue quality; this fact emphasizes the importance of making comparison with preoperative MR imaging and referring to operative report to distinguish repaired tissue versus unrepaired tendons to avoid calling these changes re-tear. New postoperative T2 hyperintensity of the capsule and pericapsular soft tissues at the level of the axillary recess may be from synovial proliferation and capsular hypervascularity.[22]

If MRA is obtained after rotator cuff repair, the presence or absence of contrast in the subacromial-subdeltoid bursa does not necessarily indicate re-tear or intact repaired tendon, respectively. Most rotator cuff repairs are not watertight, which is not required for a favorable clinical outcome[23]; therefore, contrast communicating with the subacromial-subdeltoid bursa can be normal.[12,14] Conversely, contrast may not communicate with the subacromial-subdeltoid bursa even in the presence of a recurrent full-thickness RCT following surgery secondary to fibrosis and scar tissue formation.[24]

Expected osseous changes following surgery related to bone reaction to the suture anchors include T2 signal hyperintensity of the greater tuberosity at the region of suture anchors (**Fig. 3**). This signal change can last for years following surgery in asymptomatic patients.[18] The more focal fluid-like signal surrounding the suture anchors may be seen due to hydrolysis effect of the anchors, which will ultimately be replaced by bone within the first 2 years after surgery.[12] Flattened and abnormal morphology of the greater tuberosity can be an expected postsurgical finding after surgeons create an implantation trough,[12] which can mimic Hill-Sachs impaction.

Complications

There are numerous complications of rotator cuff repair, including re-tear, dislodged or broken sutures or anchors, muscle atrophy and fatty infiltration, nerve injury, deltoid muscle dehiscence after

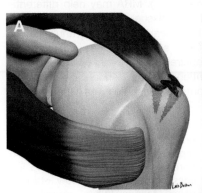
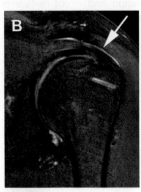
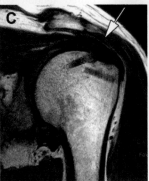

Fig. 2. 55-year-old man with prior primary RCR with intact repaired supraspinatus tendon. (*A*) Illustration of normal primary repair of rotator cuff tendon with suture anchors in the greater tuberosity without full-thickness defect. (*B*) Coronal PD with fat suppression (FS) and (*C*) coronal PD images following surgery show intact repaired tendon with expected thickening, mild irregularity and intrasubstance intermediate signal (*white arrow*); all normal postoperative findings. ([A] *Courtesy of* L. Beltran, MD, Boston, MA.)

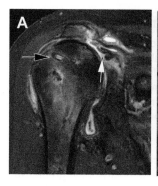
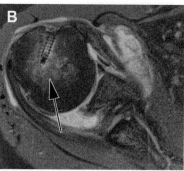

Fig. 3. 59-year-old man with prior primary RCR with full-thickness re-tear of the repaired supraspinatus tendon. (*A, B*) Coronal and axial PDFS images 4 months following surgery show delaminating full-thickness re-tear of the supraspinatus tendon (*white arrow*). Notice the expected edema-like signal of the greater tuberosity around the suture anchor (*black arrows*).

open surgery, shoulder stiffness or adhesive capsulitis, chondrolysis, and infection. The overall mean complication rate of arthroscopic repair is similar to that of open surgery, about 10.5%.[5,25] Re-tears (ranging from 11% to 94%) and shoulder stiffness (ranging from 2% to 11%) are the 2 most common complications following rotator cuff repair.[25] Among different repair techniques, the double-row suture anchor and the suture-bridge techniques have lower reported tendon re-tear rates than other techniques.[26,27] Patient age, severity of muscle atrophy and fatty infiltration, suboptimal rehabilitation, and size and location of the original tear are factors influencing the rate of re-tear.[28,29] Among these, the greatest predictive factor for re-tear is the size of the original tear in anteroposterior and mediolateral dimensions, with larger anteroposterior dimension and higher-grade of the tears posing the greatest risk of re-tear (see **Fig. 3**; **Figs. 4–6**).[29] Most re-tears are due to a failure of tendon healing as a result of poor tissue quality or fixation failure, either bony anchor pullout or suture breakage.[6,24] Loosened anchor, before being dislodged, can demonstrate osteolysis around its contour as a lobular T2 intermediate signal, which is thicker than expected after operative hydrolysis (**Fig. 7**).

The sensitivity and specificity of conventional MR imaging for postoperative rotator cuff re-tears is 84% and 91% for full-thickness tears, and 83% and 83% for partial tears, respectively.[30] MR imaging findings of rotator cuff re-tears are similar to those of original tendon tears, including a gap in the repaired tendon tissue with fluid signal or contrast material extending into or through it along with the absence of the heterogeneous repaired tendon at the expected site.[4] It is important to notice that intermediate -signal -intensity granulation tissue and scar may create the appearance of a partial-thickness or incomplete re-tear, resulting in overestimation of the degree of re-tear (see **Fig. 7**). MRA may help differentiating granulation tissue from real tear when contrast fills in the tear and not the granulation tissue (**Fig. 8**). Other secondary clues indicating failure of the repaired tendon can be obtained by paying attention to the tendon bulk at the expected footprint insertion on the greater

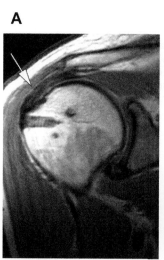
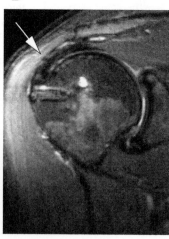

Fig. 4. 45-year-old woman with prior primary RCR and Sugaya type II intact repaired supraspinatus tendon. (*A*) Coronal PD and (*B*) coronal PDFS images following surgery show intact repaired tendon (*white arrows*) with sufficient tendon thickness and areas of high signal intensity.

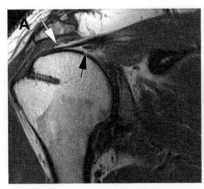
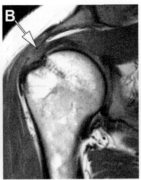

Fig. 5. Two different patients with prior primary RCR and Sugaya type III re-tear of repaired tendon. (*A*) Coronal PD image of a 47-year-old man shows insufficient thickness with less than half the thickness (*white arrow*) when compared with normal cuff and a retracted partial-thickness articular sided delaminated tear (*black arrow*). (*B*) Coronal PD image of a 44-year-old woman shows insufficient thickness and a retracted partial-thickness bursal sided tear (*white arrow*).

tuberosity, evaluating the morphology of the tendon and its myotendinous junction to assess for changes in the configuration and retraction of the repaired tendon,[4] and progression of rotator cuff muscle atrophy and fatty degeneration. Direct MRA is the most sensitive and specific technique for the diagnosis of partial-thickness or full-thickness re-tears (sensitivity 86%–100%, specificity 59%–100%);[31,32] however, it has been suggested that MRA may overestimate the tear of the repaired tendon compared with conventional MR imaging as it may accentuate small and clinically insignificant frayed edges of a repaired tendon as true defects following intraarticular contrast administration.[4,19] These clefts could be small undebrided portions of repaired tendon that would have gradually healed with time.[4]

Sugaya and colleagues[33] introduced an MR imaging-based classification system to evaluate for repaired tendon thickness and discontinuity (**Table 1**). This classification correlates well with patient functional outcomes and has shown good interobserver and intraobserver agreement for detecting full-thickness or partial-thickness re-tears of a repaired rotator cuff.[34,35]

Deep shoulder infections following arthroscopic repair are infrequently encountered, ranging from

0.3% and 1.9% (**Fig. 9**).[36,37] The most common organisms involved are *Staphylococcus aureus* and *Propionibacterium acnes*.[36,37]

IRREPARABLE ROTATOR CUFF TEARS

About 40% of all RCTs are considered massive RCTs,[38] which are particularly challenging to manage. They are usually associated with poorer clinical outcome following primary repair and have higher rate of re-tear.[39] There are variable definitions of massive RCT, which creates inconsistency in their diagnosis and treatment. Cofield's criterion[40] describing a massive tear as a 5-cm tear measured in the coronal plane and Gerber and colleague's definition of a full-thickness tear involving at least 2 adjacent tendons[41] are the most popular definitions. In massive RCT, primary repair is not always feasible because these tears are typically larger in size, have poor quality of the retracted torn tendon with scarring, and have more advanced cuff muscle atrophy and fatty degeneration. Despite recent advancement of arthroscopic primary repair,[39] massive RCTs have higher rate of re-tear ranging from 45% to 96%.[42,43] For these patients tendon debridement with option of biceps tenotomy or tenodesis can

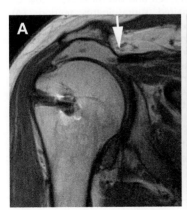
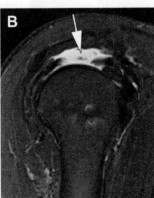

Fig. 6. 58-year-old man with prior primary RCR and Sugaya type V re-tear of repaired supraspinatus tendon. (*A*) Coronal PD and (*B*) sagittal PDFS images following surgery show full-thickness re-tear of repaired tendon with retraction (*white arrow*). Notice detached suture material in image B (*white arrow*).

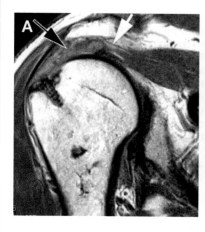
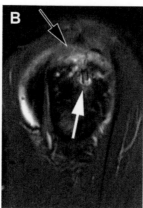

Fig. 7. 68-year-old woman with prior primary RCR and Sugaya type V re-tear of repaired supraspinatus tendon and loosened screw. (*A*) Coronal PD and (*B*) sagittal PDFS MR images following surgery show retracted full-thickness re-tear (*white arrow* in *A*), intermediate-signal-intensity scar and granulation tissue (*black arrows*) along the expected course of supraspinatus tendon, and osteolysis around one of the anchors (*white arrow* in *B*), which has slightly backed out from the cortex.

be performed mainly to achieve pain relief.[38,44] Reverse shoulder arthroplasty is a suitable choice for elderly patients with more advanced gleno-humeral arthrosis.[45,46] For the rest of these patients with irreparable massive RCT who have functional limitations and no substantial gleno-humeral arthrosis, more advanced surgical options are partial repair with augmentation procedures, including patch graft augmentation and bridging, superior capsular reconstruction (SCR),[47] and muscle tendon transfer.[47–49]

PATCH GRAFT AUGMENTATION AND BRIDGING

Grafts can be used both through open or arthroscopic techniques to augment repair of partial and full-thickness RCT if there is concern regarding healing or strength of the primary repair[50,51] or as a bridge for an irreparable defect.[52] Since its introduction in 1978,[51] studies have shown that use of graft can reinforce the primary repair in massive RCT.[38,50,53] Different graft materials, such as autograft (eg, fascia lata), allograft (eg, acellular human dermal graft), xenograft (eg, porcine dermis), and synthetic grafts (eg, poly-L-lactide acid) have been used.[38,50,51,53] For patch graft augmentation following completion of primary repair of the torn tendon, the appropriately sized graft is introduced into the joint and sutured to the underlying tendon.[54,55] Patch graft bridging is used for those with irreparable defect, usually greater than 1 cm, and insufficient excursion of the retracted torn tendon.[52] This method is used when only partial primary repair can be achieved and the graft acts as a bridge to fill the defect between the torn tendon and the footprint.[56]

Clinical outcomes partly depend on the graft material; human dermal extracellular matrix graft showed substantial reduction in postoperative re-tears,[57] while porcine grafts did not.[57] A study of arthroscopic revision rotator cuff repair with acellular human dermal allograft augmentation demonstrated 83% of patients without a re-tear and 87% without need for additional surgery at 2-year follow-up.[58] Synthetic polypropylene patch

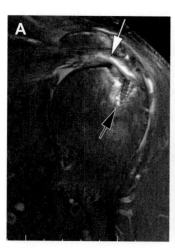
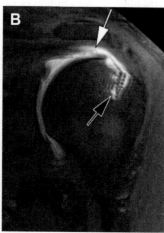

Fig. 8. 54-year-old man with prior primary RCR and full-thickness re-tear of repaired supraspinatus tendon. (*A*) Coronal PDFS arthrogram image shows intermediate-signal-intensity granulation tissue and scar (*white arrow*), which creates the appearance of a partial-thickness tear. (*B*) Coronal T1FS image reveals retracted full-thickness re-tear (*white arrow*), with contrast filling the tear gap and extends to the subdeltoid-subacromial bursa. Notice osteolysis around the anchor filled with contrast (*black arrows*).

Table 1
Classification of postoperative rotator cuff integrity using oblique coronal, oblique sagittal, and transverse T2-weighted MR images

Type I	Repaired cuff has sufficient thickness compared with normal cuff with homogenously low signal intensity
Type II	Sufficient thickness compared with normal cuff associated with partial high-intensity area
Type III	Insufficient thickness with less than half the thickness when compared with normal cuff, without discontinuity, suggesting a partial-thickness delaminated tear
Type IV	Presence of a minor discontinuity in only 1 or 2 slices on both oblique coronal and sagittal images, suggesting a small full-thickness tear
Type V	Presence of a major discontinuity observed in more than 2 slices on both oblique coronal and sagittal images, suggesting a medium- or large full-thickness tear

Data from Sugaya H, Maeda K, Matsuki K, et al. Functional and structural outcome after arthroscopic full-thickness rotator cuff repair: single-row versus dual-row fixation. Arthroscopy 2005;21(11):1307-1316.

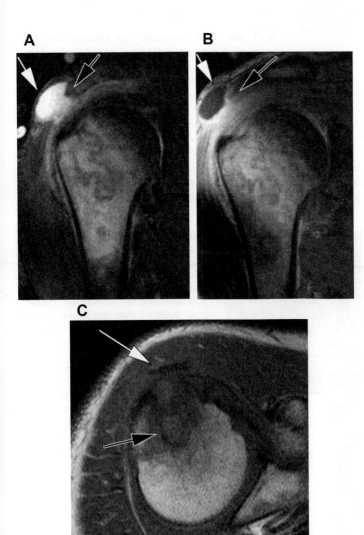

Fig. 9. 57-year-old woman who underwent open primary RCR. (*A*) Coronal T2FS and (*B*) coronal T1FS MR images following contrast administration show superficial rim enhancing abscess (*white arrow*) extending through dehiscence of the deltoid muscle (*black arrow*) from the subdeltoid bursa, which is also infected and connected to the shoulder joint through re-tear of the tendon. Notice proximal humerus osteomyelitis. (*C*) Axial PD image shows infected bone involving the anchor tract (*black arrow*). The anchor is completely dislodged (*white arrow*).

augmentation was shown to significantly improve the 3-year outcome, including function, strength, and re-tear rate following rotator cuff repair.[59] Inconsistency exists regarding rate of healing of repaired tendon when the graft is being used as an augmentation patch versus bridge,[52,55,59] although a recent systemic review reported no difference in healing and clinical outcome between the 2 methods.[51]

Normal Postoperative Imaging Findings

In a large systemic review of patients following graft augmentation and graft bridge, MR imaging was the imaging modality of choice for all patients.[51] The expected postoperative appearance is a low to intermediate heterogenous signal in the augmentation or bridging graft material with no fluid filled gap (**Fig. 10**). In the cases of augmentation, the intact graft may become imperceptible and difficult to separate from the native tendon on MR imaging.

Complication

The potential complications of patch graft are persistent or worsening pain, infection, sterile inflammatory reaction to the graft or suture material, and recurrent tear.[51] The rate of re-tear depending on the graft material ranges from 10% to 60%.[60] Patients with postoperative pain, loss of strength and limited range of motion are suspected to have graft failure and may get MR imaging to confirm the suspected graft complication. On MR imaging, the presence of full-thickness fluid cleft in the graft should be considered a recurrent tear. Based on Sugaya classification, type IV and V tendons are considered full-thickness re-tear.[60,61] Other findings suggestive of recurrent tear are laxity of the graft and progression of rotator cuff muscle fatty infiltration and atrophy over time. Rate of postoperative infection and sterile inflammatory reaction is less than 1% in a systemic review of patch graft rotator cuff repair.[51] Sterile inflammatory reaction more commonly occurs with bioabsorbable materials, such as screws or anchors and manifests as increased T2 signal, fluid accumulation and cystic changes around the implant and the anchors, with joint effusion, chondral damage and finally osteolysis.[62–64]

SUPERIOR CAPSULAR RECONSTRUCTION

SCR was first described by Mihata and colleagues[65] as an alternate treatment for symptomatic patients with irreparable massive RCT, which is ideally performed in younger patients with no significant arthrosis.[66] Originally fascia lata autograft was used for this procedure[67] but more recently dermal allograft has gained popularity, which has no donor site morbidity and has shorter operation time.[67] During SCR, the superior glenohumeral joint capsule is reconstructed by bridging the graft from the superior glenoid rim to the greater tuberosity. The reconstructed capsule,

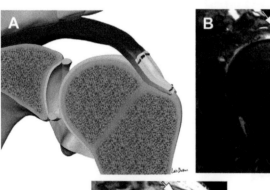
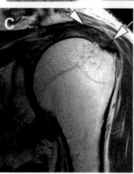

Fig. 10. 57-year-old woman with massive irreparable supraspinatus and infraspinatus tear who underwent rotator cuff debridement and patch graft augmentation. (*A*) Illustration of patch augmentation of a tear by placing graft (*yellow*) over the bursal surface of repaired tendon. (*B, C*) Postoperative coronal PD images with and without FS show intact patch graft augmentation (*white arrows*) along the bursal surface of the repaired tendon. The graft normally shows intermediate signal and fills the residual defect from bursal surface tear following debridement. ([A] *Courtesy of* L. Beltran, MD, Boston, MA.)

therefore, prevents superior humeral head translation, which could lead to rotator cuff arthropathy. Following debridement of the irreparable tendon stump, the graft is trimmed appropriately to match the defect size and then introduced through arthroscopy portals pushed to the subacromial space after applying sutures. The sutures will be tightened to the glenoid anchors usually at around 10 o'clock and 2 o'clock positions and laterally to the greater tuberosity. Side-to-side anastomosis is usually secured posteriorly to the infraspinatus tendon and often anteriorly to any residual rotator cuff tissue.[68] Two recent systemic reviews concluded that SCR results in statistically and clinically significant improvement in patient symptoms with low graft failure, complication, and reoperation rates at short-term follow-up while further studies are necessary to determine the long-term success of this technique.[69,70]

Normal Postoperative Imaging Findings

The normal postoperative MR imaging appearance of an SCR graft is a low signal and taut graft with no fluid signal discontinuity throughout its length. The graft should cover the superior humeral head (**Fig. 11**). The graft material should reach the glenoid and greater tuberosity attachments without complete or partial detachment from suture anchors. It is important to note that there are

sometimes small sutures holes in the graft more than 5 mm from the medial and lateral margins in the graft substance, which should not be interpreted as tears (**Fig. 12**).[71] The graft side-to-side attachments to the residual rotator cuff tendon if performed appear as close apposition of the graft with tendon tissue with susceptibility artifact related to suture material.

Complications

SCR re-tear can occur from the glenoid or humeral attachment and is associated with superior subluxation of the humeral head (**Figs. 13** and **14**).[61,71] In a recent study of 20 patients with SCR and MR imaging following surgery, 7 of the 11 tears occurred on the humeral side with only 1 tear on the glenoid side.[72] Performing acromioplasty at the time of SCR has been suggested to decrease the contact and aberration of the graft, lowering the risk of re-tear.[73] Tear at side-to-side anastomosis may be the only postoperative sign of partial failure of SCR.[71] Before making this diagnosis, however, it is important to refer to the operative report to ensure that side-to-side attachment was done, as they are not always performed, which can lead to a false diagnosis of side-to-side tear. Other useful secondary signs suggestive of graft failure are recurrent superior humeral subluxation and dislodged suture anchor. No other

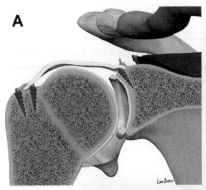
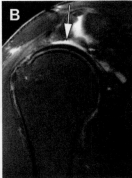
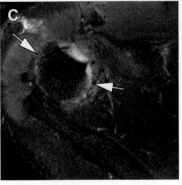

Fig. 11. 68-year-old woman with massive irreparable tear of the supraspinatus and infraspinatus tendons who had arthroscopic superior capsular reconstruction with dermal allograft. (*A*) Illustrations of superior capsular reconstruction with dermal allograft (*yellow*) bridging superior glenoid to greater tuberosity. (*B*) Coronal PDFS image shows low signal and taut graft (*arrow*) with intact humeral and glenoid attachments. The graft covers the humeral head superiorly. (*C*) Axial PDFS image shows the porous appearance of the dermal allograft (*arrows*). ([*A*] *Courtesy of* L. Beltran, MD, Boston, MA.)

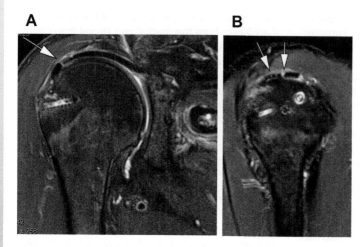

Fig. 12. 64-year-old man with massive irreparable tear of the supraspinatus and infraspinatus tendons who had arthroscopic superior capsular reconstruction with dermal allograft. (*A*) Coronal and (*B*) sagittal PDFS show low signal and taut graft with small suture holes (*arrows*), which should not be mistaken for tears.

surgical complications, such as neural injury, infection, or suture anchor problems have been reported yet.[67]

MUSCLE TENDON TRANSFER

Muscle tendon transfer is another accepted surgical alternative for symptomatic younger patients with irreparable massive RCT without glenohumeral osteoarthrosis.[50] Selection of donor tendon from several available options depends on rotator cuff structural deficit and impaired function. As general rules for this procedure, the transferred and recipient muscles should have similar excursion, tension and line of pull, transferred muscle should be expandable, and should replace only 1 function of the recipient muscle.[74,75] Latissimus dorsi (LD) and pectoralis major (PM) are the most commonly used transfer tendons. Substantial improvement in patient pain score, shoulder function, and mobility following tendon transfer has been reported.[76,77] LD transfer is typically performed in patients with massive irreparable posterosuperior RCT[76,77] via open or arthroscopically assisted procedure.[78,79] Transferred LD to the greater tuberosity acts similar to intact posterosuperior rotator cuff with external rotation and humeral head depression.[50,80] PM transfer is typically used in patients with anterosuperior irreparable massive RCT.[81–83] The sternal head force vector is closer to that of subscapularis muscle and is favored over clavicular head to simulate internal rotation.[83,84] The LD and PM tendons ultimately are attached to the greater and lesser tuberosity, respectively.

Normal Postoperative Imaging Findings

The transferred tendon is normally low to intermediate signal on MR imaging with heterogenous appearance, especially early after surgery, without fluid gap defect. The intact tendon portion of the graft may remain intermediate in signal at its humeral attachment due to scar formation.

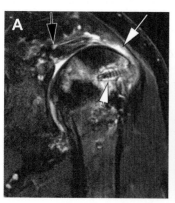
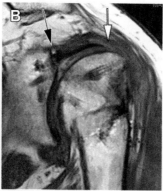

Fig. 13. 45-year-old man with massive irreparable tear of the supraspinatus and infraspinatus tendons who had arthroscopic superior capsular reconstruction with dermal allograft. (*A*) Coronal PDFS and (*B*) PD images show complete detachment of lateral margin of graft (*white arrows*) from humeral attachment, with intact medial attachment to the glenoid (*black arrows*). There is loosening of a suture anchor (*short arrow*).

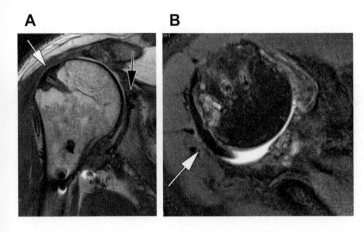

A **B**

Fig. 14. 68-year-old man with irreparable rotator cuff tear who underwent superior capsular reconstruction using dermal allograft. (*A*) Coronal PD image shows complete detachment of medial margin of graft from superior glenoid (*black arrow*), and intact humeral attachment to the anchor (*white arrow*). The graft is no longer covering the apex of the humeral head which is also elevated. (*B*) Axial PDFS image shows posteriorly displaced graft (*white arrow*).

Complications

The complications of LD transfer include infection, hematoma, injury to the neurovascular pedicle of the LD muscle, and tears of the tendon graft.[47] The most common complications of PM transfer are avulsion of the transferred tendon, supraspinatus and infraspinatus tendon tears, infection, axillary vein thrombosis, and rarely musculocutaneous nerve neuropraxia.[82,85] The transferred muscle and other muscle of the shoulder girdle should be evaluated for denervation edema and fatty infiltration as a result of nerve damage during surgery.

SUMMARY

MR imaging following rotator cuff repair can be challenging due to several factors, including altered anatomy and signal of the repaired tendon, postoperative artifacts, and new operative techniques. Familiarity with the various types of RCTs, the indications for surgery and their surgical treatments, normal postoperative MR imaging appearance, and complications specific to the surgical technique is essential for radiologists to allow an accurate and timely diagnosis following operative treatment.

DISCLOSURE

None of the authors has any disclosure.

REFERENCES

1. Colvin AC, Egorova N, Harrison AK, et al. National trends in rotator cuff repair. J Bone Joint Surg Am 2012;94(3):227–33.
2. Hurley ET, Maye AB, Mullett H. Arthroscopic rotator cuff repair. JBJS Rev 2019;7(4):e1.
3. Xu B, Chen L, Zou J, et al. The clinical effect of arthroscopic rotator cuff repair techniques: a network meta-analysis and systematic review. Sci Rep 2019;9(1):4143.
4. Kalia V, Freehill MT, Miller BS, et al. Multimodality imaging review of normal appearance and complications of the postoperative rotator cuff. Am J Roentgenol 2018;211(3):538–47.
5. Jancuska J, Matthews J, Miller T, et al. A systematic summary of systematic reviews on the topic of the rotator cuff. Orthop J Sports Med 2018;6(9). 232596711879789.
6. Pierce JL, Nacey NC, Jones S, et al. Postoperative shoulder imaging: rotator cuff, labrum, and biceps tendon. Radiographics 2016;36(6):1648–71.
7. McMenamin D, Koulouris G, Morrison WB. Imaging of the shoulder after surgery. Eur J Radiol 2008;68(1):106–19.
8. Peh WC, Chan JH. Artifacts in musculoskeletal magnetic resonance imaging: identification and correction. Skeletal Radiol 2001;30(4):179–91.
9. Dunn WR, Schackman BR, Walsh C, et al. Variation in orthopaedic surgeons' perceptions about the indications for rotator cuff surgery. J Bone Joint Surg Am 2005;87(9):1978–84.
10. Marx RG, Koulouvaris P, Chu SK, et al. Indications for surgery in clinical outcome studies of rotator cuff repair. Clin Orthop Relat Res 2009;467(2):450–6.
11. Iannotti JP. Full-thickness rotator cuff tears: factors affecting surgical outcome. J Am Acad Orthop Surg 1994;2(2):87–95.
12. Beltran LS, Bencardino JT, Steinbach LS. Postoperative MRI of the shoulder. J Magn Reson Imaging 2014;40(6):1280–97.
13. Jacobson JA, Miller B, Bedi A, et al. Imaging of the postoperative shoulder. Semin Musculoskelet Radiol 2011;15(4):320–39.
14. van der Zwaal P, Thomassen BJW, Nieuwenhuijse MJ, et al. Clinical outcome in all-arthroscopic versus mini-open rotator cuff repair in small to medium-sized

tears: a randomized controlled trial in 100 patients with 1-year follow-up. Arthroscopy 2013;29(2): 266–73.

15. Matava MJ, Purcell DB, Rudzki JR. Partial-thickness rotator cuff tears. Am J Sports Med 2005;33(9): 1405–17.

16. Chen M, Xu W, Dong Q, et al. Outcomes of single-row versus double-row arthroscopic rotator cuff repair: a systematic review and meta-analysis of current evidence. Arthroscopy 2013;29(8):1437–49.

17. Sobhy MH, Khater AH, Hassan MR, et al. Do functional outcomes and cuff integrity correlate after single- versus double-row rotator cuff repair? A systematic review and meta-analysis study. Eur J Orthop Surg Traumatol 2018;28(4):593–605.

18. Spielmann AL, Forster BB, Kokan P, et al. Shoulder after rotator cuff repair: MR imaging findings in asymptomatic individuals–initial experience. Radiology 1999;213(3):705–8.

19. Crim J, Burks R, Manaster BJ, et al. Temporal evolution of MRI findings after arthroscopic rotator cuff repair. AJR Am J Roentgenol 2010;195(6):1361–6.

20. Mohana-Borges AVR, Chung CB, Resnick D. MR imaging and MR arthrography of the postoperative shoulder: spectrum of normal and abnormal findings. Radiographics 2004;24(1):69–85.

21. Jost B, Zumstein M, Pfirrmann CWA, et al. Long-term outcome after structural failure of rotator cuff repairs. J Bone Joint Surg Am 2006;88(3):472–9.

22. Kim JN, Kwon ST, Kim KC. Early postoperative magnetic resonance imaging findings after arthroscopic rotator cuff repair: T2 hyperintensity of the capsule can predict reduced shoulder motion. Arch Orthop Trauma Surg 2018;138(2):247–58.

23. Woertler K. Multimodality imaging of the postoperative shoulder. Eur Radiol 2007;17(12):3038–55.

24. Zlatkin MB. MRI of the postoperative shoulder. Skeletal Radiol 2002;31(2):63–80.

25. Randelli P, Spennacchio P, Ragone V, et al. Complications associated with arthroscopic rotator cuff repair: a literature review. Musculoskelet Surg 2012;96(1):9–16.

26. Park MC, Tibone JE, ElAttrache NS, et al. Part II: biomechanical assessment for a footprint-restoring transosseous-equivalent rotator cuff repair technique compared with a double-row repair technique. J Shoulder Elbow Surg 2007;16(4):469–76.

27. Mihata T, Watanabe C, Fukunishi K, et al. Functional and structural outcomes of single-row versus double-row versus combined double-row and suture-bridge repair for rotator cuff tears. Am J Sports Med 2011;39(10):2091–8.

28. Goutallier D, Postel J-M, Gleyze P, et al. Influence of cuff muscle fatty degeneration on anatomic and functional outcomes after simple suture of full-thickness tears. J Shoulder Elbow Surg 2003;12(6): 550–4.

29. Le BTN, Wu XL, Lam PH, et al. Factors predicting rotator cuff retears. Am J Sports Med 2014;42(5): 1134–42.

30. Magee T, Shapiro M, Hewell G, et al. Complications of rotator cuff surgery in which bioabsorbable anchors are used. AJR Am J Roentgenol 2003; 181(5):1227–31.

31. Tudisco C, Bisicchia S, Savarese E, et al. Single-row vs. double-row arthroscopic rotator cuff repair: clinical and 3 Tesla MR arthrography results. BMC Musculoskelet Disord 2013;14(1):43.

32. Duc SR, Mengiardi B, Pfirrmann CWA, et al. Diagnostic performance of MR arthrography after rotator cuff repair. AJR Am J Roentgenol 2006;186(1): 237–41.

33. Sugaya H, Maeda K, Matsuki K, et al. Repair integrity and functional outcome after arthroscopic double-row rotator cuff repair. A prospective outcome study. J Bone Joint Surg Am 2007;89(5): 953–60.

34. Saccomanno MF, Cazzato G, Fodale M, et al. Magnetic resonance imaging criteria for the assessment of the rotator cuff after repair: a systematic review. Knee Surg Sports Traumatol Arthrosc 2015;23(2): 423–42.

35. Grant JA, Miller BS, Jacobson JA, et al. Intra- and inter-rater reliability of the detection of tears of the supraspinatus central tendon on MRI by shoulder surgeons. J Shoulder Elbow Surg 2013;22(6): 725–31.

36. Brislin KJ, Field LD, Savoie FH. Complications after arthroscopic rotator cuff repair. Arthroscopy 2007; 23(2):124–8.

37. Atesok K, MacDonald P, Leiter J, et al. Postoperative deep shoulder infections following rotator cuff repair. World J Orthop 2017;8(8):612–8.

38. Bedi A, Dines J, Warren RF, et al. Massive tears of the rotator cuff. J Bone Joint Surg Am 2010;92(9): 1894–908.

39. Henry P, Wasserstein D, Park S, et al. Arthroscopic repair for chronic massive rotator cuff tears: a systematic review. Arthroscopy 2015;31(12):2472–80.

40. Cofield RH. Subscapular muscle transposition for repair of chronic rotator cuff tears. Surg Gynecol Obstet 1982;154(5):667–72.

41. Gerber C, Fuchs B, Hodler J. The results of repair of massive tears of the rotator cuff. J Bone Joint Surg Am 2000;82(4):505–15.

42. Mellado JM, Calmet J, Olona M, et al. Surgically repaired massive rotator cuff tears: MRI of tendon integrity, muscle fatty degeneration, and muscle atrophy correlated with intraoperative and clinical findings. AJR Am J Roentgenol 2005;184(5):1456–63.

43. Galatz LM, Ball CM, Teefey SA, et al. The outcome and repair integrity of completely arthroscopically repaired large and massive rotator cuff tears. J Bone Joint Surg Am 2004;86-A(2):219–24.

44. Williams GR, Rockwood CA, Bigliani LU, et al. Rotator cuff tears: why do we repair them? J Bone Joint Surg Am 2004;86-A(12):2764–76.

45. Harreld KL, Puskas BL, Frankle MA. Massive rotator cuff tears without arthropathy: when to consider reverse shoulder arthroplasty. Instr Course Lect 2012;61:143–56.

46. Guery J, Favard L, Sirveaux F, et al. Reverse total shoulder arthroplasty survivorship analysis of eighty replacements followed for five to ten years. J Bone Joint Surg Am 2006;88(8):1742.

47. Namdari S, Voleti P, Baldwin K, et al. Latissimus dorsi tendon transfer for irreparable rotator cuff tears: a systematic review. J Bone Joint Surg Am 2012;94(10):891–8.

48. Omid R, Lee B. Tendon transfers for irreparable rotator cuff tears. J Am Acad Orthop Surg 2013;21(8): 492–501.

49. Merolla G, Chillemi C, Franceschini V, et al. Tendon transfer for irreparable rotator cuff tears: indications and surgical rationale. Muscles Ligaments Tendons J 2015;4(4):425–32.

50. Greenspoon JA, Millett PJ, Moulton SG, et al. Irreparable rotator cuff tears: restoring joint kinematics by tendon transfers. Open Orthop J 2016;10(Suppl 1: M2):266–76.

51. Ono Y, Dávalos Herrera DA, Woodmass JM, et al. Graft augmentation versus bridging for large to massive rotator cuff tears: a systematic review. Arthroscopy 2017;33(3):673–80.

52. Barber FA, Burns JP, Deutsch A, et al. A prospective, randomized evaluation of acellular human dermal matrix augmentation for arthroscopic rotator cuff repair. Arthroscopy 2012;28(1):8–15.

53. Derwin KA, Badylak SF, Steinmann SP, et al. Extracellular matrix scaffold devices for rotator cuff repair. J Shoulder Elbow Surg 2010;19(3):467–76.

54. Gilot GJ, Attia AK, Alvarez AM. Arthroscopic repair of rotator cuff tears using extracellular matrix graft. Arthrosc Tech 2014;3(4):e487–9.

55. Gilot GJ, Alvarez-Pinzon AM, Barcksdale L, et al. Outcome of large to massive rotator cuff tears repaired with and without extracellular matrix augmentation: a prospective comparative study. Arthroscopy 2015;31(8):1459–65.

56. Wong I, Burns J, Snyder S. Arthroscopic GraftJacket repair of rotator cuff tears. J Shoulder Elbow Surg 2010;19(2 Suppl):104–9.

57. Senekovic V, Poberaj B, Kovacic L, et al. Prospective clinical study of a novel biodegradable subacromial spacer in treatment of massive irreparable rotator cuff tears. Eur J Orthop Surg Traumatol 2013; 23(3):311–6.

58. Hohn EA, Gillette BP, Burns JP. Outcomes of arthroscopic revision rotator cuff repair with acellular human dermal matrix allograft augmentation. J Shoulder Elbow Surg 2018;27(5):816–23.

59. Ciampi P, Scotti C, Nonis A, et al. The benefit of synthetic versus biological patch augmentation in the repair of posterosuperior massive rotator cuff tears: a 3-year follow-up study. Am J Sports Med 2014; 42(5):1169–75.

60. Flury M, Rickenbacher D, Jung C, et al. Porcine dermis patch augmentation of supraspinatus tendon repairs: a pilot study assessing tendon integrity and shoulder function 2 years after arthroscopic repair in patients aged 60 years or older. Arthroscopy 2018; 34(1):24–37.

61. Sugaya H, Maeda K, Matsuki K, et al. Functional and structural outcome after arthroscopic full-thickness rotator cuff repair: single-row versus dual-row fixation. Arthroscopy 2005;21(11):1307–16.

62. Warden WH, Friedman R, Teresi LM, et al. Magnetic resonance imaging of bioabsorbale polylactic acid interference screws during the first 2 years after anterior cruciate ligament reconstruction. Arthroscopy 1999;15(5):474–80.

63. Müller M, Kääb MJ, Villiger C, et al. Osteolysis after open shoulder stabilization using a new bioresorbable bone anchor: a prospective, nonrandomized clinical trial. Injury 2002;33(Suppl 2): B30–6.

64. Edwards DJ, Hoy G, Saies AD, et al. Adverse reactions to an absorbable shoulder fixation device. J Shoulder Elbow Surg 1994;3(4):230–3.

65. Mihata T, McGarry MH, Pirolo JM, et al. Superior capsule reconstruction to restore superior stability in irreparable rotator cuff tears: a biomechanical cadaveric study. Am J Sports Med 2012;40(10): 2248–55.

66. Petri M, Greenspoon JA, Moulton SG, et al. Patch-augmented rotator cuff repair and superior capsule reconstruction. Open Orthop J 2016;10(Suppl 1 M7):315–23.

67. Mihata T, Lee TQ, Watanabe C, et al. Clinical results of arthroscopic superior capsule reconstruction for irreparable rotator cuff tears. Arthroscopy 2013; 29(3):459–70.

68. Adams CR, Denard PJ, Brady PC, et al. The arthroscopic superior capsular reconstruction. Am J Orthop (Belle Mead NJ) 2016;45(5):320–4.

69. Sochacki KR, McCulloch PC, Lintner DM, et al. Superior capsular reconstruction for massive rotator cuff tear leads to significant improvement in range of motion and clinical outcomes: a systematic review. Arthroscopy 2019;35(4):1269–77.

70. Catapano M, de SA D, Ekhtiari S, et al. Arthroscopic superior capsular reconstruction for massive, irreparable rotator cuff tears: a systematic review of modern literature. Arthroscopy 2019; 35(4):1243–53.

71. Samim M, Walsh P, Gyftopoulos S, et al. Postoperative MRI of massive rotator cuff tears. Am J Roentgenol 2018;211(1):146–54.

72. Denard PJ, Brady PC, Adams CR, et al. Preliminary results of arthroscopic superior capsule reconstruction with dermal allograft. Arthroscopy 2018;34(1):93–9.

73. Mihata T, McGarry MH, Kahn T, et al. Biomechanical effects of acromioplasty on superior capsule reconstruction for irreparable supraspinatus tendon tears. Am J Sports Med 2016;44(1):191–7.

74. Elhassan B, Bishop A, Shin A, et al. Shoulder tendon transfer options for adult patients with brachial plexus injury. J Hand Surg Am 2010;35(7):1211–9.

75. Elhassan BT, Wagner ER, Werthel J-D. Outcome of lower trapezius transfer to reconstruct massive irreparable posterior-superior rotator cuff tear. J Shoulder Elbow Surg 2016;25(8):1346–53.

76. El-Azab HM, Rott O, Irlenbusch U. Long-term follow-up after latissimus dorsi transfer for irreparable posterosuperior rotator cuff tears. J Bone Joint Surg Am 2015;97(6):462–9.

77. Gerber C, Rahm SA, Catanzaro S, et al. Latissimus dorsi tendon transfer for treatment of irreparable posterosuperior rotator cuff tears. J Bone Joint Surg Am 2013;95(21):1920–6.

78. Moursy M, Forstner R, Koller H, et al. Latissimus dorsi tendon transfer for irreparable rotator cuff tears: a modified technique to improve tendon transfer integrity. J Bone Joint Surg Am 2009;91(8):1924–31.

79. Petri M, Greenspoon JA, Bhatia S, et al. Patch-augmented latissimus dorsi transfer and open reduction-internal fixation of unstable os acromiale for irreparable massive posterosuperior rotator cuff tear. Arthrosc Tech 2015;4(5):e487–92.

80. Henseler JF, Nagels J, Nelissen RGHH, et al. Does the latissimus dorsi tendon transfer for massive rotator cuff tears remain active postoperatively and restore active external rotation? J Shoulder Elbow Surg 2014;23(4):553–60.

81. Galatz LM, Connor PM, Calfee RP, et al. Pectoralis major transfer for anterior-superior subluxation in massive rotator cuff insufficiency. J Shoulder Elbow Surg 2003;12(1):1–5.

82. Jost B, Puskas GJ, Lustenberger A, et al. Outcome of pectoralis major transfer for the treatment of irreparable subscapularis tears. J Bone Joint Surg Am 2003;85-A(10):1944–51.

83. Konrad GG, Sudkamp NP, Kreuz PC, et al. Pectoralis major tendon transfers above or underneath the conjoint tendon in subscapularis-deficient shoulders an in vitro biomechanical analysis. J Bone Joint Surg Am 2007;89(11):2477.

84. Gavriilidis I, Kircher J, Magosch P, et al. Pectoralis major transfer for the treatment of irreparable anterosuperior rotator cuff tears. Int Orthop 2010;34(5):689–94.

85. Shin JJ, Saccomanno MF, Cole BJ, et al. Pectoralis major transfer for treatment of irreparable subscapularis tear: a systematic review. Knee Surg Sports Traumatol Arthrosc 2016;24(6):1951–60.

Anterior Instability
What to Look for

Christopher J. Burke, MBChB[a],*, Tatiane Cantarelli Rodrigues, MD[a],
Soterios Gyftopoulos, MD, MSc[b]

KEYWORDS

- Anterior shoulder instability • Glenoid track • Glenoid bone loss • On-track and off-track lesions
- Engaging and nonengaging lesions

KEY POINTS

- The glenohumeral joint has the greatest range of motion of any major articulation, with the trade-off for this mobility being a susceptibility to injury and subsequent instability.
- Reciprocating contra-coup injuries of the humeral head and glenoid are pathognomonic for articular instability in the posttraumatic setting, usually associated with injuries to stabilizing soft tissue structures.
- The prognosis and treatment of anterior glenohumeral instability depends to a large extent on whether injury is isolated to the soft tissues or whether it also involves substantial glenoid or humeral bone loss.
- The role of imaging is centered on the identification of lesions associated with instability and lesion characterization for treatment planning.

INTRODUCTION

Anterior shoulder instability (ASI) is a common problem in the general population with incidence rates in the general US population estimated at 0.08 per 1000 person-years.[1,2]

ASI is characterized by the disruption of the dynamic and static stabilizers of the glenohumeral joint, resulting in dislocation, subluxation, and/or apprehension.[1] It represents a continuum, from an acute traumatic event causing first-time dislocation followed by repeated dislocations requiring lesser degrees of provocation at one end of the spectrum, to glenohumeral hypermobility without antecedent trauma leading to progressive instability over time at the other end of the spectrum.[3]

Imaging plays an important role in the evaluation of the ASI patient population, identifying and characterizing associated injuries for treatment planning. The purpose of this article is to review the role of various imaging modalities in the assessment of patients with ASI. Advances in 3D computed tomography (CT) and MR imaging, particularly for the quantification of bone loss is discussed, as well as concepts of engaging/nonengaging lesions and on-track/and off-track lesions.

NORMAL ANATOMY AND BIOMECHANICS

The glenohumeral joint is maintained by a complex combination of dynamic and passive stabilizers that maintain near perfect rotation of the humeral head over the central glenoid fossa during normal range of motion. The static stabilizers include the articular surface of the glenoid, the capsulolabral structures and negative intra-articular pressure, and the dynamic stabilizers are the rotator cuff, long head of biceps (LHB), deltoid, and regional musculature.[4–6]

[a] Department of Radiology, NYU Langone Health, NYU Langone Orthopedic Center, 333 East 38th Street, New York, NY 10016, USA; [b] 333 East 38th Street, New York, NY 10016, USA
* Corresponding author.
E-mail address: christopher.burke@nyulangone.org

Magn Reson Imaging Clin N Am 28 (2020) 195–209
https://doi.org/10.1016/j.mric.2019.12.004

Static Stabilizers

Articular surfaces

The glenohumeral joint is comprised of 2 articulating spherical contact surfaces: the glenoid cavity and the humeral head. The glenoid fossa covers only 25% of the humeral head surface.[7,8] This size discrepancy of the articular surfaces results in the largest range of motion of any major joint at the cost of vulnerability to trauma and potential development of instability.[7-9] The congruent articular surfaces provide stability through the negative intra-articular pressure and concavity-compression effect, which is particularly important during the midrange of glenohumeral movement when there is capsular and ligamentous laxity.[8,10]

Labroligamentous complex

The labral and ligamentous structures, specifically the inferior portions, are the main stabilizers of the glenohumeral joint with the arm at the end-range of movement that is abduction external rotation (ABER), and adduction internal rotation.[4,8,11,12] The glenoid labrum is a fibrocartilaginous structure that circumferentially covers the rim of the bony glenoid fossa, increasing the bony contact size by about one-third and improving joint surface congruity.[6,13,14] The labrum also serves as an attachment site for capsuloligamentous structures, such as the glenohumeral ligaments (GHLs), LHB, and the long head of the triceps.[6,13]

The superior, middle, and inferior GHLs are capsular bands that insert onto the labrum and adjacent glenoid rim.[11] The anterior band of the inferior glenohumeral ligament (IGHL) is critical to anterior passive joint stabilization.[3,14] It attaches to the anteroinferior labrum and primarily resists translation in the ABER position where the anteroinferior capsule becomes taut.[8,15]

Dynamic Stabilizers

The main dynamic stabilizers of glenohumeral joint are the rotator cuff, LHB, and deltoid, with additional contributions from the pectoralis major, latissimus dorsi, and periscapular muscles.[16] Centering of the humeral head on the glenoid during motion is achieved through the coordination of 2 force couples, coronal and transverse. The coronal force couple is a result of the balance of moments created by the supraspinatus working with the deltoid versus the inferior rotator cuff (infraspinatus, subscapularis, and teres minor). This is said to be balanced only if the line of action of the rotator cuff force is below the center of rotation of the humeral head so that it can oppose the moment created by the deltoid muscle. A balanced coronal force couple maintains an adequate fulcrum for the glenohumeral joint

motion. The transverse force couple is a balanced moment between the anterior subscapularis and posterior infraspinatus–teres minor muscles.

Through the midrange of motion, the capsuloligamentous structures are lax and the joint is stabilized by dynamic joint compression.[4] The primary function of the LHB is the stabilization of the glenohumeral joint in the ABER position, thereby reducing stress on the IGHL.[6] The anterior stabilizing function of the deltoid muscle is more prominent when the shoulder becomes unstable.[5] Despite this, the regional musculature and tendons alone are insufficient to maintain normal glenohumeral stability.[8]

CLINICAL SCENARIOS

Pathophysiology of Acute and Recurrent Anterior Shoulder Instability

In the vast majority of cases, ASI follows an acute traumatic event.[17,18] Fall onto an outstretched hand is a common traumatic mechanism, as is dislocation from forced ABER or a direct posterior shoulder blow.[3] Traumatic dislocation can lead to chronic instability and repeated dislocations requiring successively less force and degrees of provocation.[19] Instability can also evolve as a result of cumulative stresses related to occupational or sport-specific activities.[3,20,21]

Many factors influence the recurrence rate, such as the location and severity of structural damage, sex, and patient age at initial presentation.[22,23] Recurrent instability has been reported to occur 3 times more frequently in young men compared with women.[17,24] Only 16% of patients older than 40 years at the time of first dislocation have been reported to experience recurrent ASI, compared with 83% of patients younger than 20 years.[23]

Common Bone and Soft Tissue Findings

ASI leads to reciprocating osseous lesions of the posterosuperior humeral head and anteroinferior glenoid, due to shear forces and osteochondral compression that occur when the humeral head impacts the glenoid rim and relocates in the glenoid cavity.[16] The softer trabecular bone of the humeral head makes it more susceptible to impaction fractures, also known as Hill-Sachs (HS) lesions, after contact with the relatively more robust, wedge-shaped cortex of the anterior glenoid rim.[25]

At the time of glenohumeral dislocation, traction on the IGHL is transmitted to the labrum causing a partial or complete detachment of the labrum from the glenoid rim as well as tearing of the adjacent capsule.[3] The inferior capsulolabral complex can demonstrate various injury patterns, including soft tissue Bankart lesion, Perthes lesion, anterior labroligamentous periosteal sleeve avulsion (ALPSA), glenolabral articular disruption (GLAD) lesion (**Fig. 1**), and humeral avulsion of the glenohumeral ligament (HAGL) lesion (**Fig. 2**).[3] These capsulolabral lesions can vary depending on factors, such as the initial location of the lesion, activity level of the patient, and number of subsequent dislocations.[26,27]

Differences Between Acute and Recurrent Dislocation

The prevalence of HS lesions is reported to be 65% to 67% after initial dislocation, increasing to 84% to 93% after recurrent dislocation.[8] In arthroscopic studies, Bankart lesions, ALPSA, capsular laxity, HS lesions, glenoid rim deficiency, and

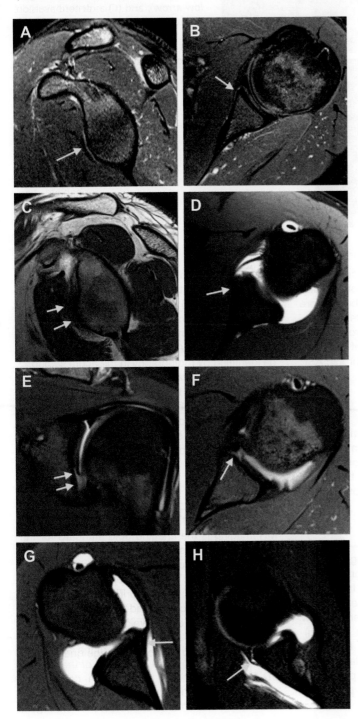

Fig. 1. Capsulolabral injuries. A 20-year-old man with history of recurrent ASI and first episode 2 years previously. (*A*) Sagittal fat-suppressed T2-weighted and (*B*) axial fat-suppressed PD-weighted images demonstrating a nondisplaced tear of the anteroinferior labrum with associated stripping of the periosteum compatible with a soft tissue Bankart lesion (*yellow arrows*). A 32-year-old man with a history of ASI. (*C*) Sagittal T1-weighted and (*D*) axial fat-suppressed T1-weighted images from an MR arthrogram demonstrate a tear of the anteroinferior labrum, which is medialized and scarred, consistent with a chronic anterior labroligamentous periosteal sleeve avulsion (ALPSA) lesion (*yellow arrows*). A 43-year-old woman with history of fall and shoulder dislocation 3 years previously. (*E*) Coronal fat-suppressed T2-weighted and (*F*) axial fat-suppressed PD-weighted images demonstrate blunting of the anteroinferior glenoid labrum with an adjacent focal full-thickness glenoid cartilage defect and delamination consistent with a glenolabral articular disruption lesion (*yellow arrows*). A 15-year-old girl with history of shoulder pain after a volleyball injury. Axial fat-suppressed T1-weighted images in the neutral (*G*) and ABER positions (*H*) from an MR arthrogram demonstrate a nondisplaced tear of the anteroinferior labrum, better visualized on the ABER sequence, with contrast extending along the base of the labrum, consistent with a Perthes lesion (*yellow arrows*).

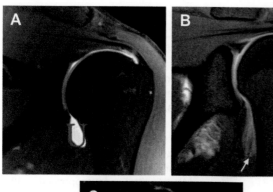

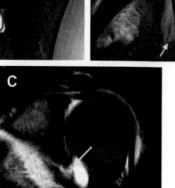

Fig. 2. Humeral avulsion of the gleno-humeral ligament. MR arthrogram coronal images demonstrating (*A*) the normal U-shaped inferior glenohumeral ligament (IGHL); (*B*) a humeral avulsion of glenohumeral ligament lesion with an inverted J-shaped morphology due to detachment of the IGHL from it humeral insertion (*yellow arrow*); and (*C*) a glenoid avulsion of the glenohumeral ligament lesion with a J-shaped morphology resulting from detachment of the IGHL from its glenoid insertion (*yellow arrow*).

greater tuberosity fractures were more common in patients with chronic repeated dislocation.[26] Rotator cuff tearing occurs in both settings but is more frequent in repeat dislocators.[26] Acute findings, such as hemarthrosis and bone marrow contusions may coexist with the sequelae of repeated dislocation in the setting of acute on chronic ASI[3] (**Table 1**).

IMAGING ALGORITHM

Accurate identification and characterization of ASI-related injuries are crucial for treatment planning and prognosis, largely depending on whether the injury(s) are isolated to the soft tissues or whether there is substantial glenoid or humeral bone loss (ie, bipolar bone loss).[28]

Radiographs

Radiographs are typically the first imaging study obtained. Following dislocation, radiographs can demonstrate the direction of humeral translation and confirm appropriate reduction.[3] The standard trauma series includes anteroposterior view (neutral or with internal/external arm rotation), scapular "Y", and axillary views.[21,29,30] If the arm cannot be abducted, a modified axillary lateral view called the Velpeau view can be performed instead of the superior-inferior axial projection view.[21]

In addition to joint alignment, radiographs can also demonstrate the typical bone injuries seen in ASI present in 95% of patients.[29] The common bony injury pattern includes an HS lesion, with or without an anteroinferior glenoid fracture (osseous Bankart lesion).[29] A total of 83% of HS lesions can be identified by radiography in the acute setting.[31] Additional radiographic projections can improve detection of these bony injuries. The Stryker notch view can help confirm the presence of HS lesions, whereas the glenoid profile view, West Point, or Bernageau views show the anteroinferior glenoid rim, thereby improving detection of glenoid lesions.[21,29]

MR Imaging

Conventional MR imaging

MR imaging is the imaging gold standard for the diagnosis of the soft tissue injuries seen in ASI and can be used to diagnose and quantify associated bone injuries.[14,31,32] Most MR imaging protocols use a combination of nonfat saturated and fat saturated T2-weighted and proton density sequences, as well as T1-weighted imaging in the axial, coronal, and sagittal oblique planes. We prefer 3T MR imaging for optimal image quality.

3D MR imaging

A 3D 2-point Dixon sequence can be added to MR examinations with minimal increase in imaging

Table 1
Most common anterior shoulder instability injuries

Clinical Scenarios	Osseous Lesions	Soft Tissue Lesions
Acute	Pathognomonic pattern of bone marrow edema Hill-Sachs	Bankart lesion Perthes lesion GLAD lesion HAGL lesion Hemarthrosis Localized extra-articular edema or hemorrhage/capsular or myotendinous injury
Chronic	Glenoid rim fracture Hill-Sachs Greater tuberosity fracture	Bankart lesion ALPSA lesion Capsular laxity Rotator cuff tear

time, allowing creation of 3D osseous models to evaluate and quantify bipolar bone injuries.[32] Glenoid bone loss (GBL) measurements performed on 3D MR imaging reconstructions have shown close correlation with measurements performed on 3D CT, the current imaging gold standard.[33–36]

MR arthrography

MR arthrography (MRA) has little or no role in the acute setting, with a joint effusion often creating an arthrographic effect.[3,31] Indications for MRA include evaluation of the labrum, glenohumeral ligaments, LHB, and rotator cuff tears.[37] The presence of gadolinium within the labrum is considered the primary criterion for diagnosing of a tear, with abnormal morphology and labral displacement typically regarded as secondary signs.[38] MRA has a sensitivity of 88% to 96% and a specificity of 91% to 98% in the evaluation of glenoid labrum lesions.[3,31]

MRA plays an important role in the assessment of younger individuals with suspected ASI, when subtle capsulolabral abnormalities may have significant influence on function, management, and prognosis.[3,39] It also has particular use in the postoperative setting of suspected recurrent labral tear.

MRA requires injection of dilute gadolinium contrast material into the joint. The injection is usually performed under fluoroscopic or ultrasound guidance using either anterior or posterior approaches. One advantage of the posterior approach is avoidance of traversing anterior

stabilizer structures, such as the anterior labrum, IGHL, or subscapularis.[37] The recommended injection volume ranges from 10 to 15 mL.[37] Occasionally in the context of a patulous capsule, the joint may accommodate a volume of up to 20 mL, but an injection greater than 15 mL carries increased risk of extra-articular leakage that may be mistaken for capsule tear.[37]

More widespread availability of 3T MR imaging with improved imaging quality has decreased the use of MRA and overall MR imaging is now more commonly than MRA. Despite this, many clinicians at our institution continue to request arthrographic imaging in the workup of ASI.

Computed Tomography

Conventional computed tomography

CT imaging is commonly performed to characterize bipolar bone loss, allowing simultaneous examination of the glenoid and humeral head.[29,40] Both 2D and 3D CT techniques are well established; however, 3D reconstructions are considered the imaging gold standard for the evaluation.[40] Most protocols include multiplanar reformats obtained from the primary axial dataset using soft tissue and osseous filters with 3D volumetric reformats.

Computed tomography arthrography

In those unable to undergo MR imaging, CT arthrography (CTA) has been shown to be reliable in detection of capsulolabral and cartilaginous injuries, with sensitivities ranging from 82% to 100% and specificities from 96% to 100%.[41] It is useful for the detection of glenoid rim fractures and humeral avulsion of the IGHL, crucial findings in preoperative planning.[41] CTA improves soft tissue evaluation compared with conventional CT and, similar to MRA, has particular use in the postoperative shoulder. Iodinated contrast material may, however, limit quantitative osseous assessment, due to similar attenuation as bone.[36]

SOFT TISSUE INJURIES
Soft Tissue Bankart Lesion

Bankart lesions are the most common of the labral injuries and include tears of both the anteroinferior labrum (3–6 o'clock) and capsule insertion/glenoid periosteum (see **Fig. 1**A, B).[9,29,42,43] The labrum may be partially or completely detached from the glenoid rim.[3] The diagnosis can be made on both noncontrast MR imaging and MRA, manifested as linear high T2 signal or contrast imbibition between the labrum and anteroinferior glenoid rim in conjunction with capsular tearing.[9,44]

Bankart labral tears demonstrate high T2-weighted fluid signal more often (92%) than T1-weighted gadolinium signal (76%) on MRA.[38] The anterior inferior labrum is the most vascular portion of the labrum thereby potentially allowing an increased capacity for healing.[38] Nacey and colleagues[38] theorized that resynovialization could cause fluid to be trapped beneath the tear possibly accounting for a higher incidence of T2-weighted fluid signal compared with superior labrum anterior and posterior (SLAP) tears, and also potentially for the concurrent lack of gadolinium within some fluid-containing Bankart tears at MRA.

Anterior Labroligamentous Periosteal Sleeve Avulsion

The ALPSA lesion is commonly seen with chronic ASI and reflects avulsion of the anterior inferior labrum and IGHL from the anterior inferior glenoid with an intact scapular periosteum.[9,44] There is a "peel back" of the anterior band of the IGHL at the glenoid attachment occurring due to the different tissue compositions of the IGHL at the attachment to the labrum and bone, with a weaker labral attachment.[9] On axial and coronal oblique MR images, an anteroinferior glenoid rim devoid of the labral tissue provides the clue for this diagnosis with further inspection revealing a medially displaced and deformed capsulolabral complex (see **Fig. 1**C, D).[3,9,44] After recurrent dislocation episodes, the avulsed capsulolabral complex can retract medially with the periosteum and heal in a displaced position, leading to recurrent ASI due to chronic persistent incompetence of the capsulolabral complex.[9] Over time, the chronically detached labrum and IGHL may synovialize and enlarge resulting in a chronic "mass-like" lesion potentially mimicking an intact capsulolabral complex at arthroscopy.[3,9]

Perthes Lesion

The Perthes lesion is a nondisplaced tear of the anteroinferior labrum and IGHL with an intact scapular periosteum.[3,9] Unlike the Bankart lesion, which is closely associated with traumatic dislocation, the Perthes lesion can result from physical overuse and repetitive microtrauma.[45] At arthroscopy, this lesion may also be overlooked because the labrum remains anatomically positioned.[46] MR imaging demonstrates a linear high signal tear of the anteroinferior labrum with an intact low signal periosteum and IGHL (see **Fig. 1**G).[46] This may be poorly conspicuous on noncontrast MR imaging where the labrum can appear normal.[3,9,46] Joint effusion or arthrographic fluid distension allows improved visualization of Perthes lesion,

usually best seen on axial images, and the lesion is often more conspicuous with the addition of oblique axial slices in the ABER position (see **Fig. 1**H).[3,9,46]

Glenolabral Articular Disruption Lesion

The GLAD lesion is a nondisplaced tear of the anterior inferior labrum accompanied by damage to the adjacent articular cartilage, including fibrillation, erosion, or delamination.[9,47] At the time of dislocation, shear forces and osseous impaction damage the articular cartilage along the anteroinferior glenoid fossa.[48] Recurrent ASI is often not the presenting complaint in these patients as the IGHL remains firmly attached to the labrum, instead patients present with pain as the result of the chondral defect.[9,48,49] On MR imaging there is a nondisplaced or minimally displaced tear of the anteroinferior labrum, with an intact periosteum and anterior band of the IGHL, associated with adjacent cartilage injury (see **Fig. 1**E, F).[49] The presence of an intra-articular effusion or contrast can improve the visualization of small chondral flaps.[44,49] With recurrent ASI episodes, chondral fragments may increase in size and detach from the glenoid fossa, resulting in intra-articular bodies and progressive cartilage loss.[24,49]

Humeral Avulsion of Glenohumeral Ligament Lesions and Other Capsulolabral Injuries

HAGL lesions have been identified in 21% of patients imaged within 7 days of an anterior dislocation episode.[50] ASI in the presence of HAGL lesions is reported to occur with a prevalence of between 2% and 9.4%.[51] On coronal MR imaging, the normal inferior capsule should appear as a U shape. With avulsion of the humeral IGHL attachment, one will see the "J" sign whereby the inferior glenohumeral recess is retracted away from the humerus (see **Fig. 2**).[9,51,52] Other MR imaging findings of a HAGL lesion include thickening and increased signal intensity of the ligament, extravasation of contrast and native joint fluid along the humeral neck.[53] There may be avulsion of an osseous fragment at the humeral insertion, referred to as a bony HAGL, occurring in 20% of HAGLs.[9,54] In such cases, CT may better demonstrate the cortical fracture or periosteal detachment.[3]

When a tear occurs at the glenoid IGHL attachment, this is described as a glenoid avulsion of the glenohumeral ligament. This demonstrates a J configuration on coronal MR imaging in the opposite direction of a HAGL lesion (see **Fig. 2**).[9,51,55] Indeed, failure of the IGHL is more frequent at its glenoid insertion (40%) or midsubstance (35%), with only 25% tearing at the humerus. Rarely, a tear may occur at the humeral IGHL attachment with a concomitant capsulolabral tear, termed the "floating" anterior IGHL.[9] SLAP lesions can be seen often in association with other more typical instability injuries, contributing to ASI secondary to the loss of stability provided by the intra-articular LHB tendon and superior labrum.[9]

Rotator Cuff Tendon Tears

Rotator cuff tendon tears in the setting of ASI are more commonly seen in middle-aged and elderly patients.[56–58] Older patients experience age-related degenerative changes of the cuff tendons and, in this population, any ASI event may damage the already-weakened rotator cuff.[58] Rotator cuff tears can also be seen in younger patients, typically athletes who endure repetitive microtrauma during overhead throwing motions or while engaging in contact sports.[58] A torn rotator cuff may cause continued dysfunction and recurrent ASI. The most commonly torn tendon is the subscapularis (**Fig. 3**).[57] The subscapularis tendon lies along the anterior aspect of the glenohumeral joint intimately associated with the anterior joint capsule, predisposing it to damage due to impaction of the anteriorly displaced humeral head.[57] Importantly, a Bankart repair is less likely to succeed with associated high-grade subscapularis tears due to its role in static and dynamic stabilization of the glenohumeral joint.[3,58,59]

In general, the clinicians at our institution do not expect terms, such as Bankart, Perthes, ALPSA, and HAGL in our reports. Instead, they prefer a detailed description of the injuries, specifying what is torn, where and if there is any displacement.

ASSESSMENT OF BONE INJURIES
Bipolar Bone Loss

Bipolar bone injuries of the glenoid and humeral head are common injuries in the setting of ASI, found in up to 80% of patients, predisposing to recurrent ASI with a cumulative effect depending on size and location.[8,29,60] Although the HS lesion is the most common imaging finding after dislocation, GBL is considered to have a greater prognostic implication due to an increasing predisposition to chronic instability with progressive GBL.[61–63] Accurate characterization and quantification of both GBL and HS lesions in the preoperative setting is therefore essential to assess prognostic potential and guide appropriate treatment.[64,65]

Glenoid bone loss

GBL can appearance in 2 forms. In the acute setting, one can see a fracture along the anterior glenoid margin (bony Bankart lesion). In the chronic setting, GBL can appear as flattening of the anterior glenoid margin due to chronic impaction and attritional change related to repeated humeral head contact.[66] A flattened glenoid has been found to predispose to recurrent ASI more often than a fractured glenoid in patients with previous Bankart repair.[66] With increasing loss of bone stock, articular incongruency creates a mechanical mismatch that predisposes to recurrent dislocation and functional disability.[64]

On radiographs, there may be irregularity and loss of the subchondral bone at the anteroinferior glenoid.[67] CT reformations may show nondisplaced fracture lines and/or small osseous fracture fragments.[3] On MR imaging and CT the first imaging sign of GBL may be straightening of the anterior glenoid rim, which can be observed even in the absence of perceptible reduction of glenoid width.[68] Enface views of the glenoid provide the best visualization of the glenoid articular surface for measurement purposes on both 2D and 3D imaging. As a result of GBL, the bony glenoid may appear as an inverted pear-shape with the inferior half of the glenoid having a shorter diameter than the superior half.[29,69,70]

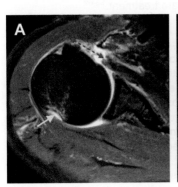 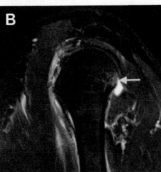

Fig. 3. Hill-Sachs lesion and supscapularis tendon tear. A 76-year-old man following ASI. (*A*) Axial fat-suppressed PD-weighted and (*B*) sagittal T2 fat-suppressed MR images demonstrating Hill-Sachs lesion (*yellow arrows*) with associated underlying bone marrow edema and a full-thickness tear of the subscapularis tendon (*red broken arrows*).

There are different methods for quantifying GBL.[71] The best-fit circle surface area method (also referred to as the "Pico method") and the glenoid width index method are the most commonly used techniques.[29,72] With the Pico method, the percentage of GBL is estimated by drawing a best-fit circle along the margins of the inferior two-thirds of glenoid with bone lesion or by measuring the contralateral glenoid.[8,29] The width measurements are made perpendicular to a line through the vertical axis of the glenoid and the missing area estimates the GBL. The ratio of width of injured glenoid: width of normal glenoid × 100 estimates the GBL.[8,29] The Pico method accurately quantifies GBL in both the anterior and anteroinferior locations[72] and is associated with recurrent dislocation when above 20%.[8,29] The glenoid width index method is a linear measurement technique representing the ratio of the maximum inferior diameter of the injured glenoid to the maximum inferior diameter of the uninjured contralateral glenoid. When interpreting the glenoid index, values of 1.0 denote normal bone stock, and values <1.0 denote GBL.[72] Compared with surface area measurements, linear measurements of glenoid bone defects have been found to overestimate bone loss.[73] These methods are not interchangeable and cannot be used with the same critical thresholds for GBL.[73]

Humeral bone loss

The prevalence of HS lesions increases from 25% in first-time dislocators to 40% to 90% in those experiencing repeated dislocations, often enlarging in size with increasing numbers of dislocations.[26] The location and orientation of the lesion depends on the position of the humeral head during dislocation and the magnitude of compressive force.[69] The HS lesion may have various appearances; deep and angular, or shallow with smooth borders.[67]

Radiographic HS lesion characteristics have been classically described as rarefaction seen medial to the lateral contour of the greater tuberosity on external rotation views; indentation or flattening of the articular surface seen on internal rotation views; and an osseous defect with the floor of the lesion best seen on tangential views.[74] CT and MR imaging may demonstrate a flattened appearance or a more concave lesion. The posterior humeral head can sometimes demonstrate a normal flattened appearance, termed the bare area, at its junction with the shaft; however, this should not be confused with an HS lesion.[75,76] An HS lesion is typically seen at or above the level of the coracoid process tip within the superior 4 to 5 mm of the humeral head margin, which should otherwise be circular on axial CT or MR images. The humeral bare area is usually located caudal to this.[67,75,76] The MR imaging appearances of an HS lesion depend on acuity, with bone marrow edema often seen in the acute setting.[3,74]

There are different ways to describe an HS lesion, including (1) subjective, (2) 3D measurements, and (3) percentage of humeral head diameter; however, there is no universally accepted measurement method.[29,77,78] Important factors include lesion size, degree of articular surface involvement, and location of the defect relative to the glenoid track.[78] Measurements of HS lesions using CT and MR imaging have shown good reliability.[29,36,71,77,78] Although CT measurements of HS lesion width have been reported to underestimate the defect size, depth measurements have been shown to be more accurate.[78]

Other bone lesions

Other less common ASI osseous injuries include coracoid process fractures, occurring in 3% to 13%, greater and lesser tuberosity fractures, occurring in 15% to 35% of dislocated shoulders.[79,80]

Engaging and Nonengaging Hill-Sachs Lesions

An engaging HS lesion was defined in 2000 by Burkhart and De Beer,[69] arthroscopically, as a significant bone defect on the humeral side that engaged the anterior glenoid rim when the arm was brought into a position of athletic function, defined as 90° abduction combined with external rotation in the range between 0° and 135°. It was an arthroscopic finding and the lesion size was not defined. In the ABER position, the glenoid rim drops into this defect causing apprehension and subluxation in mild cases or locking and dislocation in severe cases.[3,32] The prevalence of engaging HS lesions is about 7% in recurrent ASI.[81] Although the diagnosis of engagement can be made during arthroscopy, MR imaging and CT can characterize these lesions preoperatively to guide appropriate treatment.[63,69]

On-Track and Off-Track Lesions

Yamamoto and colleagues[82] introduced the glenoid track theory to emphasize the importance of bipolar bone loss evaluation to assess the risk for engagement. Subsequently in 2013, Kurokawa and colleagues,[81] using the glenoid track concept, defined an engaging HS lesion as a lesion extending beyond the medial margin of the glenoid track. The glenoid track refers to the area of posterior humeral articular surface in contact with the glenoid when the arm moves along the posterior end-range of movement with ABER positioning. The track compromises approximately 83% of the glenoid width.[8,29,83] An HS lesion that stays within the glenoid track is considered to be low risk for engagement and dislocation. An HS lesion that extends beyond the medial margin of the track is considered high risk for engagement and dislocation because there is decreased contact between the opposing bone surfaces.[8,29,83]

Di Giacomo and colleagues[84] introduced the "on-track/off-track" method, based on the glenoid track, as a technique to evaluate bipolar bone lesions and predict engagement and instability. This method is believed to improve the ability to predict engagement preoperatively, and therefore help plan optimal treatment. This is important because physical examination findings may lead to a false diagnosis of engagement related to the increased laxity afforded by torn anterior capsulolabral structures.[83]

The on-track/off-track method consists of a comparison between 2 measurements that can be performed on imaging: the HS interval and glenoid track (**Figs. 4–6**). The HS interval represents the width of the HS lesion plus the width of the intact bone bridge between the rotator cuff and the HS lesion.[84] The glenoid track is assessed using similar measurements obtained during the quantification of GBL. A best-fit circle is placed along the margins of the inferior glenoid. A horizontal line is placed within the center of the circle and extended from the posterior to the anterior margin of the circle. This line represents the estimated diameter of the intact glenoid. A second horizontal line is placed at that same level between the anterior margin of the circle and the anterior margin of the glenoid. This line represents the amount of anterior GBL. The glenoid track is calculated as $0.83 \times (D - d)$ in which D represents the

diameter of the intact glenoid in millimeters and d corresponds to the amount of GBL in millimeters (see **Figs. 4–6**).

The HS interval is composed of the HS width plus the width of the intact bone bridge (measured from the lateral margin of the HS lesion to the cuff insertion) measured in millimeters. The HS interval measurement is made on axial images at the point with the greatest medial extent of the lesion (see **Figs. 4** and **5**). Lesions are considered off-track and at risk for engagement if the HS index is greater than the glenoid track (see **Fig. 5**), whereas lesions are considered on-track and not at risk for engagement if the HS interval is less than the glenoid track (see **Fig. 4**).[83]

Clinical studies have validated the on-track/off-track method as a reliable technique to predict engagement and instability.[8,83,85] 2D MR images without 3D reconstructions have shown the on-track/off-track method to demonstrate an accuracy of 84.2% for predicting engagement.[83] MR imaging allows a more accurate estimate of the HS interval than CT, because the rotator cuff insertion is more clearly visualized.[83]

Preoperative studies have shown recurrence rates of 75% in off-track patients compared with 8% in on-track patients.[8] Locher and colleagues[86] evaluated preoperative MR imaging and/or CT scans of patients undergoing arthroscopic Bankart repair, demonstrating that an off-track HS lesion had a much higher recurrence rate of instability and need for revision surgery than an on-track HS lesion (33% vs 6%, respectively). Comparing the on-track/off-track method to GBL loss, the positive predictive value of the off-track concept to predict the recurrence was 75% compared with using a GBL of greater than 20% where the positive predictive value was 43%.[85]

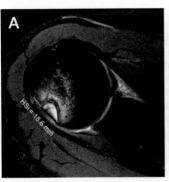 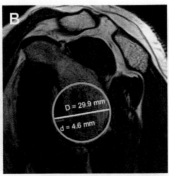

Fig. 4. On-track bipolar bone loss. A 35-year-old man with a history of ASI. (*A*) Axial fat-suppressed PD-weighted image shows a small Hill-Sachs lesion along the posterior humeral head. The Hill-Sachs interval, composed of the Hill-Sachs width (*blue line*) and bone bridge width (*orange line*) measures 18.6 mm. (*B*) Sagittal PD-weighted image shows flattening of the anterior glenoid margin. Using the best-fit circle technique (*green line*), the estimate of the intact glenoid diameter is 29.9 mm (D, *yellow line*) and amount of glenoid bone loss is 4.6 mm (d, *red line*). Using these measurements, the glenoid track was estimated to be 20.2 mm (0.83 × [29.9 – 4.6]). The Hill-Sachs interval is *less than* the glenoid track; therefore, the bipolar bone loss is characterized as *on-track*.

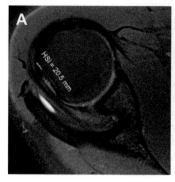
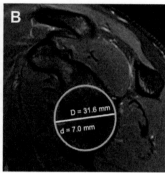

Fig. 5. Off-track bipolar bone loss. A 25-year-old man with history of recurrent ASI. (*A*) Axial fat-suppressed PD-weighted image shows a superficial broad Hill-Sachs lesion along the posterosuperior humeral head with a Hill-Sachs interval (*blue line plus orange line*) measuring 20.5 mm. (*B*) Sagittal fat-suppressed T2-weighted image shows a deficient anterior glenoid margin. Using the best-fit circle (*green line*), the intact glenoid diameter was 31.6 mm (D, *yellow line*) and glenoid bone loss 7.0 mm (d, *red line*) (0.83 × [31.6–7.0]) resulting in a glenoid track estimate of 19.2 mm. The Hill-Sachs interval is *greater than* the glenoid track; therefore, the bipolar bone loss is characterized as *off-track*.

We routinely report the size of the HS lesion, either subjectively (small, moderate, or large) or objectively (craniocaudal × transverse × anterior-posterior) and GBL (percent bone loss). We perform measurements on either 2D sagittal T1W images at the level of the glenoid surface or 3D reconstructed images of the glenoid in the en face view. MR imaging with 3D reformats are now typically ordered for ASI patients, and has all but replaced the need for pretreatment CT with 3D reformats at our institution. Measurements are performed by a radiologist and generally take between 5 and 10 minutes depending on expertise and comfort level of the reader.

TREATMENT STRATEGY

Patients without significant bone injuries typically undergo a capsulolabral repair. For those with more pronounced osseous injuries, treatment will focus on the most significant lesion, usually the glenoid.

Glenoid Bone Loss

In patients with anterior labral tearing and GBL less than 20% to 25%, the typical surgical management consists of a Bankart labral repair procedure, which involves reattachment of the torn detached labrum and IGHL to the glenoid, with reported redislocation rates of 0% to 7%.[87,88]

Historically, 20% to 25% has been accepted as the "critical" cutoff where GBL should be addressed in a primary procedure. There are, however, limited data on the impact that lesser, "subcritical" amounts of bone loss (below the 20%–25% range) have on functional outcomes and failure rates after stabilization. Recent data indicate that critical bone loss may be lower than the 20% to 25% threshold often cited. Shaha and colleagues[89] reported that GBL above 13.5% was associated with a clinically significant decrease in Western Ontario Shoulder Instability scores in a population with a high level of activity, even when not predisposing to

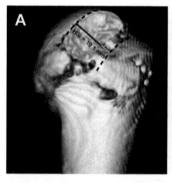
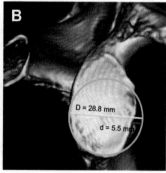

Fig. 6. On-track/off-track measurements. A 21-year-old woman with history of ASI. MR imaging 3D reconstructions demonstrate (*A*) Hill-Sachs lesion (*yellow area*) with Hill-Sachs width (*blue line*) and bone bridge width (*orange line*), resulting in a Hill-Sachs interval measuring 19.1 mm. (*B*) En face view of glenoid with a bony Bankart demonstrating the best-fit circle (*green line*) with estimates of an intact glenoid diameter, 28.8 mm (D, *yellow line*), and glenoid bone loss, 5.5 mm (d, *red line*), (0.83 × [28.8–5.5]) resulting in a glenoid track of 18.4 mm. The Hill-Sachs interval is greater than glenoid track; therefore, this bipolar bone loss is characterized as *off-track*.

recurrent ASI. High-functional demand patients, such as professional throwing athletes, may have a lower threshold for more aggressive management of mild GBL.[90] The recommended treatment may be open reduction and internal fixation for acute injuries, the Latarjet procedure for chronic injuries, and autograft or allograft procedures if a previous Latarjet procedure was unsuccessful.[90]

Greater than 25% GBL is usually treated with glenoid augmentation.[90] The preferred reconstruction approaches include the Bristow and Latarjet procedures involving an ipsilateral autologous coracoid bone block transfer.[28] The Bristow procedure transfers the lateral tip of the coracoid process. The Latarjet procedure transfers the entire horizontal coracoid pillar, and the inferior surface of the coracoid bone block, rather than the cut surface, is in contact with the glenoid vault.[91]

Humeral Bone Loss Treatment

Humeral bone defects below 20% are often managed conservatively.[90,92] An important exception is high-performance throwing athletes who require stability throughout extreme ranges of motion.[90] ASI associated with 20% to 40% humeral bone loss in acute episodes, detected within 3 to 4 weeks of the injury, can be addressed by humeroplasty to restore parameters of the HS lesion

using a size-matched bulk humeral allograft.[90,93] There is also a humeroplasty technique using percutaneous balloon and cement, similar to kyphoplasty methods.[94] For chronic injuries, remplissage has been used.[28] This surgical treatment involves tenodesis of the infraspinatus tendon and posterior glenohumeral joint capsule into the humeral HS lesion using fixation screws, thereby rendering the defect extra-articular and preventing engagement of the HS lesion with the anterior glenoid.[28,90]

The management of large humeral defects greater than 40% depends on the age and patient demand. Young active patients will require humeral reconstruction, either using cadaveric allograft or augmentation with a prosthetic cap matched to the defect size. Low-demand elderly patients are most often treated with shoulder arthroplasty.[28]

Treatment strategy for on-track/off-track lesions

Itoi[8] proposed a treatment strategy based on the on-track/off-track concept, consisting of 4 strategies (**Fig. 7**). The surgeons at our institution are not yet routinely using the on/off-track status in their treatment algorithm; however, this is widely regarded to be the suggested algorithm.

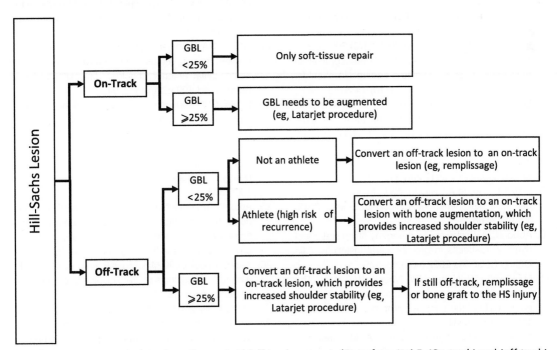

Fig. 7. Treatment strategy based on the on-track/off-track concept. (*Data from* Itoi E. 'On-track' and 'off-track' shoulder lesions. EFORT Open Rev 2017;2(8):343-351.)

SUMMARY

The radiological findings of ASI depend on the clinical scenario and differ in the setting of acute first-time dislocation versus chronic instability with repeated dislocation. MR imaging plays an important role in characterizing soft tissue injuries as well as quantifying bipolar bone loss, which affect management. Radiologists should be familiar with these techniques as well as the concepts of on-track/off-track lesions and engagement, which impact on the clinical management of ASI.

DISCLOSURE

There are no funding sources, commercial or financial conflicts of interest for any of the authors.

REFERENCES

1. Galvin JW, Ernat JJ, Waterman BR, et al. The epidemiology and natural history of anterior shoulder instability. Curr Rev Musculoskelet Med 2017;10(4):411–24.
2. Waterman B, Owens BD, Tokish JM. Anterior shoulder instability in the military athlete. Sports Health 2016;8(6):514–9.
3. Bencardino JT, Gyftopoulos S, Palmer WE. Imaging in anterior glenohumeral instability. Radiology 2013;269(2):323–37.
4. Dodson CC, Cordasco FA. Anterior glenohumeral joint dislocations. Orthop Clin North Am 2008;39(4):507–18, vii.
5. Kido T, Itoi E, Lee SB, et al. Dynamic stabilizing function of the deltoid muscle in shoulders with anterior instability. Am J Sports Med 2003;31(3):399–403.
6. Tischer T, Vogt S, Kreuz PC, et al. Arthroscopic anatomy, variants, and pathologic findings in shoulder instability. Arthroscopy 2011;27(10):1434–43.
7. Duprey S, Naaim A, Moissenet F, et al. Kinematic models of the upper limb joints for multibody kinematics optimisation: an overview. J Biomech 2017;62:87–94.
8. Itoi E. 'On-track' and 'off-track' shoulder lesions. EFORT Open Rev 2017;2(8):343–51.
9. Walz DM, Burge AJ, Steinbach L. Imaging of shoulder instability. Semin Musculoskelet Radiol 2015;19(3):254–68.
10. Abboud JA, Soslowsky LJ. Interplay of the static and dynamic restraints in glenohumeral instability. Clin Orthop Relat Res 2002;(400):48–57.
11. O'Connell PW, Nuber GW, Mileski RA, et al. The contribution of the glenohumeral ligaments to anterior stability of the shoulder joint. Am J Sports Med 1990;18(6):579–84.
12. Matsen FA, Harryman DT, Sidles JA. Mechanics of glenohumeral instability. Clin Sports Med 1991;10(4):783–8.
13. Calcei JG, Boddapati V, Altchek DW, et al. Diagnosis and treatment of injuries to the biceps and superior labral complex in overhead athletes. Curr Rev Musculoskelet Med 2018;11(1):63–71.
14. Hantes M, Raoulis V. Arthroscopic findings in anterior shoulder instability. Open Orthop J 2017;11:119–32.
15. Burkart AC, Debski RE. Anatomy and function of the glenohumeral ligaments in anterior shoulder instability. Clin Orthop Relat Res 2002;400:32–9.
16. Lippitt S, Matsen F. Mechanisms of glenohumeral joint stability. Clin Orthop Relat Res 1993;(291):20–8.
17. Cameron KL, Mauntel TC, Owens BD. The epidemiology of glenohumeral joint instability: incidence, burden, and long-term consequences. Sports Med Arthrosc Rev 2017;25(3):144–9.
18. Mazzocca AD, Brown FM Jr, Carreira DS, et al. Arthroscopic anterior shoulder stabilization of collision and contact athletes. Am J Sports Med 2005;33(1):52–60.
19. Robinson CM, Howes J, Murdoch H, et al. Functional outcome and risk of recurrent instability after primary traumatic anterior shoulder dislocation in young patients. J Bone Joint Surg Am 2006;88(11):2326–36.
20. Dumont GD, Fogerty S, Rosso C, et al. The arthroscopic Latarjet procedure for anterior shoulder instability: 5-year minimum follow-up. Am J Sports Med 2014;42(11):2560–6.
21. Dumont GD, Russell RD, Robertson WJ. Anterior shoulder instability: a review of pathoanatomy, diagnosis and treatment. Curr Rev Musculoskelet Med 2011;4(4):200–7.
22. Arciero RA, Wheeler JH, Ryan JB, et al. Arthroscopic Bankart repair versus nonoperative treatment for acute, initial anterior shoulder dislocations. Am J Sports Med 1994;22(5):589–94.
23. ROWE CR. Prognosis in dislocations of the shoulder. J Bone Joint Surg Am 1956;38-A(5):957–77.
24. Hovelius L, Saeboe M. Neer award 2008: arthropathy after primary anterior shoulder dislocation—223 shoulders prospectively followed up for twenty-five years. J Shoulder Elbow Surg 2009;18(3):339–47.
25. Antonio GE, Griffith JF, Yu AB, et al. First-time shoulder dislocation: high prevalence of labral injury and age-related differences revealed by MR arthrography. J Magn Reson Imaging 2007;26(4):983–91.
26. Yiannakopoulos CK, Mataragas E, Antonogiannakis E. A comparison of the spectrum of intra-articular lesions in acute and chronic anterior shoulder instability. Arthroscopy 2007;23(9):985–90.
27. Kim DS, Yoon YS, Yi CH. Prevalence comparison of accompanying lesions between primary and recurrent anterior dislocation in the shoulder. Am J Sports Med 2010;38(10):2071–6.

28. Beltran LS, Duarte A, Bencardino JT. Postoperative imaging in anterior glenohumeral instability. AJR Am J Roentgenol 2018;211(3):528–37.

29. Ruiz Santiago F, Martínez Martínez A, Tomás Muñoz P, et al. Imaging of shoulder instability. Quant Imaging Med Surg 2017;7(4):422–33.

30. Day MS, Epstein DM, Young BH, et al. Irreducible anterior and posterior dislocation of the shoulder due to incarceration of the biceps tendon. Int J Shoulder Surg 2010;4(3):83–5.

31. Wintzell G, Haglund-Akerlind Y, Tengvar M, et al. MRI examination of the glenohumeral joint after traumatic primary anterior dislocation. A descriptive evaluation of the acute lesion and at 6-month follow-up. Knee Surg Sports Traumatol Arthrosc 1996;4(4):232–6.

32. Gyftopoulos S, Yemin A, Mulholland T, et al. 3DMR osseous reconstructions of the shoulder using a gradient-echo based two-point Dixon reconstruction: a feasibility study. Skeletal Radiol 2013;42(3): 347–52.

33. Yanke AB, Shin JJ, Pearson I, et al. Three-dimensional magnetic resonance imaging quantification of glenoid bone loss is equivalent to 3-dimensional computed tomography quantification: cadaveric study. Arthroscopy 2017;33(4):709–15.

34. Stillwater L, Koenig J, Maycher B, et al. 3D-MR vs. 3D-CT of the shoulder in patients with glenohumeral instability. Skeletal Radiol 2017;46(3):325–31.

35. Vopat BG, Cai W, Torriani M, et al. Measurement of glenoid bone loss with 3-dimensional magnetic resonance imaging: a matched computed tomography analysis. Arthroscopy 2018;34(12): 3141–7.

36. Gyftopoulos S, Hasan S, Bencardino J, et al. Diagnostic accuracy of MRI in the measurement of glenoid bone loss. AJR Am J Roentgenol 2012;199(4): 873–8.

37. Llopis E, Montesinos P, Guedez MT, et al. Normal shoulder MRI and MR arthrography: anatomy and technique. Semin Musculoskelet Radiol 2015;19(3): 212–30.

38. Nacey NC, Fox MG, Bertozzi CJ, et al. Incidence of gadolinium or fluid signal within surgically proven glenoid labral tears at MR arthrography. Skeletal Radiol 2019;48(8):1185–91.

39. Saba L, De Filippo M. MR arthrography evaluation in patients with traumatic anterior shoulder instability. J Orthop 2017;14(1):73–6.

40. Griffith JF, Yung PS, Antonio GE, et al. CT compared with arthroscopy in quantifying glenoid bone loss. AJR Am J Roentgenol 2007;189(6):1490–3.

41. Acid S, Le Corroller T, Aswad R, et al. Preoperative imaging of anterior shoulder instability: diagnostic effectiveness of MDCT arthrography and comparison with MR arthrography and arthroscopy. AJR Am J Roentgenol 2012;198(3):661–7.

42. Palmer WE, Brown JH, Rosenthal DI. Labral-ligamentous complex of the shoulder: evaluation with MR arthrography. Radiology 1994;190(3):645–51.

43. Kompel AJ, Li X, Guermazi A, et al. Radiographic evaluation of patients with anterior shoulder instability. Curr Rev Musculoskelet Med 2017;10(4): 425–33.

44. Demehri S, Hafezi-Nejad N, Fishman EK. Advanced imaging of glenohumeral instability: the role of MRI and MDCT in providing what clinicians need to know. Emerg Radiol 2017;24(1):95–103.

45. Gerber C, Nyffeler RW. Classification of glenohumeral joint instability. Clin Orthop Relat Res 2002;(400):65–76.

46. Wischer TK, Bredella MA, Genant HK, et al. Perthes lesion (a variant of the Bankart lesion): MR imaging and MR arthrographic findings with surgical correlation. AJR Am J Roentgenol 2002;178(1):233–7.

47. Waldt S, Burkart A, Imhoff AB, et al. Anterior shoulder instability: accuracy of MR arthrography in the classification of anteroinferior labroligamentous injuries. Radiology 2005;237(2):578–83.

48. Neviaser TJ. The GLAD lesion: another cause of anterior shoulder pain. Arthroscopy 1993;9(1):22–3.

49. Sanders TG, Tirman PF, Linares R, et al. The glenolabral articular disruption lesion: MR arthrography with arthroscopic correlation. AJR Am J Roentgenol 1999;172(1):171–5.

50. Liavaag S, Stiris MG, Svenningsen S, et al. Capsular lesions with glenohumeral ligament injuries in patients with primary shoulder dislocation: magnetic resonance imaging and magnetic resonance arthrography evaluation. Scand J Med Sci Sports 2011;21(6):e291–7.

51. Carlson CL. The "J" sign. Radiology 2004;232(3): 725–6.

52. Melvin JS, Mackenzie JD, Nacke E, et al. MRI of HAGL lesions: four arthroscopically confirmed cases of false-positive diagnosis. AJR Am J Roentgenol 2008;191(3):730–4.

53. Wang W, Huang BK, Sharp M, et al. MR arthrogram features that can be used to distinguish between true inferior glenohumeral ligament complex tears and iatrogenic extravasation. AJR Am J Roentgenol 2019;212(2):411–7.

54. Bui-Mansfield LT, Taylor DC, Uhorchak JM, et al. Humeral avulsions of the glenohumeral ligament: imaging features and a review of the literature. AJR Am J Roentgenol 2002;179(3):649–55.

55. Mannem R, DuBois M, Koeberl M, et al. Glenoid avulsion of the glenohumeral ligament (GAGL): a case report and review of the anatomy. Skeletal Radiol 2016;45(10):1443–8.

56. Itoi E, Tabata S. Rotator cuff tears in anterior dislocation of the shoulder. Int Orthop 1992;16(3):240–4.

57. Gyftopoulos S, Carpenter E, Kazam J, et al. MR imaging of subscapularis tendon injury in the setting of

anterior shoulder dislocation. Skeletal Radiol 2012; 41(11):1445–52.

58. Gombera MM, Gomberawalla MM, Sekiya JK. Rotator cuff tear and glenohumeral instability: a systematic review. Clin Orthop Relat Res 2014;472(8): 2448–56.

59. Morag Y, Jamadar DA, Miller B, et al. The subscapularis: anatomy, injury, and imaging. Skeletal Radiol 2011;40(3):255–69.

60. Arciero RA, Parrino A, Bernhardson AS, et al. The effect of a combined glenoid and Hill-Sachs defect on glenohumeral stability: a biomechanical cadaveric study using 3-dimensional modeling of 142 patients. Am J Sports Med 2015;43(6):1422–9.

61. Itoi E, Lee SB, Berglund LJ, et al. The effect of a glenoid defect on anteroinferior stability of the shoulder after Bankart repair: a cadaveric study. J Bone Joint Surg Am 2000;82(1):35–46.

62. Lo IK, Parten PM, Burkhart SS. The inverted pear glenoid: an indicator of significant glenoid bone loss. Arthroscopy 2004;20(2):169–74.

63. Burns DM, Chahal J, Shahrokhi S, et al. Diagnosis of engaging bipolar bone defects in the shoulder using 2-dimensional computed tomography: a cadaveric study. Am J Sports Med 2016;44(11):2771–7.

64. Piasecki DP, Verma NN, Romeo AA, et al. Glenoid bone deficiency in recurrent anterior shoulder instability: diagnosis and management. J Am Acad Orthop Surg 2009;17(8):482–93.

65. Shah AS, Karadsheh MS, Sekiya JK. Failure of operative treatment for glenohumeral instability: etiology and management. Arthroscopy 2011;27(5): 681–94.

66. Gyftopoulos S, Albert M, Recht MP. Osseous injuries associated with anterior shoulder instability: what the radiologist should know. AJR Am J Roentgenol 2014;202(6):W541–50.

67. Vande Berg B, Omoumi P. Dislocation of the shoulder joint—radiographic analysis of osseous abnormalities. J Belg Soc Radiol 2016;100(1):89.

68. Lee RK, Griffith JF, Tong MM, et al. Glenoid bone loss: assessment with MR imaging. Radiology 2013;267(2):496–502.

69. Burkhart SS, De Beer JF. Traumatic glenohumeral bone defects and their relationship to failure of arthroscopic Bankart repairs: significance of the inverted-pear glenoid and the humeral engaging Hill-Sachs lesion. Arthroscopy 2000;16(7):677–94.

70. Di Giacomo G, de Gasperis N, Scarso P. Bipolar bone defect in the shoulder anterior dislocation. Knee Surg Sports Traumatol Arthrosc 2016;24(2): 479–88.

71. Walter WR, Samim M, LaPolla FWZ, et al. Imaging quantification of glenoid bone loss in patients with glenohumeral instability: a systematic review. AJR Am J Roentgenol 2019;1–10. https://doi.org/10. 2214/AJR.18.20504.

72. Bois AJ, Fening SD, Polster J, et al. Quantifying glenoid bone loss in anterior shoulder instability: reliability and accuracy of 2-dimensional and 3-dimensional computed tomography measurement techniques. Am J Sports Med 2012;40(11): 2569–77.

73. Bakshi NK, Cibulas GA, Sekiya JK, et al. A clinical comparison of linear- and surface area-based methods of measuring glenoid bone loss. Am J Sports Med 2018;46(10):2472–7.

74. Workman TL, Burkhard TK, Resnick D, et al. Hill-Sachs lesion: comparison of detection with MR imaging, radiography, and arthroscopy. Radiology 1992;185(3):847–52.

75. Sandstrom CK, Kennedy SA, Gross JA. Acute shoulder trauma: what the surgeon wants to know. Radiographics 2015;35(2):475–92.

76. Massengill AD, Seeger LL, Yao L, et al. Labrocapsular ligamentous complex of the shoulder: normal anatomy, anatomic variation, and pitfalls of MR imaging and MR arthrography. Radiographics 1994; 14(6):1211–23.

77. Assunção JH, Gracitelli MEC, Borgo GD, et al. Tomographic evaluation of Hill-Sachs lesions: is there a correlation between different methods of measurement? Acta Radiol 2016;58(1):77–83.

78. Kodali P, Jones MH, Polster J, et al. Accuracy of measurement of Hill-Sachs lesions with computed tomography. J Shoulder Elbow Surg 2011;20(8): 1328–34.

79. McLaughlin HL, MacLellan DI. Recurrent anterior dislocation of the shoulder. II. A comparative study. J Trauma 1967;7(2):191–201.

80. Cottalorda J, Allard D, Dutour N, et al. Fracture of the coracoid process in an adolescent. Injury 1996; 27(6):436–7.

81. Kurokawa D, Yamamoto N, Nagamoto H, et al. The prevalence of a large Hill-Sachs lesion that needs to be treated. J Shoulder Elbow Surg 2013;22(9): 1285–9.

82. Yamamoto N, Itoi E, Abe H, et al. Contact between the glenoid and the humeral head in abduction, external rotation, and horizontal extension: a new concept of glenoid track. J Shoulder Elbow Surg 2007;16(5):649–56.

83. Gyftopoulos S, Beltran LS, Bookman J, et al. MRI evaluation of bipolar bone loss using the on-track off-track method: a feasibility study. AJR Am J Roentgenol 2015;205(4):848–52.

84. Di Giacomo G, Itoi E, Burkhart SS. Evolving concept of bipolar bone loss and the Hill-Sachs lesion: from "engaging/non-engaging" lesion to "on-track/off-track" lesion. Arthroscopy 2014;30(1):90–8.

85. Shaha JS, Cook JB, Rowles DJ, et al. Clinical validation of the glenoid track concept in anterior glenohumeral instability. J Bone Joint Surg Am 2016; 98(22):1918–23.

86. Locher J, Wilken F, Beitzel K, et al. Hill-Sachs off-track lesions as risk factor for recurrence of instability after arthroscopic bankart repair. Arthroscopy 2016;32(10):1993–9.

87. Rowe CR, Zarins B, Ciullo JV. Recurrent anterior dislocation of the shoulder after surgical repair. Apparent causes of failure and treatment. J Bone Joint Surg Am 1984;66(2):159–68.

88. Millett PJ, Horan MP, Martetschlager F. The "bony Bankart bridge" technique for restoration of anterior shoulder stability. Am J Sports Med 2013;41(3):608–14.

89. Shaha JS, Cook JB, Song DJ, et al. Redefining "critical" bone loss in shoulder instability: functional outcomes worsen with "subcritical" bone loss. Am J Sports Med 2015;43(7):1719–25.

90. Ramhamadany E, Modi CS. Current concepts in the management of recurrent anterior gleno-humeral joint instability with bone loss. World J Orthop 2016;7(6):343–54.

91. Giles JW, Degen RM, Johnson JA, et al. The Bristow and Latarjet procedures: why these techniques should not be considered synonymous. J Bone Joint Surg Am 2014;96(16):1340–8.

92. Porter DA, Birns M, Hobart SJ, et al. Arthroscopic treatment of osseous instability of the shoulder. HSS J 2017;13(3):292–301.

93. Kazel MD, Sekiya JK, Greene JA, et al. Percutaneous correction (humeroplasty) of humeral head defects (Hill-Sachs) associated with anterior shoulder instability: a cadaveric study. Arthroscopy 2005;21(12):1473–8.

94. Stachowicz RZ, Romanowski JR, Wissman R, et al. Percutaneous balloon humeroplasty for Hill-Sachs lesions: a novel technique. J Shoulder Elbow Surg 2013;22(9):e7–13.

Posterior Shoulder Instability: What to Look for

Domenico Albano, MD[a,b], Carmelo Messina, MD[a,c], Luca Maria Sconfienza, MD, PhD[a,c],*

KEYWORDS

- MR imaging - Magnetic resonance arthrography - Shoulder - Instability - Labrum - Glenoid

KEY POINTS

- Glenoid dysplasia and retroversion increase the risk of posterior shoulder instability and can be associated with a compensatory hypertrophy of the cartilage and the posterior labrum.
- Flattening and/or retroversion of the chondrolabral portion of the glenoid reduce the containment of the glenohumeral joint and may contribute to posterior shoulder instability.
- Posterior shoulder dislocation can result in bone lesions, such as reverse bony Bankart and McLaughlin fracture, which may predispose to posterior shoulder instability.
- Posterior labral tears can be observed in patients with posterior shoulder instability, including reverse Bankart, Kim lesion, and posterior labrocapsular periosteal sleeve avulsion.
- Posterior translation of the humeral head and posterior capsular laxity, seen at magnetic resonance arthrography by increased area of the posterior capsular pocket, can be observed in posterior shoulder instability.

INTRODUCTION

Posterior shoulder instability is less common than anterior instability and accounts for as much as 10% of all cases of shoulder instability.[1] Clinical picture of posterior instability is generally less evident, being therefore challenging to diagnose and often overlooked. Patients generally do not report a clear sensation of instability but just vague pain, weakness, and/or joint clicking, with a rare history of an acute traumatic event associated to symptom onset.[2] Different causal mechanisms have been associated with this condition, including acute trauma, microtrauma, or nontraumatic mechanisms. Repetitive microtrauma to the posteroinferior capsulolabral complex can lead to posterior instability, especially in soldiers, climbers, weight-lifters, swimmers, and those playing overhead sport activities.[3] A purely traumatic event less commonly leads to this condition. A posterior dislocation generally is not the starting point of posterior instability as opposed to an anterior shoulder dislocation.[4] Lastly, posterior instability can arise and progress to become clinically evident in patients with generalized joint laxity and multidirectional shoulder instability or anatomic abnormalities involving the glenoid, humeral head, posterior capsule, and labrum, which can predispose to shoulder instability.[2]

In this setting, imaging has a crucial role in the detection of posteroinferior capsulolabral complex and bony/soft tissue abnormalities that reduce joint stability. Magnetic resonance (MR) arthrography (MRA) is essential to show subtle capsulolabral and ligamentous findings.[5,6] This review describes

[a] IRCCS Istituto Ortopedico Galeazzi, Via Riccardo Galeazzi 4, Milano 20161, Italy; [b] Sezione di Scienze Radiologiche, Dipartimento di Biomedicina, Neuroscienze e Diagnostica Avanzata, Università degli Studi di Palermo, Via del Vespro 127, Palermo 90127, Italy; [c] Dipartimento di Scienze Biomediche per la Salute, Università degli Studi di Milano, Via Pascal 36, Milano 20133, Italy
* Corresponding author. Unità Operativa di Radiologia Diagnostica e Interventistica, IRCCS Istituto Ortopedico Galeazzi, Via Riccardo Galeazzi 4, Milano 20161, Italy.
E-mail address: io@lucasconfienza.it

Magn Reson Imaging Clin N Am 28 (2020) 211–221
https://doi.org/10.1016/j.mric.2019.12.005
1064-9689/20/© 2019 Elsevier Inc. All rights reserved.

the pathologic MR features of posterior instability and the underlying joint abnormalities predisposing to this condition.

MAGNETIC RESONANCE TECHNIQUE

MRA is regarded as the gold-standard imaging modality for shoulder instability.[5] Indeed, the injection of paramagnetic contrast agent into the joint allows for capsule distension and better visualization of intraarticular structures. However, standard MR can be considered after trauma, because capsular distension is ensured by joint effusion.[7] The increasing use of 3T MR scanners has raised the issue of the actual role of MRA. In fact, in a previous study on 150 shoulder scans at 3T, MRA has shown to be more accurate than standard MR in the detection of superior labrum anterior and posterior tears, with nonnegligible impact on patient management, but no significant differences were observed in the diagnosis of posterior labral tears.[8] Generally, up to 20 cc of gadolinium-based contrast agent is injected with anterior or posterior approach before MRA,[9] and images acquisition should be performed within 1 hour to avoid excessive contrast resorption.[10] Fluoroscopy is still the preferred guidance to inject the shoulder joint, followed by ultrasound.[5,11,12] For what concerns MRA sequences, there is no consensus on the best imaging protocol, although fat-suppressed spin echo T1-weighted images are acquired on the 3 planes— with the shoulder in neutral position—with one nonfat-saturated T1-weighted (for bone injuries and muscle trophism) and one fluid sensitive sequence (for bone marrow edema and bursitis).[6] In the setting of posterior shoulder instability, some investigators suggest to add an axial sequence in internal rotation of the shoulder to put into tension the posterior capsulolabral and ligamentous structures.[7]

ANATOMY
Glenoid and Humeral Head

Only one-third of the humeral head articulates with the glenoid, which allows the glenohumeral joint to have the largest range of motion of any joint in the human body.[13] The stability of this joint results from the balance of static and dynamic stabilizers acting in different ways. The bony structures of the glenoid and humeral head are static stabilizers whose anatomy is crucial to compensate the relative instability of the joint. When dealing with MR examinations of patients with posterior shoulder instability, the bony morphologic features of the joint should be thoroughly assessed, including glenoid version, shape, inclination, depth, and size, as well as humeral head morphology, position, and version.[14]

The normal glenoid fossa is pear shaped, with a mean width of 25 mm, a mean height of 35 mm, and retroversion with respect to the scapular body ranging from 0° to 7°, although a mild anteversion can be seen in stable shoulders of healthy controls. The normal glenoid is also tilted from superomedial to inferolateral by about 15° with deep concave shape in the caudal portion and flat shape in the cranial portion.[15–18] The humeral head is almost spherical, with a larger radius in the superior portion and centered in the glenoid fossa in normal conditions.[18] The shoulder girdle muscles stabilize the shoulder joint forcing the convex head of the humerus against the concave surface of the glenoid fossa. This mechanism is defined as the concavity/compression phenomenon, and any abnormalities or bone loss (eg, humeral compression fractures, glenoid fractures, or dysplasia) can alter this stabilizing effect.[19,20]

Capsulolabral Ligamentous Complex

The labrum is a round or triangular fibrocartilage, with a thickness of about 3 to 4 mm, attached to the peripheral rim of the glenoid.[21] The labrum contributes to joint stability because it increases the glenoid depth by one-third, thereby increasing its contact area with the humeral head and limiting its anterior and posterior translation (**Fig. 1**A, B).[22] Further, the labrum protects the articular cartilage from shear injuries and is site of insertion of important stabilizers including the glenohumeral ligaments and the long head of the biceps tendon.[23] Although the anterior part of the labrum, especially the superior portion, is a frequent site of anatomic variants such as sublabral foramen and sulcus, the posterior labrum is more consistent.[24] The posterior labrum, however, does have variability in its bony attachment with a medialized insertion that can be observed in up to 40% of patients, which can be misinterpreted for a labral tear.[25]

The posterior capsule, which includes the capsular area from the intraarticular tract of the long head of the biceps tendon to the inferior glenohumeral ligament (IGHL), is the thinnest and weakest part of shoulder joint capsule.[26] It, however, plays a crucial role in joint stability and is one of the primary posterior shoulder stabilizers together with the IGHL, especially at 90° abduction.[27] Different measurements to assess the capsular area and width on MRA have been proposed with the attempt of identifying imaging

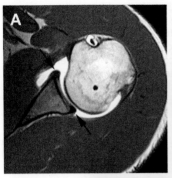
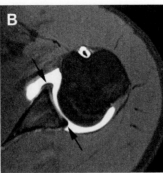
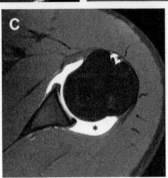

Fig. 1. Left shoulder MRA of a 25-year-old female patient. (A) Axial T1-weighted and (B) fat-saturated T1-weighted images acquired in neutral position of the upper limb show the normal appearance of the labrum (arrows), presenting as a hypointense triangular structure attached to the peripheral rim of the glenoid and increasing the glenoid depth. When MRA is performed with the upper limb in external rotation, (C) an increased posterior capsular area (asterisk) in the axial fat-saturated T1-weighted image can be seen.

features to help in the diagnosis of posterior shoulder instability, which is discussed later.[28] When using these measurements, the volume of contrast media injected into the joint and the position of the humerus must be taken into consideration because a large variability in contrast distribution and capsular width can be observed when MR images are acquired in internal versus external rotation of the arm (**Fig. 1**C).

MAGNETIC RESONANCE FINDINGS OF POSTERIOR INSTABILITY
Glenoid and Humeral Head

Glenoid dysplasia is a developmental abnormality, probably related to a defect of ossification of the inferior glenoid precartilage, presenting with bony deficiency of the scapular neck and the posteroinferior portion of the glenoid fossa.[29] It can present in isolation or in association with other abnormalities in syndromic disorders.[29] Glenoid dysplasia has a wide range of imaging findings with variable degree of severity. Hypoplasia of the scapular neck and humeral head with varus deformity of humeral neck can be detected.[30] The glenoid fossa can show an irregular surface with flattening of both glenoid and humeral articular surfaces.[31] The posteroinferior glenoid deficiency can present with 2 different appearances of the glenoid: "lazy J" type, with rounding posteroinferior glenoid rim (**Fig. 2**), and "delta" type, with sharp triangular

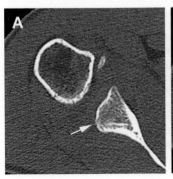
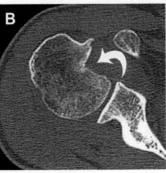

Fig. 2. Right shoulder computed tomography (CT) of a 35-year-old male patient with posteroinferior glenoid deficiency presenting with "lazy J" appearance with rounding posteroinferior glenoid rim (A, arrow). The same patient showed an impaction fracture (B, curved arrow) of the lesser tuberosity (reverse Hill-Sachs or McLaughlin lesion).

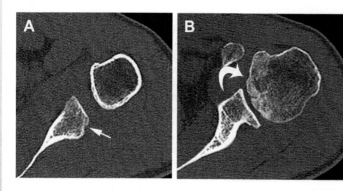

Fig. 3. Left shoulder of the same patient of Fig. 2 with sharp triangular ("delta" type) posteroinferior bony defect (A, arrow). A McLaughlin lesion is recognized also in the left shoulder (B, curved arrow).

posteroinferior bony defect (Fig. 3).[32,33] Although in some cases these 2 patterns can be difficult to differentiate,[28] it is important to identify any developmental articular surface deficiency in this region that can serve as a *wake-up call* to search for any associated findings. Indeed, MR findings frequently observed in glenoid dysplasia include a compensatory hypertrophy of the cartilage, often with chondral fissures, and hypertrophy of the posterior labrum, which can present low-to-intermediate signal intensity and round or triangular shape.[30,34] Based on the MR appearance, glenoid dysplasia can be graded as (1) mild, when the defect of the posterior glenoid is detected in just 1 or 2 axial images, with regular appearance of posterior labrum; (2) moderate, when posterior glenoid insufficiency is observed in more axial slices and posterior labrum is hypertrophic; or (3) severe, when the entire posteroinferior glenoid is abnormal and the labrum is markedly hypertrophic (Fig. 4A).[30,31] The insufficiency of the posterior glenoid can also be caused or increased by the degree of glenoid retroversion, with increased retroversion resulting in greater posterior instability.[28] For every 1° increase in retroversion, the risk of posterior shoulder instability increases by 15% to 17%.[28,35] Another bony finding that can be observed in this setting is posterior translation of the humeral head, which has been associated with posterior instability and posterior labral tears (Fig. 4B).[28,33]

Aside from developmental abnormalities of bony structures, posttraumatic bone injuries of both glenoid and humeral head can potentially lead to posterior shoulder instability and should be reported. Reverse bony Bankart is a fracture of the posteroinferior glenoid rim (Fig. 5) related to posterior shoulder dislocation and predisposing to further dislocations due to a reduction of glenoid articular surface, similarly to anterior instability resulting from anterior glenoid bone loss.[36] Posterior dislocation can also cause an impaction fracture of the lesser tuberosity, referred to as a reverse Hill-Sachs or McLaughlin lesion, which increases the risk of instability when more than 30% of articular surface is involved or

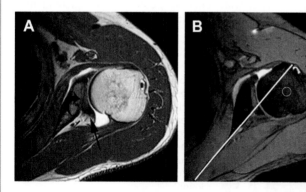

Fig. 4. Left shoulder MRA of a 29-year-old male patient with history of multiple posterior subluxations. (A) Axial T1-weighted image in external rotation of the upper limb and (B) gradient-echo T2-weighted image in neutral position of the upper limb show a retroverted and dysplastic glenoid with bony deficiency of the posteroinferior portion of the glenoid fossa (curved arrow) and compensatory hypertrophy of the cartilage and the posterior labrum (arrow). Also note the posterior translation of the humeral head, as shown by the position of the center of the humeral head (circle) as compared with the scapular line (white line) that is drawn tangential to ventral surface of scapular body.

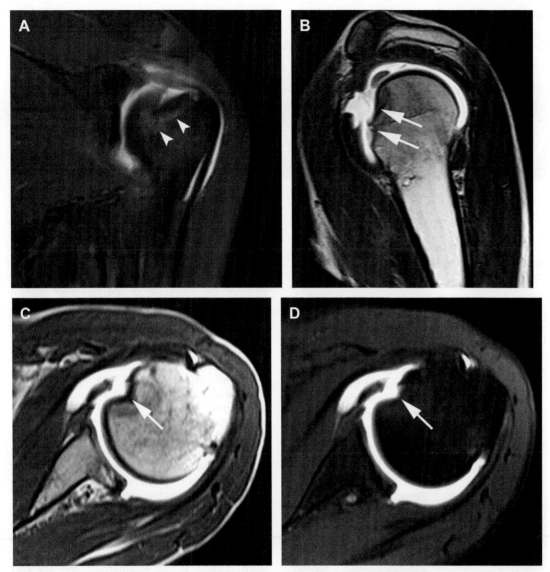

Fig. 5. Left shoulder MRA of a 42-year-old male patient with history of recent traumatic posterior shoulder dislocation. (*A*) Coronal fat-saturated proton density–weighted, (*B*) sagittal T1-weighted, (*C*) axial T1-weighted, and (*D*) axial fat-saturated T1-weighted images show the impaction fracture (*arrows*) of the lesser tuberosity (McLaughlin lesion), with bone marrow edema due to the recent trauma (*A, arrowheads*).

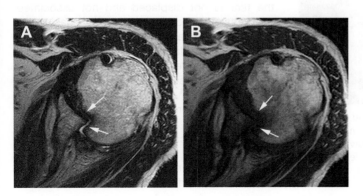

Fig. 6. Left shoulder MR of a 62-year-old male patient with history of multiple traumatic posterior shoulder dislocations and limited range of motion. (*A*) Axial T2-weighted and (*B*) T1-weighted images show a deep engaging reverse Hill-Sachs fracture (*arrows*).

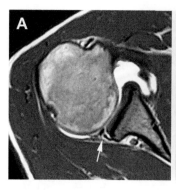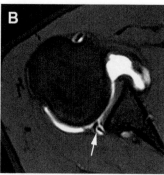

Fig. 7. Right shoulder MRA of a 27 year-old female patient with atraumatic pain. (A) Axial T1-weighted and (B) fat-saturated T1-weighted images show a reverse Bankart lesion presenting as a detachment of the posteroinferior labrum with avulsion of the periosteum (arrows), which is better depicted in the fat-saturated image.

when there are associated injuries of the posterior capsulolabral ligamentous complex (**Figs. 6 and 7**).[36,37]

Capsulolabral Ligamentous Complex

The version and height of the chondrolabral portion of the glenoid should also be evaluated in patients with posterior or multidirectional shoulder instability. A flattening of the posterior labrum, where it is thinner than the anterior labrum, results in decreased glenoid depth and increased retroversion (**Fig. 8**). As demonstrated by Kim and colleagues,[38] this finding

is associated with decreased contact between the humeral head and glenoid and posterior shoulder instability. Although it is still unclear whether the flattening of the posterior labrum is a cause or a consequence of posterior instability and whether it plays a critical role in posterior instability, this finding should be evaluated in MR examination of patients with this condition.

Posterior labral tears are less frequent in patients with posterior instability than anteroinferior labral tears in patients with anterior instability.[39,40] It has been shown, however, that posterior labral tears do result in posterior translation of the humeral head, with larger tears predisposing to posterior instability.[41] Different kinds of posterior labral tears can be encountered, including reverse Bankart lesion, Kim lesion, and posterior labrocapsular periosteal sleeve avulsion (POLPSA).[36] The reverse Bankart lesion is a detachment of the posteroinferior labrum with avulsion of the periosteum similar to its counterpart the Bankart lesion (anteroinferior labral tear) (**Fig. 9**).[42] This lesion leads to laxity of posterior IGHL and posterior capsule and can be associated with a reverse bony Bankart with avulsion of posteroinferior glenoid bony rim.[21] Generally, the tear is not displaced and not associated with adjacent chondral injuries.[43] Occasionally, a posterior Bankart lesion can be associated to a posterior paralabral cyst, which can extend into the spinoglenoid notch with or without signs of compression neuropathy of the suprascapular nerve.[44] Although the paralabral cyst and nerve entrapment can be easily recognized by ultrasound,[45] early related muscle edematous changes can be detected only using MR.[44] The Kim lesion is an incomplete and concealed posteroinferior labrum tear. It presents as a superficial tear between the labrum

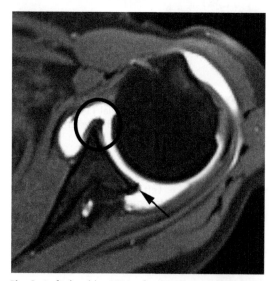

Fig. 8. Left shoulder MRA of a 40-year-old female patient. Axial fat-saturated T1-weighted image shows flattening of the posterior labrum (arrow), where it is thinner than the anterior labrum (circle), resulting in decreased glenoid depth and increased retroversion.

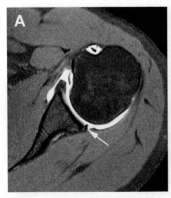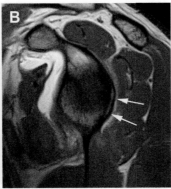

Fig. 9. Left shoulder MRA of a 22-year-old female patient with history of posterior shoulder subluxations. (*A*) Axial fat-saturated T1-weighted and (*B*) sagittal T1-weighted images show a Kim lesion presenting as an incomplete and concealed posteroinferior labrum tear between the labrum and the cartilage layer without complete avulsion (*arrows*).

and the cartilage layer without complete avulsion (see **Fig. 9**).[46] This type of lesion can also appear as a flattened posterior labrum, increasing glenoid retroversion, as described earlier.[38,46] The POLPSA lesion results from the stripping of the posteroinferior labrum from the posterior glenoid rim with an intact periosteum (**Fig. 10A–C**).[47] If the periosteal sleeve is filled with fibrous tissue, intraarticular contrast may not undercut the lesion in MRA examinations (**Fig. 10D**).

It has been established that insufficiency of the posterior capsular ligamentous structures is associated with recurrent posterior subluxations.[48] The posterior band of the IGHL can be injured from posterior microtraumatic instability or after traumatic posterior dislocations, with tears being located at the glenoid insertion, in midsubstance of the ligament, or at the humeral insertion, which is also referred to as a posterior humeral avulsion of the glenohumeral ligament.[49] The higher frequency of injury at the humeral insertion of this ligament compared with that of its anterior counterparts is probably related to the fact that the posterior band is the thinnest and weakest portion of the IGHL complex.[49,50] In addition to injuries of the joint capsule, it is important to search for MRA findings of capsular laxity. Patients with posterior and multidirectional instability generally present with an increased capsular volume at MRA.[51] Different methods to identify capsular laxity on MRA have been proposed: (1) linear sagittal measurement from the coracoid to the posterior capsule on the sagittal-oblique sequence in the slice with the maximum posterior capsular distension; (2) linear axial measurement from the lesser tuberosity to the posterior capsule on the axial sequence in the slice with the largest posterior capsule distension; (3) sagittal and axial capsular area on the sagittal-oblique

and axial sequences, respectively, with largest amount of contrast agent; and (4) axial posterior capsular area on the axial sequence with the maximum posterior distension.[28,51] In particular, the axial area of the posterior capsular pocket has been reported as strongly associated with posterior shoulder instability (see **Fig. 10**).[28] These measurements can be seen as time-consuming but can be helpful to identify critical findings associated with posterior shoulder instability. Another imaging feature that can be observed in overhead throwers with posterior shoulder pain and instability is the Bennett lesion, an ossification of the posterior capsule at its glenoid insertion.[52] This feature is believed to be the result of a chronic stress-related traction injury of the posterior band of the IGHL and appears as a linear or curvilinear ossification adjacent to the posteroinferior glenoid rim.[52]

Injury to labroligamentous structures outside of the posterior shoulder may also contribute to posterior instability. A potential role of coracohumeral and superior glenohumeral ligament injuries in posterior instability has been postulated, although contradictory data have been reported.[14,53–55] Investigators have reported increased posteroinferior shoulder instability after sectioning the rotator interval capsule in cadaveric specimens.[54] Conversely, in other studies no improvement of posterior instability has been reported after arthroscopic rotator interval closure.[55]

Muscles

Dynamic shoulder stabilizers including the rotator cuff, long head of the biceps tendon, and deltoid muscle are the most important dynamic stabilizers in preventing posterior shoulder dislocations and may contribute to instability, thereby requiring a thorough evaluation.[14] The

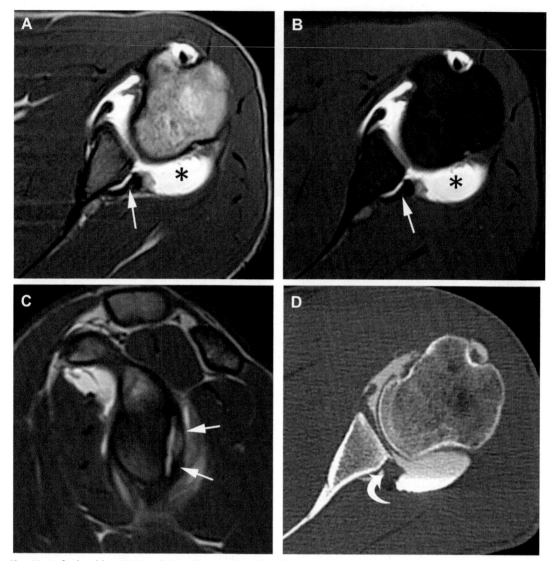

Fig. 10. Left shoulder MRA and CT arthrography of a 22-year-old male patient with posterior shoulder insta-bility. (A) Axial T1-weighted, (B) axial fat-saturated T1-weighted, and (C) sagittal T1-weighted MRA images show a POLPSA lesion resulting from the stripping of the posteroinferior labrum from the glenoid rim with intact periosteum (arrows). Also note the pathologic increase of the axial area of the posterior capsular pocket (A, B, asterisk). (D) Axial CT arthrography performed 1 month later shows the periosteal sleeve filled by fibrous tissue (curved arrow).

rotator cuff and scapular muscles contribute to the concavity-compression of the glenohumeral joint. In particular, the subscapularis should be carefully evaluated in patients with posterior instability, as it is the most important rotator cuff muscle counteracting posterior translation of the humeral head.[56] The extra-rotator muscles act as posterior compressors. In cases of traumatic posterior shoulder dislocations, iso-lated injuries of the infraspinatus or teres minor can also be observed due to the intimate association of these structures with the poste-rior capsule.[57] Although it is often unclear whether the cuff tears are related to the trauma or to the acquired instability, the diagnosis of cuff injuries has important implications. Indeed, cuff tears and glenohumeral instability are closely related, with posterosuperior cuff tears having shown a correlation with the number of dislocations.[58]

MR findings of posterior shoulder instability are summarized in **Table 1**.

Table 1
Magnetic resonance findings of posterior shoulder instability

Structure	MR Findings
Glenoid	• Flat articular surface • Hypoplasia • Retroversion • Posteroinferior deficiency ("lazy J" or "delta" type) • Reverse bony Bankart lesion
Humeral head	• Flat articular surface • Hypoplasia • Varus humeral neck • Posterior translation • Reverse Hill-Sachs (McLaughlin)
Posterior labrum	• Flattened labrum • Reverse Bankart lesion • Kim lesion • POLPSA
Capsule and ligaments	• Posterior IGHL tear • Bennett lesion • Posterior capsular area

SUMMARY

MR and MRA allow for a comprehensive evaluation of patients with posterior shoulder instability. This condition can be the result of developmental abnormalities or micro/macrotraumatic injuries and often presents with nonspecific findings on clinical examination. Imaging examinations are crucial for accurate diagnosis and appropriate patient management. Radiologists should be aware of common MR imaging features that can be encountered in patients with posterior shoulder instability including abnormalities of the glenoid and humeral head and posterior capsulolabral ligamentous complex.

DISCLOSURE

Authors have no commercial or financial conflict of interests to disclose related to the present article. Authors also did not receive any funding for this article.

REFERENCES

1. Antosh IJ, Tokish JM, Owens BD. Posterior shoulder instability. Sports Health 2016;8:520–6.
2. Provencher MT, LeClere LE, King S, et al. Posterior instability of the shoulder: diagnosis and management. Am J Sports Med 2011;39:874–86.
3. Cho JH, Chung NS, Song HK, et al. Recurrent posterior shoulder instability after rifle shooting. Orthopedics 2012;35:e1677–9.
4. Hawkins RJ, McCormack RG. Posterior shoulder instability. Orthopedics 1988;11:101–7.
5. Sconfienza LM, Albano D, Messina C, et al. How, when, why in magnetic resonance arthrography: an International Survey by the European Society of Musculoskeletal Radiology (ESSR). Eur Radiol 2018;28:2356–68.
6. Bellelli A, Silvestri E, Barile A, et al. Position paper on magnetic resonance imaging protocols in the musculoskeletal system (excluding the spine) by the Italian College of Musculoskeletal Radiology. Radiol Med 2019;124:522–38.
7. Farber JM, Buckwalter KA. Sports-related injuries of the shoulder: instability. Radiol Clin North Am 2002; 40:235–49.
8. Magee T. 3-T MRI of the shoulder: is MR arthrography necessary? Am J Roentgenol 2009;192:86–92.
9. Jacobson JA, Lin J, Jamadar DA, et al. Aids to successful shoulder arthrography performed with a fluoroscopically guided anterior approach. Radiographics 2003;23:373–8.
10. Omoumi P, Teixeira P, Lecouvet F, et al. Glenohumeral joint instability. J Magn Reson Imaging 2011; 33:2–16.
11. Sconfienza LM, Adriaensen M, Albano D, et al. Clinical indications for image-guided interventional procedures in the musculoskeletal system: a Delphi-based consensus paper from the European Society of Musculoskeletal Radiology (ESSR)—part I, shoulder. Eur Radiol 2019. https://doi.org/10.1007/s00330-019-06419-x.
12. Sconfienza LM, Chianca V, Messina C, et al. Upper limb interventions. Radiol Clin North Am 2019;57: 1073–82.
13. Warner JJ, Caborn DN, Berger R, et al. Dynamic capsuloligamentous anatomy of the glenohumeral joint. J Shoulder Elbow Surg 1993;2:115–33.
14. Tannenbaum EP, Sekiya JK. Posterior shoulder instability in the contact athlete. Clin Sports Med 2013;32: 781–6.
15. Saha AK. Dynamic stability of the glenohumeral joint. Acta Orthop Scand 1971;42:491–505.
16. Saha AK. Mechanism of shoulder movements and a plea for the recognition of the "zero" position of the glenohumeral joint. Clin Orthop Relat Res 1983;173:3–10.
17. Saygi B, Karahan N, Karakus O, et al. Analysis of glenohumeral morphological factors for anterior shoulder instability and rotator cuff tear by magnetic resonance imaging. J Orthop Surg (Hong Kong) 2018;26. 2309499018768100.
18. Inui H, Sugamoto K, Miyamoto T, et al. Evaluation of three-dimensional glenoid structure using MRI. J Anat 2001;199:323–8.
19. Lippitt SB, Vanderhooft JE, Harris SL, et al. Glenohumeral stability from concavitycompression: a quantitative analysis. J Shoulder Elbow Surg 1993;2:27.

20. Sekiya JK, Wickwire AC, Stehle JH, et al. Hill-Sachs defects and repair using osteoarticular allograft transplantation: biomechanical analysis using a joint compression model. Am J Sports Med 2009;37: 2459.

21. De Coninck T, Ngai SS, Tafur M, et al. Imaging the Glenoid Labrum and Labral Tears. Radiographics 2016;36:1628–47.

22. Bencardino JT, Beltran J. MR imaging of the glenohumeral ligaments. Radiol Clin North Am 2006; 44(4):489–502.

23. Zlatkin MB, Sanders TG. Magnetic resonance imaging of the glenoid labrum. Radiol Clin North Am 2013;51:279–97.

24. Gustas CN, Tuite MJ. Imaging update on the glenoid labrum: variants versus tears. Semin Musculoskelet Radiol 2014;18:365–73.

25. Nourissat G, Radier C, Aim F, et al. Arthroscopic classification of posterior labrum glenoid insertion. Orthop Traumatol Surg Res 2014;100:167–70.

26. Pagnani MJ, Warren RF. Stabilizers of the glenohumeral joint. J Shoulder Elbow Surg 1994;3:173.

27. O'Brien SJ, Schwartz RS, Warren RF, et al. Capsular restraints to anterior-posterior motion of the abducted shoulder: a biomechanical study. J Shoulder Elbow Surg 1995;4:298.

28. Galvin JW, Parada SA, Li X, et al. Critical findings on magnetic resonance arthrograms in posterior shoulder instability compared with an age-matched controlled cohort. Am J Sports Med 2016;44: 3222–9.

29. Currarino G, Sheffield E, Twickler D. Congenital glenoid dysplasia. Pediatr Radiol 1998;28:30–7.

30. Harper KW, Helms CA, Haystead CM, et al. Glenoid dysplasia: incidence and association with posterior labral tears as evaluated on MRI. AJR Am J Roentgenol 2005;184:984–8.

31. Abboud JA, Bateman DK, Barlow J. Glenoid dysplasia. J Am Acad Orthop Surg 2016;24:327–36.

32. Edelson JG. Localized glenoid hypoplasia. An anatomic variation of possible clinical significance. Clin Orthop Relat Res 1995;321:189–95.

33. Weishaupt D, Zanetti M, Nyffeler RW, et al. Posterior glenoid rim deficiency in recurrent (atraumatic) posterior shoulder instability. Skeletal Radiol 2000;29: 204–10.

34. Munshi M, Davidson JM. Unilateral glenoid hypoplasia: unusual findings on MR arthrography. AJR Am J Roentgenol 2000;175:646–8.

35. Owens BD, Campbell SE, Cameron KL. Risk factors for posterior shoulder instability in young athletes. Am J Sports Med 2013;41:2645–9.

36. Shah N, Tung GA. Imaging signs of posterior glenohumeral instability. AJR Am J Roentgenol 2009;192: 730–5.

37. Yun G, Kang Y, Ahn JM, et al. Posterior decentering of the humeral head on shoulder MR arthrography: significant association with posterior synovial proliferation. AJR Am J Roentgenol 2017;208: 1297–303.

38. Kim SH, Noh KC, Park JS, et al. Loss of chondrolabral containment of the glenohumeral joint in atraumatic posteroinferior multidirectional instability. J Bone Joint Surg Am 2005;87:92–8.

39. Papendick L, Savoie FI. Anatomy-specific repair techniques for posterior shoulder instability. J South Orthop Assoc 1995;4:169–76.

40. Altchek D, Warren R, Wickiewicz T, et al. Arthroscopic labral débridement. Am J Sports Med 1992;20:702–6.

41. Tung GA, Hou DD. MR arthrography of the posterior labrocapsular complex: relationship with glenohumeral joint alignment and clinical posterior instability. AJR Am J Roentgenol 2003;180: 369–75.

42. Fitzpatrick D, Grubin J. Navigating the alphabet soup of labroligamentous pathology of the shoulder. Am J Orthop 2016;45:58–60.

43. Harish S, Nagar A, Moro J, et al. Imaging findings in posterior instability of the shoulder. Skeletal Radiol 2008;37:693–707.

44. Albano D, Chianca V, Zappia M, et al. Imaging of usual and unusual complication of rotator cuff repair. J Comput Assist Tomogr 2019;43:359–66.

45. Sconfienza LM, Albano D, Allen G, et al. Clinical indications for musculoskeletal ultrasound updated in 2017 by European Society of Musculoskeletal Radiology (ESSR) consensus. Eur Radiol 2018;28: 5338–51.

46. Kim SH, Ha KI, Yoo JC, et al. Kim's lesion: an incomplete and concealed avulsion of the posteroinferior labrum in posterior or multidirectional posteroinferior instability of the shoulder. Arthroscopy 2004;20: 712–20.

47. Farshad-Amacker NA, Jain Palrecha S, Farshad M. The primer for sports medicine professionals on imaging: the shoulder. Sports Health 2013;5: 50–77.

48. Petersen S. Conservative management of shoulder injuries: posterior shoulder instability. Orthop Clin North Am 2000;31:263–74.

49. Bigliani LU, Pollock RG, Soslowsky LJ, et al. Tensile properties of the inferior glenohumeral ligament. J Orthop Res 1992;10:187–97.

50. Ticker JB, Bigliani LU, Soslowsky LJ, et al. Inferior glenohumeral ligament: geometric and strain-rate dependent properties. J Shoulder Elbow Surg 1996;5:269–79.

51. Dewing CB, McCormick F, Bell SJ, et al. An analysis of capsular area in patients with anterior, posterior, and multidirectional shoulder instability. Am J Sports Med 2008;36:515–22.

52. Ferrari JD, Ferrari DA, Coumas J, et al. Posterior ossification of the shoulder: the Bennett lesion—

etiology, diagnosis, and treatment. Am J Sports Med 1994;22:171–5.

53. Cole BJ, Rodeo SA, O'Brien SJ, et al. The anatomy and histology of the rotator interval capsule of the shoulder. Clin Orthop Relat Res 2001;390:129–37.

54. Harryman DT II, Sidles JA, Harris SL, et al. The role of the rotator interval capsule in passive motion and stability of the shoulder. J Bone Joint Surg Am 1992;74:53–66.

55. Mologne TS, Zhao K, Hongo M, et al. The addition of rotator interval closure after arthroscopic repair of either anterior or posterior shoulder instability: effect on glenohumeral translation and range of motion. Am J Sports Med 2008;36:1123–31.

56. Blasier RB, Soslowsky LJ, Malicky DM, et al. Posterior glenohumeral subluxation: active and passive stabilization in a biomechanical model. J Bone Joint Surg Am 1997;79:433.

57. Waldt S, Brügel M. Classification of normal labral variants and labral injuries. Radiologe 2015;55:211–20.

58. Porcellini G, Paladini P, Campi F, et al. Shoulder instability and related rotator cuff tears: arthroscopic findings and treatment in patients aged 40 to 60 years. Arthroscopy 2006;22:270–6.

Postoperative MR Imaging in Shoulder Instability and Intra-articular Damage

Christoph Stern, MD[a,b], Samy Bouaicha, MD[b,c], Filippo Del Grande, MD[d], Reto Sutter, MD[a,b],*

KEYWORDS

- Postoperative MR imaging • Shoulder instability • Labral repair • Latarjet • Bone block procedures
- Hill-Sachs repair

KEY POINTS

- Postoperative MRI after soft tissue repairs for shoulder instability shows an altered appearance of the labrum and/or the capsule as a normal finding and needs to be distinguished from recurrent pathology.
- After glenoid augmentation procedures the shape of the glenoid varies in appearance depending on the surgical procedure performed and can be best evaluated on MRI or CT.
- After humeral bone loss procedures including surgical disimpaction of a humeral head impaction or allograft augmentation as well as remplissage procedure either MRI or CT is most suitable for the postoperative evaluation depending on the amount of metallic hardware used.

INTRODUCTION

MR imaging of the postoperative shoulder is challenging and radiologists are increasingly confronted with this task because of a growing number of instability procedures performed.[1] Exact knowledge of the anatomy and labral variants is essential to interpret the postoperative situation where the radiologist is confronted with altered anatomic structures. The radiologist must be familiar with different surgical techniques for correct interpretation of image findings. Furthermore, close collaboration with the referring surgeon aids in establishing the final diagnosis, because of intraoperative complications or divergent procedures that are only known by the surgeon.

Besides altered anatomy and different appearance of the operated labrum, the radiologist is faced with artifacts from metallic hardware or abrasion, which can compromise MR image quality and interpretation. With the use of metal artifact reduction techniques MR image quality is improved substantially. Nevertheless, the radiologist must be familiar with alternative imaging modalities, in particular computed tomography (CT) arthrography, and has to judge its usage depending on the specific postoperative situation.

Surgery for shoulder instability is performed in patients with recurrent shoulder instability and includes anatomic soft tissue repairs, bone augmentation procedures at the anterior and posterior glenoid rim, and humeral bone loss procedures.

[a] Radiology, Balgrist University Hospital, Forchstrasse 340, Zurich 8008, Switzerland; [b] Faculty of Medicine, University of Zurich, Zurich, Switzerland; [c] Department of Orthopaedic Surgery, Balgrist University Hospital, Forchstrasse 340, Zurich 8008, Switzerland; [d] Department of Radiology, Ospedale Regionale di Lugano, Via Tesserete 46, Lugano 6900, Switzerland
* Corresponding author. Radiology, Balgrist University Hospital, Forchstrasse 340, Zurich 8008, Switzerland.
E-mail address: Reto.Sutter@balgrist.ch

Magn Reson Imaging Clin N Am 28 (2020) 223–242
https://doi.org/10.1016/j.mric.2019.12.006
1064-9689/20/© 2019 Elsevier Inc. All rights reserved.

The goal of the surgical therapy is to repair capsulolabral damage, augment glenoidal and/or humeral bone loss, and last but not least to restore shoulder stability and function.

This article focuses on capsulolabral surgery, bone block transfers, and humeral bone loss procedures in patients with shoulder instability and their postoperative imaging evaluation. Surgical procedures and common complications are explained, and expected and pathologic imaging findings at postoperative MR imaging and other imaging modalities are shown.

POSTOPERATIVE IMAGING

Evaluation of the postoperative shoulder usually starts with radiographs to get an impression of what type of surgical procedure was performed, to evaluate any screws or anchors and to assess the joint position and any osseous abnormalities.

To evaluate the labrum, ligaments, and capsule MR imaging is the preferred imaging modality because of its superior soft tissue contrast in the preoperative and postoperative setting. Sensitivity for detection of pathologic changes of these anatomic structures is higher after intravenous administration of gadolinium-based contrast material and best with intra-articular injection of contrast material (MR arthrography).[2,3] However, in the postoperative situation MR image quality is strongly compromised in the presence of metallic hardware and/or intraoperative abrasions depending on the surgical procedure performed. The type, size, and orientation of metallic hardware influence the severity of magnetic susceptibility artifacts. Titanium-based hardware create little to moderate geometric distortion, signal loss, or signal pile-up, whereas stainless steel and cobalt-chrome implants cause severe artifacts, which may obscure surrounding structures or mimic pathology (eg, a false-positive labral retear).[3–5] Insufficient fat suppression is another problem that is caused by metallic hardware.

Therefore, MR imaging techniques should be implemented to reduce magnetic susceptibility artifacts to a minimum, such as the short tau inversion recovery (STIR) and short tau inversion recovery with optimized inversion pulse (STIR WARP)[6] sequence or the Dixon technique[7] instead of spectral fat saturation techniques, an increase of the receiver bandwidth and matrix size, and usage of thin sections and lower magnetic field strength (if available). Gradient echo sequences are more prone to magnetic susceptibility than fast spin echo sequences and should be avoided. For cases of strong metal artifacts specially designed vendor-specific sequences, such as slice encoding for metal artifact correction (SEMAC) or multiacquisition variable-resonance image combination (MAVRIC), are used if available.[5,8–13] **Table 1** shows the MR arthrography imaging protocol, which is routinely used in our institution for the evaluation of the preoperative shoulder and also postoperatively after soft tissue repair surgery without or with only little metallic hardware. For all other postoperative cases with implanted metallic hardware a different MR arthrography protocol is used (**Table 2**).

If MR imaging and MR arthrography is contraindicated (eg, pacemaker or claustrophobia) or severely compromised by metal artifacts, CT arthrography is good alternative imaging method to evaluate the postoperative labrum and intra-articular structures.[2]

Ultrasound as a further alternative is suitable to evaluate the postoperative shoulder, especially for the static and dynamic investigation of the rotator cuff. However, global assessment of the labrum, cartilage, and bone is restricted because of only partial visibility.[9]

CAPSULOLABRAL PROCEDURES
Surgical Procedures

In patients with anterior shoulder dislocation usually an avulsion of the anteroinferior labrum and attached capsule occur, where the anterior band of the inferior glenohumeral ligament acts as the main passive stabilizer anteriorly. Because of the inherent lack of osseous stability of the glenohumeral joint, persistent instability, especially in young individuals, is associated with disruption of these soft tissue stabilizers.[14,15] When anatomic restoration is the goal of a surgical procedure the capsulolabral tissue is reattached at the glenoid rim (widely called Bankart repair) using different anchor systems. Within the last two decades arthroscopic techniques have mainly replaced open procedures and are considered as gold standard today. Implants for capsulolabral repair may differ in size and material and type of anchorage within the glenoid bone. Knotted and knotless, single, or double loaded suture-anchors are available. For successful surgical outcomes, it is important to firmly reattach the usually inferiorly and medially displaced anterior band of the inferior glenohumeral ligament at the anatomic position on the glenoid (3–4 o'clock in a right shoulder) and secure the repair with a minimum of three anchors (**Fig. 1**).[16–18]

In rare cases of posterior instability with a structural deficiency of the posterior capsulolabral complex similar fixation techniques with the same types of implants are used. Reattachment of the posterior labrum may also be

Table 1
Standard MR arthrography imaging protocol for the postoperative shoulder

Sequence	FOV	Slice Thickness (mm)	Number of Slices	Slice Gap (mm)	Matrix	TE (ms)	TR (ms)	Flip Angle	Receiver Bandwidth (Hz/Px)	Parallel Imaging Acceleration Factor (Grappa)	Duration (mm:ss)
Coronal oblique T1 TSE FS	160 × 160	3	19	0.6	384 × 384	11	461		191	1	03:34
Coronal oblique PD TSE FS	160 × 160	4	20	0.8	384 × 384	34	2200		260	1	03:46
Sagittal oblique T1 TSE	160 × 160	4	29	0.8	384 × 384	11	450		191	2	02:25
Sagittal oblique T2 TSE FS	160 × 160	4	23	0.8	256 × 256	71	3800		260	1	03:19
Axial 3D Trufi FS	180 × 180	1.7	52	0	512 × 512	5	11	28°	199	1	03:43

This protocol is readily used after soft tissue repairs and rotator cuff repairs without or with only little metallic hardware.
Abbreviations: 3D, three-dimensional; FOV, field of view; FS, fat saturation; PD, proton density; TE, echo time; TR, repetition time; TSE, turbo spin echo.

Table 2
MR arthrography imaging protocol for the postoperative shoulder with metal artifact reduction

Sequence	FOV	Slice Thickness (mm)	Number of Slices	Slice Gap (mm)	Matrix	TE (ms)	TR (ms)	TI (ms)	Receiver Bandwidth (Hz/Px)	Parallel Imaging Acceleration Factor (Grappa)	Duration (mm:ss)
Coronal oblique T1 TSE Dixon (IP/W)	160 × 160	3	19	0.6	384 × 384	12	578		250	2	03:08
Coronal oblique PD TSE Dixon (IP/W)	160 × 160	4	20	0.8	384 × 384	41	2900		250	2	03:22
Sagittal oblique T1 TSE high BW	160 × 160	4	29	0.8	384 × 384	10	450		395	2	02:25
Sagittal oblique STIR WARP	170 × 170	4	23	0.8	256 × 256	47	4000	170	300	1	03:50
Axial PD TSE Dixon (IP/W)	160 × 160	3	23	0.6	384 × 384	41	3330		250	2	03:51

This protocol is specially tailored for shoulders with larger metal screws, as typically seen in Latarjet procedures. In cases with total shoulder arthroplasty, the protocol is further adapted with through-plane distortion correction (eg, slice encoding for metal artifact correction) to reduce the metal artifacts even further.

Abbreviations: BW, bandwidth; FOV, field of view; IP, in-phase image; PD, proton density; STIR WARP, short tau inversion recovery with optimized inversion pulse; TE, echo time; TI, inversion time; TR, repetition time; TSE, turbo spin echo; W, water-only image.

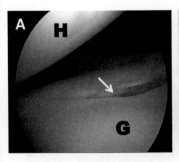 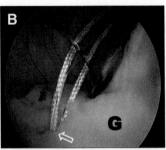

Fig. 1. Arthroscopic anteroinferior Bankart repair. (*A*) Arthroscopic view from posterior to anterior in a left shoulder shows an extensive tear of the anteroinferior labrum (*arrow*). (*B*) Arthroscopic Bankart repair: a suture anchor is placed over a rigid canula into the anterior glenoid rim (*arrow*). C, canula; G, glenoid; H, humerus. (*Courtesy of* K. Wieser, MD, Zurich, Switzerland.)

performed in cases of degenerative paralabral cyst formation where the labrum is surgically detached to decompress the cyst and is reattached thereafter. Soft tissue procedures of the glenohumeral capsule without involvement of the glenoid or humerus, such as capsular plication or shift, are a sparse surgical entity nowadays. In cases where the (inferior) capsule is ripped off its attachment at the humeral head, called humeral avulsion of the glenohumeral ligament (HAGL), the ligament/capsular pouch is anatomically reattached along the anatomic neck of the humerus using the same anchor systems as for Bankart repairs.

When the avulsion of the capsulolabral complex includes a small bone chip of the glenoid rim it is called a bony Bankart lesion. In these cases, when a soft tissue repair is still indicated, the bone fragment is reduced and incorporated in the soft tissue repair.[19] Larger posttraumatic bony defects are considered to be true fractures of the glenoid and not an avulsion injury. Their treatment may differ depending on size and location of the fracture.[20]

Imaging Evaluation: Expected Postoperative Findings

The anatomy and morphology of the postoperative labrum and capsuloligamentous structures can best be evaluated on MR imaging and MR arthrography. On sagittal oblique images the extent of labral repair is best visualized according to the distribution of metallic or bioabsorbable suture anchors along the glenoid rim (**Fig. 2**). The axial and coronal oblique image plane are best suited to evaluate the postoperative labrum, which may be altered in contour, shape, and signal intensity. The normal repaired labrum is firmly reattached to the glenoid rim at its anatomic position without undermining fluid or contrast material, and has a hypointense signal and a more rounded and blunted shape because of suturing (see **Fig. 2**). A little fraying or thickening of the

labrum with intermediate signal intensity is a common postoperative appearance and should not be mistaken for a pathology.[8,21,22] Adjacent perilabral scar tissue with or without susceptibility artifacts from abrasion is a common finding (**Fig. 3**). Major substance loss of the labrum should always be correlated with the surgical procedure performed to distinguish normal postoperative change from a new labral defect. After repair of a superior labral anterior posterior (SLAP) tear the same imaging criteria can be applied as for a Bankart repair. A smaller and blunted superior labrum is a common finding after debridement depending on how much labral tissue was resected. Fraying and substance loss are typical findings of the remaining superior labrum after tenotomy and/or tenodesis of the long head of the biceps tendon (see **Fig. 2**).[5,8]

In cases where a small bone chip of the glenoid rim (anterior or posterior) was reattached together with the labrum, the chip should be closely adapted to the glenoid with no step at the articular surface and with no entrance of fluid or contrast material. The reconstructed bony glenoid is best evaluated on sagittal oblique T1-weighted MR images or on reformatted sagittal oblique CT images and should resemble the typical pear shape of the glenoid (**Fig. 4**). Scarring or granulation tissue around the postoperative labrum is a frequent and expected finding.

Depending on the capsular procedure performed capsular thickening together with susceptibility artifacts are typical postoperative findings. Evaluation of the postoperative capsule volume is best in conjunction with preoperative images (see **Fig. 4**).

After repair of a HAGL the inferior glenohumeral ligament should be continuously visible and maybe thickened. Suture anchors at the humeral head-neck junction are visible after reattachment (**Fig. 5**). There might be a spilling of contrast material in the quadrilateral space at MR or CT arthrography, which should not be called a pathologic finding in the postoperative setting after HAGL repair.

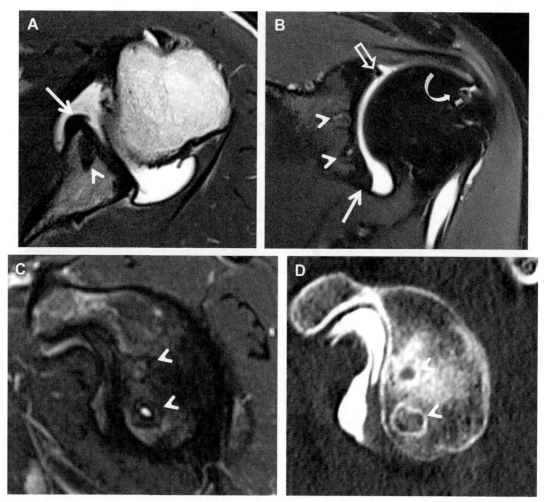

Fig. 2. Normal anteroinferior Bankart repair. A 29-year-old man with previous anteroinferior labrum repair and tenodesis of the long head of the biceps tendon. (*A*) Axial proton density MR arthrogram and (*B*) coronal oblique fat-suppressed proton density MR arthrogram show a smooth, little rounded, and hypointense anteroinferior labrum with little scarring (*solid arrow*) as an expected normal postoperative finding. No fraying, fragmentation, or fluid cleft is visible. After tenotomy of the long biceps tendon substance loss and some fraying of the superior labrum (*open arrow* in *B*) is an expected normal postoperative appearance. Note bioabsorbable anchor (*curved arrow* in *B*) of the biceps tenodesis in the superior humeral head. Distribution of bioabsorbable suture anchors (*arrowheads* in *A–D*) after anteroinferior labral repair and glenoid shape is best evaluated on sagittal oblique images (*C*, sagittal oblique short tau inversion recovery image after arthrography; *D*, reformatted sagittal oblique CT arthrogram). No glenoid bone loss is visible.

Common Complications

Any larger amount of fluid or contrast material within the labral substance or undermining the labrum after repair is indicative of a recurrent tear (**Fig. 6**). A failed labral repair should also be considered in case of a displaced or absent labrum.[8,9] Evaluation criteria is applied to the anterior, posterior, and superior labrum. In the postoperative shoulder after instability repair surgery, sensitivity of anterior labral, posterior labral, and superior labral anterior posterior tear was 80%, 81%, and 71%, respectively, for conventional noncontrast MR imaging according to a study by Magee.[2] MR arthrography can increase sensitivity up to 100% for each pathology because of fluid distention of the joint and demarcation of a retear, which may be masked by granulation tissue with intermediate signal intensity on conventional MR images.[2] The use of abduction and external rotation (ABER) positioning during MR imaging acquisition can further increase the sensitivity of a labral retear anteroinferiorly.[23] After repair of a bony Bankart lesion, undercutting fluid or contrast material between the bone chip and the glenoid bone is suspicious of nonhealing or

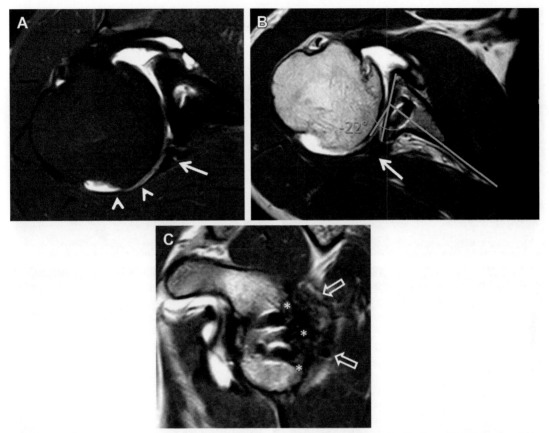

Fig. 3. Normal posterior Bankart repair. A 31-year-old man with previous posterior Bankart repair after posterior instability. (*A*) Axial fat-suppressed proton density MR arthrogram and (*B*) axial T1-weighted MR arthrogram after labral repair show a thick posterior labrum with scarring and mild intermediate signal intensity, triangular in shape and with no fluid cleft (*solid arrow* in *A* and *B*), which is consistent with an intact repair. (*B*) There is approximately 22° glenoid retroversion and elongation of the posterior joint capsule with posterior subluxation of the humeral head (*arrowheads* in *A*). (*C*) Sagittal oblique proton density MR arthrogram shows irregular margins of the posterior glenoid rim (*asterisks*) with adjacent scarring and small susceptibility artifacts from abrasion (*arrows*). (*A–C*) Note metal anchors in the posterior glenoid with moderate susceptibility artifacts.

persistent/recurrent instability (**Fig. 7**), although interposition of granulation tissue can be a normal finding, indicative of fibrous healing (see **Fig. 4**).

CT arthrography as an alternative imaging method has an accuracy comparable with noncontrast MR imaging for cases that preclude MR imaging assessment because of severe metallic artifacts or MR imaging contraindications.[2] Susceptibility artifacts can simulate false-positive labral tears on postoperative shoulder MR imaging[3]; hence, CT arthrography may help in clarifying equivocal cases.

After capsular procedures substantial capsular fraying at the glenoid or humeral attachment is suspicious of an insufficient repair. Detachment of the inferior glenohumeral ligament or a gap in the capsule demonstrate a failed repair, with a significant amount of fluid or contrast material next to the defect being a common finding. Capsular

elongation or a failed repair are associated with incongruent articulation of the humeral head, which can lead to recurrent labral tears, cartilage defects, or premature osteoarthritis and should be mentioned in the report.

As a further complication osteolysis can occur around suture anchors, especially with bioabsorbable anchors, which are designed to dissolve and may resorb over time.[22] Ultrasound-guided needle placement with injection of local anesthetics and corticosteroids or platelet-rich plasma may be an effective treatment option for symptomatic anchors in selected cases (**Fig. 8**).

Furthermore, suture anchors can loosen and protrude from the drill holes, eventually leading to rapid mechanical cartilage damage, particularly on the humeral side. Completely displaced anchors are visible as free bodies within the joint and are prone to cause synovitis.

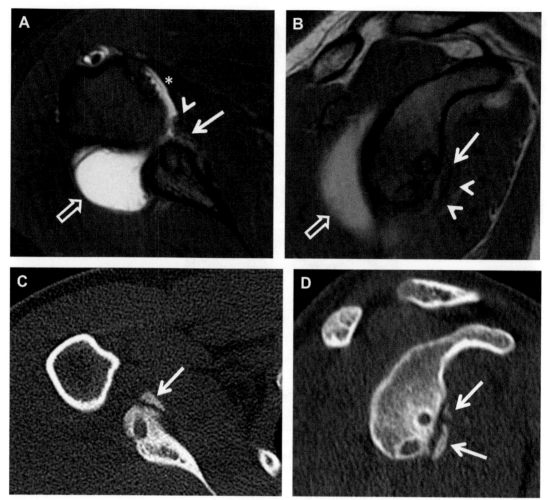

Fig. 4. Anteroinferior bony Bankart repair with fibrous healing and capsular shift procedure. An 18-year-old man with previous repair of an anteroinferior bony Bankart lesion and tightening of the anterior joint capsule (capsular shift). (*A*) Axial fat-suppressed proton density MR arthrogram and (*B*) sagittal oblique T1-weighted MR arthrogram show the readapted anteroinferior labrum (*arrowheads*) and bone chips (*solid arrows*), which are better visualized in the (*C*) axial and (*D*) reformatted sagittal oblique CT image. No contrast material is seen on MR images between the glenoid and the slightly displaced bone chips with sclerotic margins, which is consistent with fibrous healing. The anterior capsule is thickened after capsular shift procedure (*asterisk* in *A*) with reduced volume of the anterior recess. Note relative widening of the posterior recess (*open arrow*).

Focal cartilage defects can arise postoperatively because of cartilage degeneration or are caused by iatrogenic damage during surgery (**Fig. 9**).

GLENOID BONE LOSS PROCEDURES
Surgical Procedures

Unstable shoulders might not only have an insufficient joint capsule but also lack of bony support of the anterior or posterior glenoid rim. These defects are either the result of a single traumatic event or because of chronic instability with gradual attrition of the glenoidal bone stock. Even small bone losses may result in unfavorable surgical results when they are not addressed with augmentation of the deficient glenoid socket.[24] Different (auto-) graft options for glenoid augmentation are available. Most surgeons use either the coracoid as a local bone block transfer (Latarjet procedure or Bristow-Latarjet procedure) or a graft from the iliac crest (bicortical or tricortical/J-graft). The graft must be placed flush to the glenoid surface and is usually fixed with two screws. Other fixation techniques, including endobutton systems or press-fit implantation with the J-graft, have been described. Malpositioning of the graft too medial (persistent instability) or too lateral (early osteoarthritis) must be avoided.[25] For all of the previously

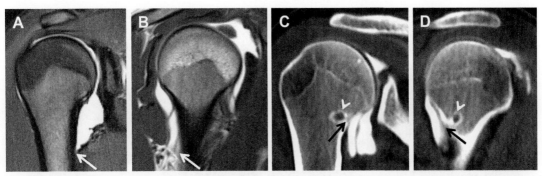

Fig. 5. Posterior HAGL repair. A 19-year-old woman with history of posterior labrum repair (not shown) and repair of a posterior humeral avulsion of the glenohumeral ligament (PHAGL). (*A*) Preoperative coronal oblique fat-suppressed proton density MR arthrogram and (*B*) sagittal oblique T1-weighted MR arthrogram show a PHAGL lesion (*white arrows*). In the (*C*) postoperative reformatted coronal oblique and (*D*) sagittal oblique CT arthrogram the posterior band of the inferior glenohumeral ligament is reattached to the humeral neck (*black arrows*) with a bioabsorbable suture anchor (*arrowheads*).

mentioned grafts, open and arthroscopic surgical techniques are described; however, open techniques are currently more frequent. With open techniques, different surgical approaches to the shoulder joint are performed. Anterior bone blocks are fixed to the glenoid via take down or split of the subscapular tendon/muscle or through the rotator interval. Posterior fixation usually requires a deltoid split and deep dissection of the plane between the infraspinatus and teres minor muscle. When posterior instability is associated with posterior glenoid dysplasia, an open wedge osteotomy (Scott) with or without additional graft (J-graft) insertion may be performed.[26]

Imaging Evaluation: Expected Postoperative Findings

The goal of bone block procedures is to augment a significant glenoidal bone defect or a dysplastic posterior glenoid and to restore glenohumeral stability. Depending on the surgical procedure performed, there is a variable appearance of the postoperative osseous glenoid. Glenoid shape is evaluated best on sagittal oblique images, whereas the axial imaging plane is best suited for the articular surface. MR imaging and CT are used with CT being superior to evaluate the osseous anatomy.

After the Latarjet procedure the transferred tip of the coracoid process is visible at the anteroinferior glenoid and is firmly attached by fixation screws. The coracoid transfer should be flush with the articular surface of the glenoid without medial or lateral offset. The conjoint tendon (short head of the biceps and coracobrachialis), which is not detached, descends from the apex of the transferred coracoid process and passes through a horizontal incision of the inferior subscapularis tendon. Because of this procedure the conjoint tendon

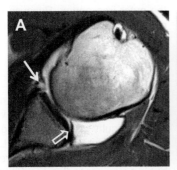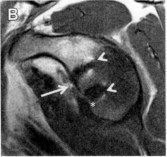

Fig. 6. Recurrent labral tear. A 36-year-old man with history of anteroinferior labrum repair and recurrent shoulder dislocations. (*A*) Axial proton density MR arthrogram and (*B*) sagittal oblique T1-weighted MR arthrogram show a fragmented and frayed anteroinferior labrum with interposition of contrast material (*solid arrow*), consistent with a recurrent tear. An additional posterior labrum tear is seen (*open arrow* in A). There is moderate glenoid bone loss anteroinferiorly (*asterisk*). Note metal anchors in the anteroinferior glenoid with little susceptibility artifacts (*arrowheads*).

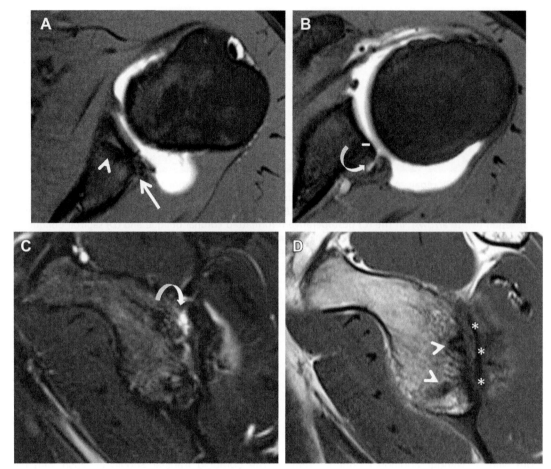

Fig. 7. Posterior bony Bankart repair with partial nonhealing. A 26-year-old man with history of a posterior labrum repair with refixation of a small bone chip after posterior instability. (*A*, *B*) Axial fat-suppressed three-dimensional TRUFI MR arthrogram and (*C*) sagittal oblique fat-suppressed T2-weighted MR arthrogram: after repair the inferior part of the bone chip is readapted (*arrow* in *A*), whereas there is a cleft with contrast material filling (*arrow* in *B* and *C*) superiorly, consistent with nonhealing. The humeral head is decentered posteriorly and there is cartilage thinning at the posterior glenoid (*solid line* in *B*). (*D*) Sagittal oblique T1-weighted MR arthrogram demonstrates the superiorly slightly displaced shell-like posterior bony Bankart fragment (*asterisks*). Note bioabsorbable anchors in the posterior glenoid (*arrowheads* in *A* and *D*).

acts as a sling to further stabilize the joint and to prevent anterior redislocation (**Figs. 10** and **11**).[5,8,21,27] Scar tissue is found in proximity to the subscapularis split.

Similarly to the Latarjet procedure a bone block from the iliac crest (bicortical or tricortical) is fixed firmly to the anterior or posterior glenoid by screws without offset to stabilize the joint (**Fig. 12**).[28,29]

A J-bone graft is used for a more anatomic reconstruction of the glenoid in contrast to the nonanatomic Latarjet procedure. The J-shaped bicortical iliac crest bone graft that is inserted into an artificial crevice after glenoid osteotomy is visible at the anterior or posterior glenoid rim with MR imaging and CT. The bone graft slightly differs in trabecular texture from the native glenoid bone and is demarcated by a thin sclerotic line at the periphery representing

the outer iliac cortex. Because the J-bone graft is primarily stable after correct positioning usually no screw fixation is necessary (**Fig. 13**).[30]

Common Complications

Positioning and osseous integration of the bone graft can best be evaluated with CT and with more difficulty with MR imaging. Nonunion of the transferred coracoid tip after Latarjet procedure or of the iliac bone block is infrequently observed but is not necessarily associated with instability.[31] Additional osteolysis or loosening of the fixation screws, however, raise suspicion of an insufficient procedure with persistent or recurrent instability and can predispose to impingement of adjacent tendons (**Fig. 14**). A fracture of the fixation screws

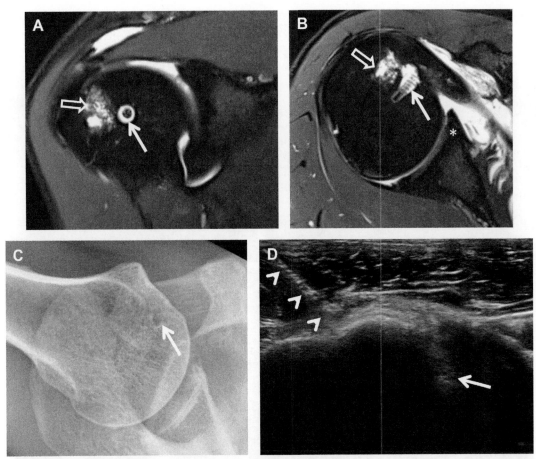

Fig. 8. Osteolysis around interference screw after biceps tenodesis. A 40-year-old man with history of labrum repair and tenodesis of the long head of the biceps tendon. (*A*) Coronal oblique and (*B*) axial fat-suppressed proton density MR arthrogram show osteolysis (*hyperintense rim*) around the bioabsorbable interference screw (*solid arrow*) in the superior intertubercular sulcus after biceps tenodesis with adjacent intraosseous ganglia (*open arrow*). After repair the anteroinferior labrum is slightly scarred (*asterisk* in *B*). (*C*) In the axial radiograph, osteolysis is also visible around the radiolucent interference screw with a thin rim of sclerosis (*arrow*). (*D*) Transverse gray scale ultrasound image shows ultrasound-guided needle placement (*arrowheads*) at the superior intertubercular sulcus for injection of corticosteroid and local anesthetics, which resulted in pain relief. Note hyperechoic area caused by interference screw (*arrow*).

is usually associated with dislocation of the graft (**Fig. 15**), although graft dislocation can also occur with an intact but displaced screw (**Fig. 16**). Another complication is fragmentation or partial resorption of the transferred bone graft, which can lead to insufficient glenohumeral stability or uncovering of portions of the screws. The exposed hardware parts can cause irritation or impingement of surrounding soft tissues or even result in pseudobursa formation (**Fig. 17**).

HUMERAL BONE LOSS PROCEDURES
Surgical Procedures

With glenohumeral dislocation especially after trauma, a humeral head impaction fracture may occur posteriorly (anterior dislocation) or anteriorly (posterior dislocation). With anteroinferior dislocation the corresponding osseous lesion at the posterosuperior aspect of the humeral head is called a Hill-Sachs lesion.

In cases with large Hill-Sachs lesions or combined anterior glenoid bone loss and significant humeral impaction (so-called bipolar bone loss), the humeral head is at risk to engage with the glenoid during external rotation, which can lead to recurrent dislocation of the shoulder. Whether a Hill-Sachs lesion engages with the glenoid depends on the size and the location of the humeral head impaction zone and the size of the residual articular surface of the glenoid and is predicted using the on-track/off-track method, which is described in detail elsewhere in this issue.[32]

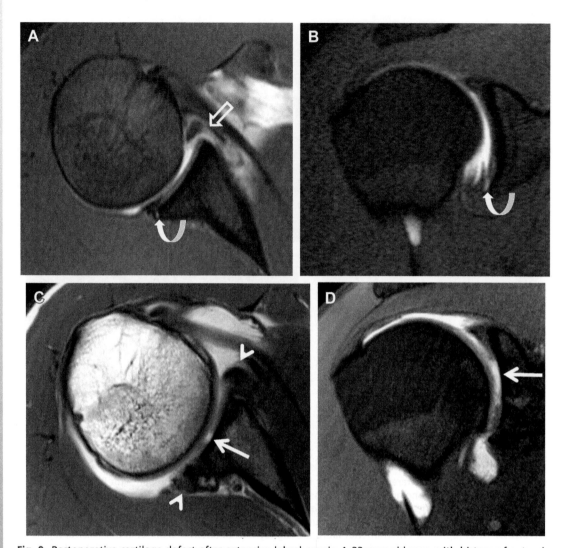

Fig. 9. Postoperative cartilage defect after extensive labral repair. A 32-year-old man with history of extensive labral repair (4–9 o'clock). (*A*) Preoperative axial fat-suppressed T1-weighted MR arthrogram and (*B*) coronal oblique fat-suppressed T1-weighted MR arthrogram show a large labrum tear anteroinferior (*open arrow* in *A*), and inferior (*curved arrow* in *B*) extending to posterior (*curved arrow* in *A*). No glenoid cartilage defect is visible preoperatively. (*C*) Postoperative axial T1-weighted and (*D*) coronal oblique fat-suppressed T1-weighted MR arthrogram show a deep cartilage defect at the center of the glenoid (*arrow*). Note thickened and irregular anterior and posterior labrum after repair (*arrowheads* in *C*).

On-track lesions usually do not need bone augmentation procedures, whereas off-track lesions often have continued instability if bone loss is not addressed. The goal of augmenting glenoid bone loss with a bone block procedure is to transform an off-track lesion into an on-track lesion and prevent recurrent instability.

Humeral bone loss is addressed surgically by either disimpaction of the impacted area with a bone tamper in an acute setting or filling the defect with an allograft in the chronic setting to restore the normal contour and sphericity of the humeral head.[33,34] Alternatively, the infraspinatus tendon

is surgically fixed into the defect using suture anchors (referred to as remplissage procedure) to fill the bony defect.[35] In rare cases of anterior humeral bone loss with posterior dislocation, the same principles may be applied.

Imaging Evaluation: Expected Postoperative Findings

Depending on the surgical procedure performed and the amount of metallic hardware used either CT or MR imaging is most suitable to evaluate the postoperative situation.

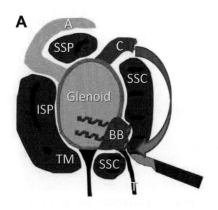

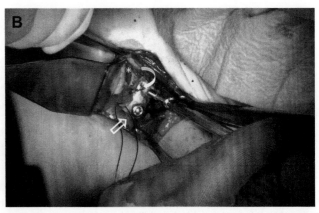

Fig. 10. Latarjet procedure. (*A*) Sagittal illustration. The tip of the coracoid process (C) is cut and transferred to the anteroinferior glenoid through a horizontal incision of the inferior one-third of the subscapularis tendon. The conjoint tendon (T; short head of the biceps and coracobrachialis), which is not detached from the transferred bone block, acts as a sling to further stabilize the joint and to prevent anterior redislocation. Fixation screws are used to secure the bone graft to the anteroinferior glenoid. (*B*) Surgical situs in a right shoulder: the transferred coracoid bone graft is fixed flush to the anteroinferior glenoid surface using two partially threaded screws. *Asterisk,* glenohumeral joint space; *curved arrow,* coracoid bone block; *open arrow,* conjoint tendon; A, acromion; BB, bone block; ISP, infraspinatus; SSC, subscapularis; SSP, supraspinatus; TM, teres minor. (*Courtesy of* K. Wieser, MD, Zurich, Switzerland.)

After a remplissage procedure, MR imaging best demonstrates the fixation of the posterior joint capsule and infraspinatus tendon into the Hill-Sachs lesion, which renders the defect extra-articular and tightens the posterior joint capsule. The transfer is secured by one or more suture anchors. With an intact remplissage, there should be no significant amount of fluid or contrast material between the posterior humeral head defect and the attached infraspinatus tendon.[5,8,21,35,36]

Some localized scar tissue is an expected postoperative finding (**Fig. 18**).

CT with or without secondary three-dimensional reconstruction of the osseous structures is most appropriate to assess the reconstructed humeral head contour and sphericity after disimpaction in the acute setting or after humeral head allograft augmentation in the chronic setting. If available a comparison with preoperative images is advantageous. In the normal postoperative setting, the

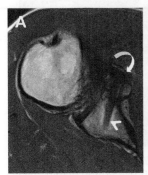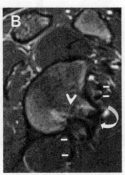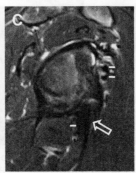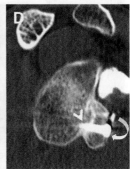

Fig. 11. Latarjet procedure. A 29-year-old man with previous coracoid bone block transfer to the anteroinferior glenoid (Latarjet procedure). Anteroinferior glenoid augmentation with a coracoid bone block is demonstrated in the (*A*) axial proton density MR image, (*B*, *C*) sagittal oblique short tau inversion recovery with optimized inversion pulse (STIR WARP) image, and (*D*) reformatted sagittal oblique CT arthrogram: the tip of the coracoid process is cut and transferred together with the conjoint tendon to the anteroinferior glenoid rim through an artificial split of the inferior one-third of the subscapularis tendon (*solid lines* in *B* and *C* show tendon slips of the subscapularis). The transferred bone graft (*curved arrow* in *A*, *B* and *D*) is firmly attached to the anteroinferior glenoid by screws (*arrowhead* in *A*, *B* and *D*) without offset and is fused. The conjoint tendon (*open arrow* in *C*), which is not detached from the transferred coracoid tip, acts as a sling to further stabilize the joint and to prevent anterior redislocation. Note moderate susceptibility artifacts caused by screws.

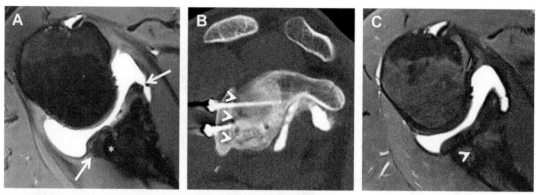

Fig. 12. Posterior bone block procedure. A 22-year-old man with history of extended labral repair (4–9 o'clock) and posteroinferior bone block stabilization after recurrent posterior instability. (*A*) Axial fat-suppressed three-dimensional TRUFI MR arthrogram shows a thickened anterior and posterior labrum with inhomogeneous signal intensity (*arrows*) after extensive repair and dysplasia of the posteroinferior glenoid (*asterisk*). (*B*) Postoperatively after bone block procedure because of recurrent instability reformatted sagittal oblique CT arthrogram demonstrates a tricortical bone graft from the iliac crest firmly attached to the posteroinferior glenoid and secured with fixation screws. The bone graft is completely fused with the posterior glenoid (*arrowheads* in *B*), which is also visible in the axial fat-suppressed proton density MR arthrogram (*arrowhead* in *C*). There is a smooth outline of the augmented articular surface of the glenoid.

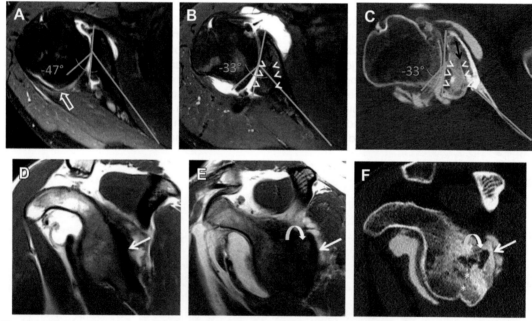

Fig. 13. J-bone graft. A 40-year-old man with history of posterior glenoid osteotomy and J-bone graft because of massive glenoid dysplasia with strong retroversion. (*A*) Preoperative axial fat-suppressed proton density MR arthrogram shows a massive dysplasia of the posterior glenoid with strong retroversion of −47° and posterior subluxation of the humeral head (*arrow*). Retroversion reduced to −33° after posterior glenoid osteotomy (Scott procedure) and insertion of a J-bone graft (*arrowheads* in *B* and *C*) in the artificial crevice. The bone graft is demarcated in the (*B*) postoperative axial fat-suppressed proton density MR arthrogram and in the (*C*) postoperative axial CT arthrogram by a slightly different trabecular texture and a thin sclerotic line at the periphery (*black arrows*). (*D, E*) Sagittal oblique T1-weighted MR arthrogram shows the augmented posterior glenoid after J-bone graft (*solid arrow* in *E*) as compared with the preoperative dysplastic posterior glenoid (*arrow* in *D*). (*F*) In the postoperative reformatted sagittal oblique CT arthrogram the J-bone graft (*solid arrow*) is fused with the posterior glenoid (*asterisks*). Note cystic changes in the posterosuperior glenoid (*curved arrow* in *E* and *F*) caused by osteoarthritis.

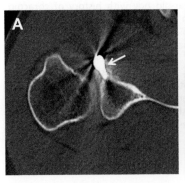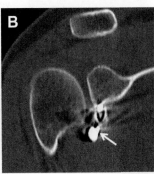

Fig. 14. Screw loosening after Latarjet procedure. A 26-year-old patient with pain 8 months after coracoid bone graft transfer to the anteroinferior glenoid (Latarjet procedure). (*A*) Axial and (*B*) reformatted coronal oblique CT images show loosening of the inferior screw with partial backing out anteriorly (*arrow*) that predisposes to impingement of the inferior subscapularis tendon. Findings are suspicious of an insufficient Latarjet procedure with persistent or recurrent instability.

fracture fragments or allograft should be firmly attached to the proximal humerus with intact screws such that the osseous surfaces are aligned without step off and the normal convex contour of the humeral head is restored (**Fig. 19**).

Common Complications

Similar complications can occur after humeral head allograft augmentation as with glenoid augmentation procedures including nonunion, necrosis, or fragmentation of the allograft and partial graft resorption with associated loosening, fracture, or dislocation of the fixation screws.

With a remplissage, a dehiscence of the infraspinatus tendon from the Hill-Sachs defect with interposition of a significant amount of fluid or contrast material is suspicious for a failure. The presence of new bone marrow edema adjacent to the Hill-Sachs lesion is also suspicious for a failed procedure with recurrent anterior dislocation.[21] Lastly, anchor dislocation is another complication after remplissage, usually resulting in insufficiency.

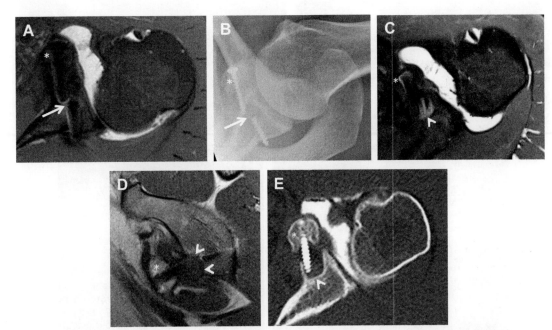

Fig. 15. Hardware failure and osteolysis after Latarjet procedure. A 36-year-old man with previous coracoid bone graft augmentation of the anteroinferior glenoid (Latarjet procedure). (*A*) Axial fat-suppressed proton density MR arthrogram shows a broken screw (*arrow*) after transfer of the coracoid tip to the anteroinferior glenoid, which is also shown in the axial radiograph (*arrow* in *B*). In the follow-up 3 years later osteolysis developed around the broken screw thread in the anterior glenoid bone as depicted in the axial fat-suppressed proton density MR arthrogram (*arrowhead* in *C*) and sagittal oblique T1-weighted MR arthrogram (*arrowheads* in *D*), which is also shown in the axial CT arthrogram (*arrowhead* in *E*). Note anterior dislocation of the bone block (*asterisk* in *A–E*).

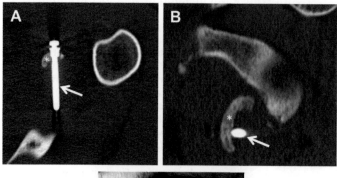

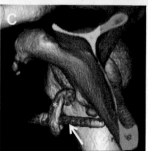

Fig. 16. Hardware and graft dislocation after Latarjet procedure. A 17-year-old boy with history of coracoid tip transfer to the anteroinferior glenoid (Latarjet procedure). (*A*) Axial CT image, (*B*) reformatted sagittal oblique CT image, and (*C*) three-dimensional CT osseous reconstruction show an anterior dislocation of the intact fixation screw (*arrow*) together with the C-shaped bone graft (*asterisk*) from the anteroinferior glenoid.

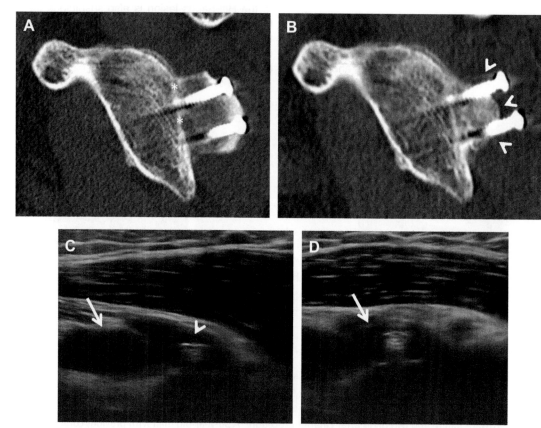

Fig. 17. Partial bone block resorption with pseudobursa formation. A 30-year-old man with previous posterior bone block procedure after recurrent instability. (*A*) Reformatted sagittal oblique CT image shows a posterior glenoid augmentation with an iliac bone graft, which is fixed to the posterior glenoid rim by screws and is fused (*asterisks*). (*B*) In the follow-up reformatted sagittal oblique CT image 9 months later, there is partial resorption of the bone block around the screw heads (*arrowheads*), which consequently exposes the proximal portion of the screws. (*C*) Longitudinal and (*D*) transverse gray scale ultrasound image show a hypoechoic fluid collection (*arrow*) surrounding the screw heads (*arrowhead*) underneath the infraspinatus muscle, which is consistent with pseudobursa formation.

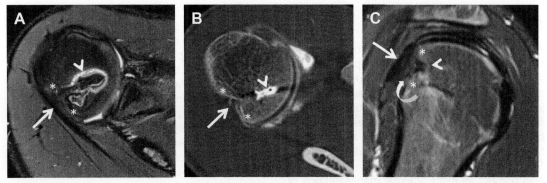

Fig. 18. Remplissage. A 29-year-old man with previous remplissage after a large Hill-Sachs lesion. (A) Axial fat-suppressed proton density MR image, (B) axial CT arthrogram, and (C) sagittal oblique STIR WARP image show a remplissage procedure with fixation of the posterior joint capsule and the infraspinatus tendon (*solid arrow*) into a large Hill-Sachs lesion (in between *asterisks*) secured by a suture anchor (*arrowhead*). There is little granulation tissue (*curved arrow* in C) but no contrast agent or fluid between the infraspinatus tendon and the Hill-Sachs defect, which is consistent with an intact remplissage. Note little susceptibility artifacts caused by metal anchor.

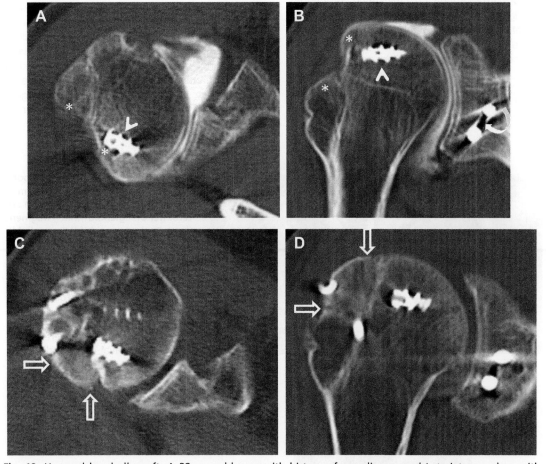

Fig. 19. Humeral head allograft. A 32-year-old man with history of remplissage and Latarjet procedure with recurrent instability. (A) Axial and (B) reformatted coronal oblique CT arthrogram show a large Hill-Sachs defect in the posterior humeral head (in between *asterisks*). Note metal anchor after previous remplissage (*arrowhead*) and fixation screws in the glenoid after Latarjet procedure (*curved arrow*). In the postoperative axial (C) and reformatted coronal oblique (D) CT image the large Hill-Sachs lesion is filled with a convex-shaped femoral head allograft (*arrows*) and fixated by screws. No step off is visible after reconstruction of the humeral head contour and sphericity. The allograft is partially fused with the humeral head.

GENERAL COMPLICATIONS

As with any other invasive procedure, joint infection is a rare but devastating complication after instability surgery of the shoulder, usually occurring in the early postoperative period. A large joint effusion with massive, sometimes nodular synovitis and adjacent soft tissue edema is suspicious for septic arthritis. A joint aspiration is, however, necessary for definitive diagnosis. Soft tissue abscesses or septic bursitis can also present as extra-articular manifestations of infection.[8,22]

Adhesive capsulitis is another well-known complication after shoulder surgery, including instability surgery, and is sometimes difficult to differentiate from infection, especially in the early postoperative period. Signs that may indicate the presence of adhesive capsulitis at MR imaging and MR arthrography are a thickened coracohumeral ligament, fibrovascular infiltration of the rotator interval, a thickened joint capsule at the level of the rotator interval and/or axillary recess, and reduced volume of the axillary recess. Furthermore, pericapsular edema may coexist (**Fig. 20**).[37–40] If performing arthrography, additional useful hints that adhesive capsulitis may be present are painful injection with increased

resistance and decreased intra-articular volume of the injected contrast material. For equivocal cases, joint aspiration is necessary to exclude infection from the differential diagnosis. Most cases of adhesive capsulitis are treated nonsurgically with physical therapy with or without intra-articular corticosteroid injection.

Postoperatively, adhesions might form, which can be an incidental finding without clinical significance or can cause symptoms like a snapping phenomenon, pain, or a reduced range of motion (**Fig. 21**). In some cases, adhesiolysis may be necessary.

Another potential complication is injury to the axillary nerve during instability surgery, because of its close proximity to the inferior joint structures. Depending on the site of injury, denervation edema is observed in the deltoid and/or teres minor muscle in the acute stage, whereas atrophy and/or fatty infiltration is visible in the chronic stage.[8,22]

A reported rare complication after shoulder arthroscopy is diffuse chondrolysis with cartilage loss within 1 year thereafter, mainly observed in young patients. High volume and high dose of intra-articular local anesthetics during surgery and foreign body reaction to anchors are reported risk factors for diffuse chondrolysis.[5,8,9]

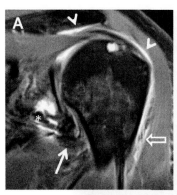
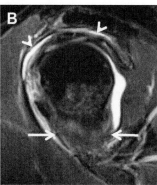
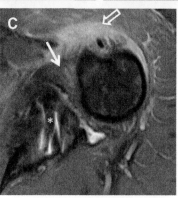

Fig. 20. Adhesive capsulitis after bony Bankart repair. A 65-year-old man with history of screw fixation of an anteroinferior glenoid rim fragment (bony Bankart repair). (*A*) Coronal oblique fat-suppressed proton density MR image, (*B*) sagittal oblique STIR image, and (*C*) axial fat-suppressed proton density MR image show a thickened inferior capsule with little adjacent edema (*solid arrows*) and restricted volume of the axillary recess, consistent with adhesive capsulitis. There is additional subacromial-subdeltoid bursitis (*arrowheads* in *A* and *B*) with adjoining soft tissue edema (*open arrow* in *A* and *C*). Note fixation screws in the anteroinferior glenoid with susceptibility artifacts (*asterisk* in *A* and *C*).

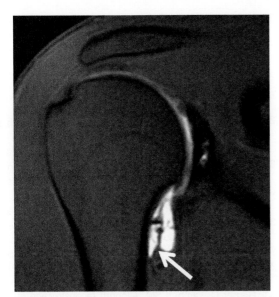

Fig. 21. Postoperative adhesions. A 31-year-old man with history of posterior Bankart repair after posterior instability. Coronal oblique fat-suppressed T1-weighted MR arthrogram shows band-like adhesions in the axillary recess, which formed postoperatively (*arrow*).

Insufficiency of the subscapularis that can occur after open surgical procedures using anterior surgical approaches for instability repair has become a rare finding with the increase in arthroscopic techniques, which have mostly replaced open Bankart procedures and obviate subscapularis tendon detachment or incision. Few cases of subscapularis insufficiency, however, have been reported after a Latarjet procedure.[22,41,42]

Lastly, even after successful instability surgery, new or progressive osteoarthritis may arise caused by microinstability or macroinstability of the shoulder related to altered biomechanics. Soft tissue repairs of shoulder instability may fail, which necessitates conversion to a bone augmentation procedure. Although some complications of bone augmentation procedures have been reported in this article, generally bone augmentation procedures have an excellent clinical outcome, and recurrent instability after surgery is less common than for soft tissue repairs.[43]

SUMMARY

MR imaging of the postoperative shoulder after instability surgery is a challenging task. The radiologist must be familiar with the different surgical techniques that are used including soft tissue repairs and bone augmentation procedures and the altered anatomy, expected postoperative findings, and common complications of these different procedures to accurately differentiate normal postoperative changes from true postoperative pathology. Additionally, the radiologist must also be knowledgeable in selecting the most appropriate imaging techniques and protocols to minimize artifacts from orthopedic hardware and be able to provide diagnostic images and add value to patient care.

DISCLOSURE STATEMENT

The authors have nothing to disclose.

REFERENCES

1. Bonazza NA, Liu G, Leslie DL, et al. Trends in surgical management of shoulder instability. Orthop J Sports Med 2017;5(6). 2325967117712476.
2. Magee T. Imaging of the post-operative shoulder: does injection of iodinated contrast in addition to MR contrast during arthrography improve diagnostic accuracy and patient throughput? Skeletal Radiol 2018;47(9):1253–61.
3. Wagner SC, Schweitzer ME, Morrison WB, et al. Shoulder instability: accuracy of MR imaging performed after surgery in depicting recurrent injury–initial findings. Radiology 2002;222(1):196–203.
4. Hargreaves BA, Worters PW, Pauly KB, et al. Metal-induced artifacts in MRI. AJR Am J Roentgenol 2011;197(3):547–55.
5. Beltran LS, Bencardino JT, Steinbach LS. Postoperative MRI of the shoulder. J Magn Reson Imaging 2014;40(6):1280–97.
6. Ulbrich EJ, Sutter R, Aguiar RF, et al. STIR sequence with increased receiver bandwidth of the inversion pulse for reduction of metallic artifacts. AJR Am J Roentgenol 2012;199(6):W735–42.
7. Low RN, Austin MJ, Ma J. Fast spin-echo triple echo Dixon: initial clinical experience with a novel pulse sequence for simultaneous fat-suppressed and nonfat-suppressed T2-weighted spine magnetic resonance imaging. J Magn Reson Imaging 2011;33(2):390–400.
8. Pierce JL, Nacey NC, Jones S, et al. Postoperative shoulder imaging: rotator cuff, labrum, and biceps tendon. Radiographics 2016;36(6):1648–71.
9. McMenamin D, Koulouris G, Morrison WB. Imaging of the shoulder after surgery. Eur J Radiol 2008;68(1):106–19.
10. Bancroft LW, Wasyliw C, Pettis C, et al. Postoperative shoulder magnetic resonance imaging. Magn Reson Imaging Clin N Am 2012;20(2):313–25, xi.
11. Zanetti M, Hodler J. MR imaging of the shoulder after surgery. Radiol Clin North Am 2006;44(4):537–51, viii.

12. Sutter R, Hodek R, Fucentese SF, et al. Total knee arthroplasty MRI featuring slice-encoding for metal artifact correction: reduction of artifacts for STIR and proton density-weighted sequences. AJR Am J Roentgenol 2013;201(6):1315–24.

13. Koch KM, Lorbiecki JE, Hinks RS, et al. A multispectral three-dimensional acquisition technique for imaging near metal implants. Magn Reson Med 2009;61(2):381–90.

14. Hovelius L, Augustini BG, Fredin H, et al. Primary anterior dislocation of the shoulder in young patients. A ten-year prospective study. J Bone Joint Surg Am 1996;78(11):1677–84.

15. Kralinger FS, Golser K, Wischatta R, et al. Predicting recurrence after primary anterior shoulder dislocation. Am J Sports Med 2002;30(1):116–20.

16. Itoigawa Y, Itoi E, Sakoma Y, et al. Attachment of the anteroinferior glenohumeral ligament-labrum complex to the glenoid: an anatomic study. Arthroscopy 2012;28(11):1628–33.

17. Mauro CS, Voos JE, Hammoud S, et al. Failed anterior shoulder stabilization. J Shoulder Elbow Surg 2011;20(8):1340–50.

18. Randelli P, Ragone V, Carminati S, et al. Risk factors for recurrence after Bankart repair a systematic review. Knee Surg Sports Traumatol Arthrosc 2012; 20(11):2129–38.

19. Sugaya H, Takahashi N. Arthroscopic osseous Bankart repair in the treatment of recurrent anterior glenohumeral instability. JBJS Essent Surg Tech 2016;6(3):e26.

20. Maquieira GJ, Espinosa N, Gerber C, et al. Non-operative treatment of large anterior glenoid rim fractures after traumatic anterior dislocation of the shoulder. J Bone Joint Surg Br 2007;89(10): 1347–51.

21. Beltran LS, Duarte A, Bencardino JT. Postoperative imaging in anterior glenohumeral instability. AJR Am J Roentgenol 2018;211(3):528–37.

22. Woertler K. Multimodality imaging of the postoperative shoulder. Eur Radiol 2007;17(12):3038–55.

23. Sugimoto H, Suzuki K, Mihara K, et al. MR arthrography of shoulders after suture-anchor Bankart repair. Radiology 2002;224(1):105–11.

24. Shahab JS, Cook JB, Song DJ, et al. Redefining "critical" bone loss in shoulder instability: functional outcomes worsen with "subcritical" bone loss. Am J Sports Med 2015;43(7):1719–25.

25. Willemot L, De Boey S, Van Tongel A, et al. Analysis of failures after the Bristow-Latarjet procedure for recurrent shoulder instability. Int Orthop 2019; 43(8):1899–907.

26. Ortmaier R, Moroder P, Hirzinger C, et al. Posterior open wedge osteotomy of the scapula neck for the treatment of advanced shoulder osteoarthritis with posterior head migration in young patients. J Shoulder Elbow Surg 2017;26(7):1278–86.

27. Lafosse L, Lejeune E, Bouchard A, et al. The arthroscopic Latarjet procedure for the treatment of anterior shoulder instability. Arthroscopy 2007;23(11): 1242.e1-5.

28. Ranalletta M, Tanoira I, Bertona A, et al. Autologous tricortical iliac bone graft for failed Latarjet procedures. Arthrosc Tech 2019;8(3):e283–9.

29. Schwartz DG, Goebel S, Piper K, et al. Arthroscopic posterior bone block augmentation in posterior shoulder instability. J Shoulder Elbow Surg 2013;22(8):1092–101.

30. Auffarth A, Schauer J, Matis N, et al. The J-bone graft for anatomical glenoid reconstruction in recurrent posttraumatic anterior shoulder dislocation. Am J Sports Med 2008;36(4):638–47.

31. Gupta A, Delaney R, Petkin K, et al. Complications of the Latarjet procedure. Curr Rev Musculoskelet Med 2015;8(1):59–66.

32. Itoi E. 'On-track' and 'off-track' shoulder lesions. EFORT Open Rev 2017;2(8):343–51.

33. Gerber C, Lambert SM. Allograft reconstruction of segmental defects of the humeral head for the treatment of chronic locked posterior dislocation of the shoulder. J Bone Joint Surg Am 1996;78(3):376–82.

34. Re P, Gallo RA, Richmond JC. Transhumeral head plasty for large Hill-Sachs lesions. Arthroscopy 2006;22(7):798.e1-4.

35. Boileau P, O'Shea K, Vargas P, et al. Anatomical and functional results after arthroscopic Hill-Sachs remplissage. J Bone Joint Surg Am 2012;94(7):618–26.

36. Park MJ, Garcia G, Malhotra A, et al. The evaluation of arthroscopic remplissage by high-resolution magnetic resonance imaging. Am J Sports Med 2012; 40(10):2331–6.

37. Mengiardi B, Pfirrmann CW, Gerber C, et al. Frozen shoulder: MR arthrographic findings. Radiology 2004;233(2):486–92.

38. Lee MH, Ahn JM, Muhle C, et al. Adhesive capsulitis of the shoulder: diagnosis using magnetic resonance arthrography, with arthroscopic findings as the standard. J Comput Assist Tomogr 2003;27(6):901–6.

39. Chi AS, Kim J, Long SS, et al. Non-contrast MRI diagnosis of adhesive capsulitis of the shoulder. Clin Imaging 2017;44:46–50.

40. Emig EW, Schweitzer ME, Karasick D, et al. Adhesive capsulitis of the shoulder: MR diagnosis. AJR Am J Roentgenol 1995;164(6):1457–9.

41. Maynou C, Cassagnaud X, Mestdagh H. Function of subscapularis after surgical treatment for recurrent instability of the shoulder using a bone-block procedure. J Bone Joint Surg Br 2005;87(8):1096–101.

42. Scheibel M, Habermeyer P. Subscapularis dysfunction following anterior surgical approaches to the shoulder. J Shoulder Elbow Surg 2008;17(4):671–83.

43. Bessiere C, Trojani C, Carles M, et al. The open Latarjet procedure is more reliable in terms of shoulder stability than arthroscopic Bankart repair. Clin Orthop Relat Res 2014;472(8):2345–51.

Thrower's Shoulder: An Approach to MR Imaging Interpretation

Faysal Altahawi, MD, Joshua M. Polster, MD*

KEYWORDS

- Thrower's shoulder • Shoulder MR imaging • SLAP • Labrum

KEY POINTS

- Throwers typically have chronic changes or remote injuries in the labrum and rotator cuff, which can make interpretation challenging.
- 3 T MR image is the standard for diagnosing labral pathology in throwers. Intra-articular gadolinium is particularly useful with 1.5 T MR imaging and on postoperative patients.
- The late-cocking phase of throwing is implicated in the posterosuperior pattern of injury in the labrum and rotator cuff by biceps–labral anchor peel-back torsional forces and posterosuperior impingement.
- A sublabral sulcus should be thin and smooth without extension posterior to the biceps anchor.
- Increased cleft width and depth, posterior or intralabral extension, or irregular labral margins suggest a tear.

INTRODUCTION

Throwing athletes are at risk for shoulder injuries, particularly baseball pitchers.[1–3] Although the biomechanics of overhand pitching has been highly studied and reviewed, an understanding of mechanics can aid musculoskeletal radiologists in piecing together the most relevant shoulder MR imaging findings in a manner that will allow orthopedic or sports medicine physicians to make management decisions. Throwers commonly have chronic changes or remote injuries in the shoulder, which can make interpretation particularly challenging because the lines between adaptive or pathologic changes can be blurred, and many professional throwing athletes can have known asymptomatic abnormal imaging findings (**Fig. 1**). It is often in difficult cases, however, where the musculoskeletal radiologist can provide the most value. In this article, we aim to focus on the challenges of interpreting shoulder MR imaging in the throwing athlete with an approach formed by evidence-based literature and clinical experience, with a particular focus on superior labrum tears.

IMAGING TECHNIQUE

Optimizing technique is a prerequisite for any radiologic examination and can also be of utmost importance in the MR imaging evaluation of the thrower's shoulder. Several considerations must be applied to tailor the examination to the thrower while implementing a practical protocol to a radiologist's practice.

Anatomic considerations of imaging include small curved structures with variable orientation, some of which have tension on them in the standard imaging positions, but none of which experience the physical forces of throwing at the time of imaging. High spatial resolution in multiple planes or even 3-dimensional imaging helps to account for the small size and orientation of the structures.

Cleveland Clinic Foundation, 9500 Euclid Avenue, A21, Cleveland, OH 44195, USA
* Corresponding author.
E-mail address: polstej@ccf.org

Magn Reson Imaging Clin N Am 28 (2020) 243–255
https://doi.org/10.1016/j.mric.2019.12.007

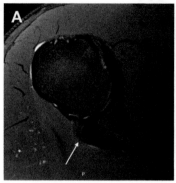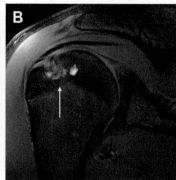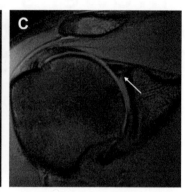

Fig. 1. Asymptomatic 21-year old pitcher after Major League Baseball draft with chronic changes seen in throwers including (*A*) a Bennett lesion (*arrow*) with posterior capsular thickening, (*B*) reactive cystic changes in the greater tuberosity (*arrow*) relating to chronic internal impingement, and (*C*) asymptomatic signal abnormalities in the posterior/superior labrum (*arrow*).

Additionally, high tissue contrast optimizes differentiation between normal and abnormal tissues as well as between joint fluid and the structure being evaluated. Imaging structures in both resting and stressed states would capture more of the dynamic forces in the shoulder.

The current standard for optimal resolution is 3 T MR imaging. The greater spatial resolution and contrast-to-noise ratio that can be achieved with 3 T imaging has been demonstrated to translate to higher diagnostic accuracy when compared with 1.5 T for labral pathology regardless of the use of intra-articular gadolinium.[4] Although there may be limited availability of 3 T MR imaging at some practices, 1.5 T imaging may also be preferred in some cases when there is metal-related susceptibility artifact, which is more pronounced at 3 T. With increasing adoption of 3 T MR imaging, there are ongoing innovations in shoulder MR imaging that can be clinically useful, but are not yet in widespread use, including 3-dimensional isotropic imaging and accelerated imaging.[5,6]

As with most musculoskeletal MR imaging examinations, fat-saturated fluid-sensitive sequences such as proton density and T2-weighted sequences are standard to any shoulder MR imaging protocol, because they maximize the contrast of bright joint fluid against darker tendinous, ligamentous, or cartilaginous structures. Intra-articular gadolinium injection can further enhance tissue contrast by creating high signal in the joint fluid against these darker structures on T1 sequences, with the benefit of adding joint fluid, which may reveal tears by distension that may otherwise be difficult to appreciate. MR arthrography has indeed demonstrated greater diagnostic accuracy than conventional MR imaging for the diagnosis of superior labral tears and rotator cuff tears at 1.5 T.[4,7] However, the contrast benefits of MR arthrography become equivocal at 3 T

imaging, with studies demonstrating marginal or no benefit for some labral tears.[4,8,9] The use of abduction and external rotation (ABER) positioning during MR imaging acquisition can partially reproduce some of the positioning and forces of throwing and may be beneficial in diagnosing related pathology.[10–12]

There are limitations to shoulder MR imaging.[13] Some of the limitations are practically modifiable and some are not. The ideal clinical MR imaging study for evaluation of a superior labral tear with regard to accuracy is currently a 3 T MR imaging evaluation performed after intra-articular gadolinium injection with an additional ABER position sequence. However, it is unlikely for the majority of clinical musculoskeletal radiologists to obtain all of these ideal conditions on every athlete. One study has found routine 3 T shoulder MR imaging to be the most cost-effective evaluation for SLAP tears over MR arthrography, although in the absence of 3 T MR imaging, 1.5 T MR arthrography was more cost effective than routine 1.5 T shoulder MR imaging.[14] Similarly, ABER positioning requires repositioning in the MR imaging scanner and increases scan time.[15] At our institution, most athletes are typically evaluated at a dedicated sports health center where they are scanned on a 3 T MR imaging system with multichannel shoulder coils using standard 2-dimensional multiplanar acquisitions. ABER positioning is not routinely performed unless specifically requested by the radiologists and arthrograms are only performed in a minority of patients when requested by the ordering physician.

THROWING BIOMECHANICS

Throwing mechanics are generally broken down into 6 phases: windup, stride, arm cocking, acceleration, deceleration, and follow-through[16,17](**Fig. 2**). The transition from when the arm is almost fully cocked and beginning to accelerate forward is typically considered the phase of greatest shoulder stresses.[18] Here, the shoulder has reached the maximal ABER position, and the largest direct and centrifugal forces are acting as the primary muscles engage and the arm begins accelerating forward. At this point the arm is transitioning very quickly from external rotation to internal rotation with direct, tensile, and rotational forces acting on the tendons, including torsional forces acting on the biceps-superior labral complex at the supraglenoid tubercle.[19] There are similar and associated shearing forces on the labrum, capsule, and rotator cuff.[18]

Injuries and chronic changes in the thrower's shoulder can largely be appreciated by understanding the anatomic relationships and acting forces at this phase. There are felt to be 2 primary mechanisms for superior labral injuries in the thrower's shoulder: (1) the peel-back phenomenon and (2) posterosuperior impingement, also termed internal impingement (**Fig. 3**). The peel-back mechanism is related to the torsional forces at the biceps anchor in the ABER position causing the posterosuperior labrum to be stripped or peeled away from the glenoid posterior to the biceps anchor.[3,20] Additionally, because the ABER position is maximized there is a resultant posterosuperior impingement characterized by compression of the posterior supraspinatus or anterior infraspinatus tendon articular surface and the posterosuperior labrum between the greater tuberosity and the posterosuperior glenoid.[21] When the force of impingement in this position becomes supraphysiologic and is chronically repeated, this can also lead to rotator cuff and labral injuries and reactive osseous and capsular changes[19,22] (see **Fig. 1**). Some of the chronic changes of thrower's shoulder may be considered adaptive, acting to maximize external rotation in throwers to allow greater pitching velocity, but can also amplify both posterosuperior impingement and torsional forces on the biceps and superior labrum.

SUPERIOR LABRAL TEARS

Superior labral tears usually involve the region near the origin of the long head biceps tendon where the tendon is confluent with the superior labrum. As such, tears often extend anterior and posterior to it, and are referred to as superior labrum anterior to posterior (SLAP) tears.[23] This term can be a misnomer, however, as even within the clinical subclassifications of SLAP tears, the anterior and posterior involvement is not necessary.[24,25] Therefore, in our clinical use, we tend to avoid the term SLAP, and simply refer to these as superior labral tears and describe the extent and nature of tear involvement.

Labral Imaging Considerations

Labral tears can present challenges to radiologists given the small size, curved anatomy, and anatomic variation. Similar to knee menisci on the tibiae, the labral fibrocartilage is normally low signal on fluid sensitive and T1 sequences, is triangular in cross-sectional shape, and curves along

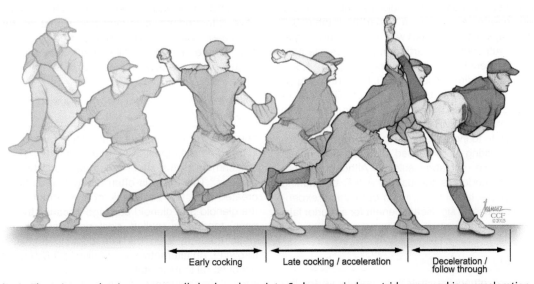

Fig. 2. Throwing mechanics are generally broken down into 6 phases: windup, stride, arm cocking, acceleration, deceleration, and follow-through. (Reprinted with permission, Cleveland Clinic Center for Medical Art & Photography © 1998-2019. All Rights Reserved.)

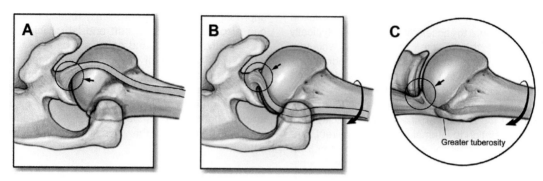

Fig. 3. The biceps anchor from above. Contrast (*A*) the lack of biceps–labral tension in neutral position (*arrow*) with (*B*) the external rotation position (*curved arrow*) in late cocking, which creates tension and a peel-back effect on the superior biceps–labral complex (*small arrow*). (*C*) Posterosuperior impingement impinges the rotator cuff and labrum between the greater tuberosity and posterosuperior glenoid margin (*small arrow*). (Reprinted with permission, Cleveland Clinic Center for Medical Art & Photography © 1998-2019. All Rights Reserved.)

the curvature of the glenoid rim and articular cartilage edge. Although some labral tears represent clefts into the substance of the labrum in an appearance analogous to meniscus tears, many are detachments of the labrum from the underlying bone as represented by fluid separating the labrum from the bone (**Fig. 4**).

Superior labral tears are best identified on coronal oblique images because these images provide the most orthogonal cross-section of the labral-bone interface at the level of the biceps anchor. Depending on the extent of the tear, anterior and posterior extensions may be best seen on axial images. In some cases, sagittal or axial sequences may be useful for identifying displaced labral fragments (**Fig. 5**). The 3 T magnetic field strength has been shown to be an important factor affecting diagnostic accuracy for superior labrum tears, with greater accuracy on nonarthrographic 3 T MR imaging as compared with 1.5 T MR arthrography.[4] Although MR arthrography has demonstrated benefit in studies including at 1.5 T imaging, studies evaluating 3 T MR arthrography for superior labral tears have actually demonstrated decreased specificity as compared with conventional 3 T MR imaging.[4,8] This may presumably relate to increased false positives on arthrography relating to increased distention of variant anatomy (ie, sublabral sulcus). Although limited literature endorses the use of ABER positioning for superior labral tears,[8,12] in our clinical experience there is no significant benefit for superior labral tears in throwers.

Imaging Considerations after Labral Repair

Although otherwise limited in usefulness for the labrum, sagittal images can have some usefulness for positional cross-referencing in the case of prior

labral repair by identifying the intraosseous location of suture anchors on non–fat-suppressed imaging, such as T1-weighted images (**Fig. 6**). For evaluation in the case of prior labral repair, assessment of the integrity of the repair is best performed on images directly orthogonal to the glenoid rim and labrum at the level of repair. Although often not feasible, ideal imaging planes to evaluate the repair include customized planes orthogonal to the labrum–glenoid junction prescribed based on the location of the anchors as identified on the sagittal images. The use of 3-dimensional sequences allow multiplanar reformatting after acquisition to create such planes,[6] although we do not routinely use these modalities at our institution. In the case of assessing the postoperative labrum, an MR arthrogram may be of particular use in distinguishing the frequently seen postoperative intermediate fluid-sensitive signal at the labrum–glenoid junction from a true recurrent tear, where a contrast-filled cleft between the labrum and bone is seen (see **Fig. 6**).

Distinguishing Superior Labral Tears from Anatomic Variants

The most common superior labral tear overall and in throwers is a type II SLAP tear, characterized by detachment of the superior labrum from the glenoid.[23,26] This injury is often thought of as being created with the peel-back of the labrum from the glenoid and glenoid cartilage because the biceps tendon is pulled posteriorly and twists when the arm is in the late cocking phase of throwing. An alternative mechanism of posterosuperior labral tears in athletes is by direct injury with internal impingement. A labral tear is demonstrated on MR imaging as a fluid or contrast signal, typically linear and separating the labrum from the

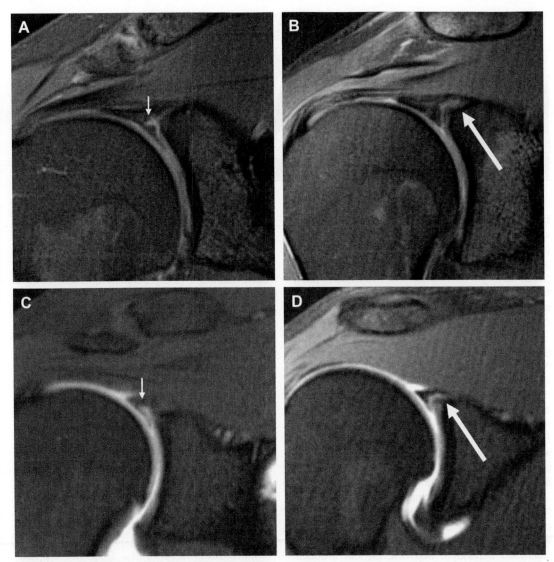

Fig. 4. (*A, B*) Superior labral tears are readily identified on routine 3 T MR imaging and (*C, D*) with intra-articular gadolinium injection. (*A, C, small arrows*) Extension of signal into the substance of the labrum away from the glenoid articular surface or (*B, D, large arrows*) following the contour of the glenoid is indicative of a labral tear rather than a sublabral sulcus.

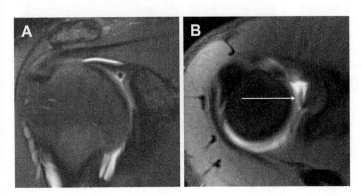

Fig. 5. (*A*) A superior labral tear is well demonstrated on coronal images, but (*B*) the displaced fragment (*arrow*) is better appreciated on the axial images.

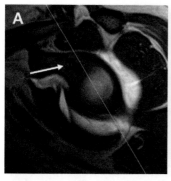
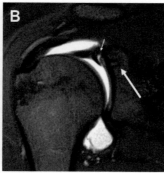

Fig. 6. (*A*) Sagittal T1-weighted image of a 3 T MR arthrography demonstrating a labral repair anchor along the superior labrum (*large arrow*) with cross-reference (*cross-reference line*). (*B*) The cross-referenced coronal oblique arthrogram image demonstrates a superior labral retear (*small arrow*), with contrast undercutting the superior labrum at the repair anchor (*large arrow*) following the glenoid contour. This finding was confirmed on arthroscopy.

bone or sometimes as clefts of increased signal extending into the substance of the labrum[3,20,24] (see **Fig. 4**). Sometimes the increased signal intensity of the cleft on fluid-sensitive sequences may not be as bright as the joint fluid. In throwers, tears tend to extend posterior to the biceps attachment, in keeping with the other posterosuperior injury patterns of throwing injury.[26]

A common challenge for the radiologist is distinguishing a superior labral tear from the sublabral recess, an anatomic variant[25] (**Fig. 7**). Fluid or contrast signal entering the labral substance rather than paralleling the glenoid rim is a specific sign of a labral tear,[25] however, may not be sensitive in the case of throwers with detached labral tears. Fluid beneath the base of the labrum, particularly when shallow, small, smooth, and not extending posterior to the biceps anchor, may represent a sublabral sulcus (also termed a sublabral recess).

There are several imaging findings that can help to distinguish a type II tear from a sulcus more confidently[25] (**Fig. 8**). The typical sublabral recess is less than 2 mm in width with smooth margins, so increased separation from the glenoid articular surface greater than 2 mm (2.5 mm on MR arthrograms) and irregular margins are more suggestive of a tear.[25,27] Articular cartilage signal, typically intermediate, should also not be confused for tear, and is also typically less than 2 mm. Similarly, a cleft of increased signal that separates the labrum from the glenoid and follows the glenoid contour medially is suggestive of a tear when the cleft is more than 5 mm deep.[28,29] Signal extension posterior to the biceps anchor has classically been considered an indicator of a tear over a variant (**Fig. 9**); however, this is no longer considered a reliable indicator of a tear in isolation.[25]

Labral tears can also emerge from a sublabral recess.[28] The presence of a labral tear extending into the labral substance with a sulcus can result in a double Oreo cookie appearance with 2 bands of brighter signal relating to the sulcus or recess and the tear.[29] The sublabral foramen and the

Buford complex extending along the anterior labrum are more widely appreciated and easier to identify owing to the typical anterior superior locations and characteristic appearance; as such, labral tears are rarely diagnosed where there is labrum–glenoid separation isolated to the 1 to 3 o'clock anterior positions[25]; labral separation extending below these bounds or past the biceps anchor, however, is indicative of a labral tear. The presence of a paralabral cyst can confirm the presence of a tear or be the first indicator to the radiologist that a labral tear is present (**Fig. 10**).

Labral Tear Characterization and Management Considerations

Although simply identifying the presence of a labral tear in a thrower is valuable information for a clinician, characterizing a tear accurately can also provide clinical insight for management

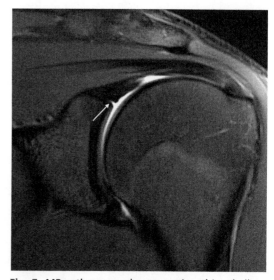

Fig. 7. MR arthrogram demonstrating thin, shallow, smoothly marginated signal that does not extend posterior to the biceps anchor (*arrow*), with no tear demonstrated at surgery.

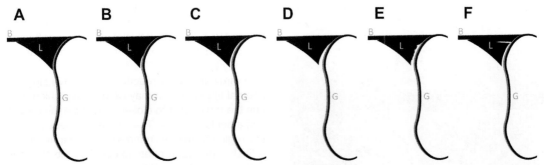

Fig. 8. The biceps–labral anchor on coronal view. (*A*) Lack of signal deep to or within the superior labrum indicates a normal appearance of the superior labrum. (*B*) Signal relating to a sublabral sulcus is typically thin, smoothly marginated, and does not extend posterior to the biceps anchor. Labral tears can be more confidently identified as more of the following findings are identified: (*C*) cleft extends deeper along the glenoid (>5 mm), (*D*) width of the cleft is >2 mm (2.5 mm for arthrograms), (*E*) irregular labral margins, (*F*) if signal extends into the substance of the labrum, or if the cleft extends posterior to the biceps anchor. B, biceps; G, glenoid; L, labrum.

decisions. It is notable that fraying of the superior labrum, manifested on MR imaging by mildly increased nonlinear signal and irregular margins, is classified as a SLAP type I tear.[23,25] Because there is no glenoid detachment, these are typically treated conservatively.

The identification and distinction of type III and type IV tears can also present an important challenge for the radiologist[13] (**Fig. 11**). SLAP type III is defined as a bucket handle superior labral tear involving the substance of the labrum and sparing the biceps–labral anchor. SLAP type IV lesions, in contrast, are bucket handle superior labral tears consisting of detachment of the labrum and anchor from the glenoid rim and extension into the long head of the biceps tendon. Although the distinction is typically descriptive rather than categorical in clinical reports, identifying detachment from the glenoid over intrasubstance tearing, as well as extension into the biceps anchor, is important for a surgeon to determine whether to repair a labrum rather than debride if intervening surgically. Surgical intervention for intrasubstance SLAP type I and type III tears is typically debridement and for

detached SLAP type II and IV tears is typically repair.[13,30,31] Exceptions are of course present, with debridement of SLAP IV lesions sometimes preferred if more than one-half of the biceps–labral complex remains anchored and repair of type III lesions sometimes considered in peripheral tears in the red–red zone of the labrum, similar to knee menisci.[31]

Characterizing extensions to the posterior and anterior labrum is typically a straightforward task for the radiologist, with typical extension to the posterior–superior labrum for throwers. Notably, however, throwers can have isolated posterosuperior labral tears without involving the biceps anchor–superior labrum complex, presumably related to a posterosuperior impingement mechanism.[19] These tears typically coexist with the posterior capsular thickening that is often seen in throwers and usually is contiguous with the labrum. Similar to rotator cuff tears, an abnormal labral signal is common in throwing athletes with or without symptoms, particularly if they have had prior surgery (see **Fig. 1**). Perilabral edema can be used as an indicator for acute labral pathology and therefore can be useful for

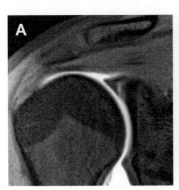

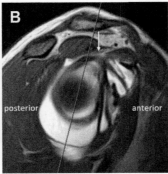

Fig. 9. (*A*) Surgically proven superior labral tear with sublabral signal on MR arthrogram coronal images extending deep and (*B*) posterior to the biceps anchor (*arrow*) when cross-referenced on sagittal images (*line*).

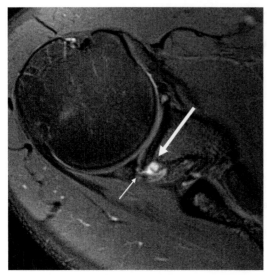

Fig. 10. A paralabral cyst indicates the presence of a labral tear. This patient has a posterior–superior labral tear with small paralabral cyst (*large arrow*) and small communicating neck (*small arrow*).

detecting acute injury in throwers with baseline labral abnormalities, when present[19] (**Fig. 12**). Surgical intervention is typically reserved for failed nonsurgical intervention.

ROTATOR CUFF

Rotator cuff tears in throwers are classically partial thickness articular surface tears centered at the junction of the supraspinatus and infraspinatus tendons, and are believed to be related to posterosuperior impingement in the extreme ABER positioning of late cocking phase[20] (**Fig. 13**). Although shoulder MR imaging typically has high sensitivity for full-thickness rotator cuff tears, sensitivity for partial thickness tears that can be seen in throwers is only moderate.[13] Similar to superior labral tears, MR arthrography has higher overall accuracy than routine noncontrast shoulder MR imaging at 1.5 T

and similar accuracy at 3 T, with higher sensitivity and lower specificity for arthrography at 3 T.[7,9] The use of ABER for partial thickness rotator cuff tears has demonstrated mixed results in the literature, but may be helpful[12,19,32,33] (**Fig. 14**).

In throwers, other reactive or adaptive signs of internal impingement may be present, which may cue the radiologist to closely scrutinize the rotator cuff articular surface. The partial thickness tears in this region have been referred to as adaptive, but it is likely more appropriate to consider the changes that occur with repetitive trauma from impingement as expected changes that may or may not be symptomatic.[27,34] Whether on conventional MR imaging or MR arthrography, the fluid or contrast signal should extend from the undersurface into the tendon substance. An important distinction for such partial thickness tears that should be relayed to clinician when identified is whether more or less than 50% of the tendon thickness is involved, because any surgical treatment typically involves debridement when less than 50% is involved and may involve completion of the tear and repair in higher grade tears.[13] Furthermore, identification of delamination or flap components can push the treatment decision toward surgery and is important for operative planning, because these tear components may be treated with different surgical techniques, such as layer-to-layer suturing for delamination.[13]

Similar to other findings encountered in the throwing athlete, rotator cuff tearing can be seen in asymptomatic throwers.[34,35] Acute rotator cuff injuries may also occur, and can be recognized with acute myotendinous edema or other acute injuries.[19] In addition to superior rotator cuff tendon tearing, throwers may also present with inferior myotendinous subscapularis injuries, as opposed to the typical superior subscapularis tendon tearing more commonly seen in the general population[36] (**Fig. 15**). Adaptive osseous changes in the thrower's shoulder that maximize external rotation such as humeral torsion may be protective for

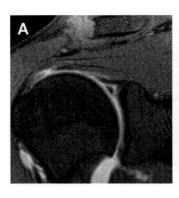

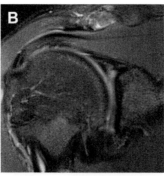

Fig. 11. Bucket handle superior labral tears can involve (*A*) the substance of the labrum (SLAP III) or (*B*) extend into the biceps anchor (SLAP IV).

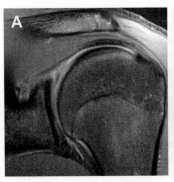
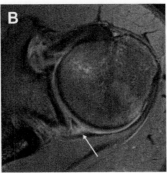

Fig. 12. (*A*) Superior labral tear with (*B*) posterior extension and perilabral edema (*arrow*).

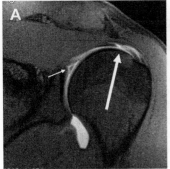
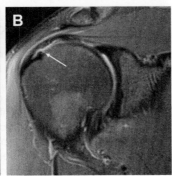

Fig. 13. (*A*) A high-grade partial thickness articular surface supraspinatus tendon tear (*large arrow*) with some delamination was not intervened on at the time of surgery performed for a bucket handle superior labral tear (*small arrow*) in this thrower. (*B*) Similarly, this partial thickness articular surface supraspinatus tear (*arrow*) in a professional baseball pitcher was treated nonoperatively.

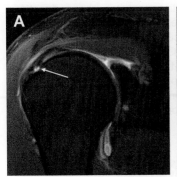
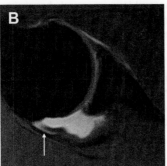

Fig. 14. (*A*) Partial thickness articular surface supraspinatus tear (*arrow*) is identified on neutral coronal images. (*B*) On ABER positioning, a delamination component is appreciated (*arrow*).

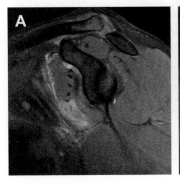
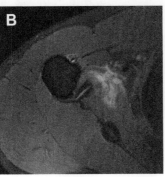

Fig. 15. (*A*) Sagittal and (*B*) axial MR images demonstrating an acute grade II myotendinous subscapularis strain in a pitcher.

subscapularis tears as less force is needed to achieve angular velocity.[36] Throwing athletes rarely return to the pre-injury playing level after rotator cuff surgery.[19] As such, surgical intervention is typically reserved as a last resort for athletes failing nonoperative management.

LONG HEAD OF THE BICEPS TENDON

Torsional and tensile forces on the biceps tendon with throwing predispose throwers to long head of biceps tendinosis and partial thickness tears.[37] Accuracy for the identification of tendinosis and partial thickness tears has historically been low with MR imaging.[38] In addition to small anatomic size, the inconsistent and oblique and curved course of the biceps tendon as it extends from the intra-articular portion originating at the biceps–labral complex anchor over the lesser tuberosity turning into the intertubercular groove makes it particularly difficult to image owing to partial volume averaging and magic angle artifacts. Inconsistencies also arise from differences in humeral rotational positioning and anatomy at the time of imaging, with throwers predisposed to increased humeral torsion in the throwing arm, which increases the difficulty in achieving consistent positioning during imaging.[39]

The appearance on MR imaging of biceps tendinopathy can include diameter change, contour irregularity, and alteration of normal low signal intensity (**Fig. 16**). Similar to other pathologies in the shoulder, 3 T imaging is useful, with studies achieving better accuracies for biceps tendon pathology on MR imaging when 2 of these findings are present at 3 T MR imaging.[40] The tendon is best assessed in cross-section perpendicular to its course, which would be on the sagittal sequences for the intra-articular portion and on the axial sequences for the intertubercular portion. Internal rotation of the humerus and extension of the elbow increases the portion of the tendon in the extra-articular portion, which may improve diagnosis in this area.[13] Frequent presence of magic-angle in the biceps tendon can be improved by evaluating the tendon on sequences with longer echo times and with ABER positioning. The course of the biceps should be closely assessed for dislocation or medial perching on the lesser tuberosity, which might be seen coincident with subscapularis tendon tearing. Despite the best efforts, some symptomatic biceps tendinopathy will remain hidden on MR imaging.

CHRONIC CHANGES IN THROWERS

Much of the chronic changes seen in throwers on MR imaging can be understood as adaptive or reactive changes related to maximizing external rotation in the late cocking phase. For radiologists, being familiar with the constellation of these typically asymptomatic findings can help to differentiate them from symptomatic throwing related injuries (see **Fig. 1**).

In the soft tissues, often times the most striking distinguishing feature of a thrower's shoulder MR imaging is the posterosuperior capsular thickening and shortening, which acts to shift the humeral head in the posterosuperior direction, allowing greater external rotation before internal impingement occurs[19] (see **Fig. 1**). By contrast, the anterior capsule is stretched and looser to accommodate this motion. The posteroinferior capsule is also typically involved in the thickening and tightening, in part related to the traction forces on the posteroinferior capsule during follow-through and deceleration.[26] As

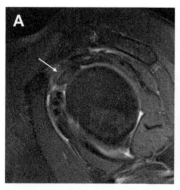 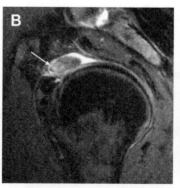 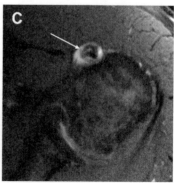

Fig. 16. (*A*) Tendinosis of the intra-articular long head of biceps tendon (*arrow*) is identified on sagittal 3 T MR imaging images with enlargement and increased signal. (*B*) A different patient with similar background tendinosis also demonstrating partial thickness tearing (*arrows*) in the (*B*) intra-articular and (*C*) intertubercular long head of biceps tendon.

mentioned, there can be associated isolated posterior labral tears in throwers. Although these changes occur to maximize external rotation, they can also be associated with a glenohumeral internal rotation deficit, a clinical examination finding rather than an imaging finding. This deficit is typically treated with stretching, but has been treated with capsulotomy and labral repair for failed conservative measures.[19]

Characteristic chronic bony changes can also be seen in throwers. When the posterior glenoid capsular insertion becomes ossified, it is termed a Bennett lesion (see **Fig. 1**). This can be readily identified radiographically and on computed tomography scans and is very common in baseball pitchers.[19] Any prior or coincident imaging may therefore be useful because it can be difficult to identify ossification from thickened capsule on fat-saturated MR imaging sequences. Other osseous changes include glenoid retroversion and humeral torsion (**Fig. 17**). Glenoid retroversion manifests in pitchers as focally convex morphology of the posterior or posterior–superior glenoid, but has not demonstrated a protective effect on injury.[22] Humeral torsion describes the axial rotational relationship between the proximal and distal humerus at the articular surfaces. In pitchers, humeral torsion is commonly asymmetric, allowing maximal external rotation at the elbow relative to the shoulder in the dominant arm, an adaptation felt to be protective against the incidence and severity of shoulder injuries in professional pitchers.[38] Reactive changes can also occur in the posterior humeral head related to internal impingement, including remodeling, subcortical cyst formation, bone marrow edema, and cortical flattening.[19]

SUMMARY

An understanding of the biomechanics of throwing can help the radiologist to identify a thrower on MR imaging and tailor the search pattern to throwing-related injuries. Many of the changes and injuries associated with a thrower's shoulder are related to achieving maximal external rotation in the late cocking phase of throwing. Torsional forces at the biceps anchor in this phase are related to the posterosuperior labral tearing pattern seen in throwers. Internal impingement also occurs in throwers and is associated with partial thickness tears of the superior rotator cuff. Interpretation of imaging findings in throwers is difficult, particularly because some abnormal findings may be asymptomatic and some symptomatic pathology may have no imaging correlate. The optimization of imaging techniques and familiarity with which findings may be pathologic and relevant to the thrower's symptoms will maximize the value of the radiologist's interpretation.

DISCLOSURE

The authors have no commercial or financial conflicts of interest to disclose.

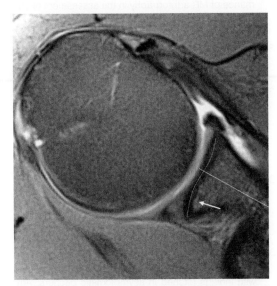

Fig. 17. Focal glenoid retroversion in throwers is typically along the posterior or posterosuperior glenoid, and is demonstrated by loss of the perpendicular relationship between the posterior glenoid surface (*dotted line*) and scapular axis (*solid line*), and the convex contour of the posterior glenoid articular surface (*arrow*).

REFERENCES

1. Andrews JR, Carson WG, Mcleod WD. Glenoid labrum tears related to the long head of the biceps. Am J Sports Med 1985;13(5):337–41.
2. Walch G, Boileau P, Noel E, et al. Impingement of the deep surface of the supraspinatus tendon on the posterosuperior glenoid rim: an arthroscopic study. J Shoulder Elbow Surg 1992;1(5):238–45.
3. Burkhart S, Morgan C. The peel-back mechanism: its role in producing and extending posterior type II SLAP lesions and its effect on SLAP repair rehabilitation. Arthroscopy 1998;14(6):637–40.
4. Symanski JS, Subhas N, Babb J, et al. Diagnosis of superior labrum anterior-to-posterior tears by using MR imaging and MR arthrography: a systematic review and meta-analysis. Radiology 2017;285(1): 101–13.
5. Gottsegen CJ, Merkle AN, Bencardino JT, et al. Advanced MRI techniques of the shoulder joint: current applications in clinical practice. Am J Roentgenol 2017;209(3):544–51.

6. Altahawi F, Subhas N. 3D MRI in musculoskeletal imaging: current and future applications. Curr Radiol Rep 2018;6(8):27.

7. de Jesus JO, Parker L, Frangos AJ, et al. Accuracy of MRI, MR arthrography, and ultrasound in the diagnosis of rotator cuff tears: a meta-analysis. Am J Roentgenol 2009;192(6):1701–7.

8. Ajuied A, McGarvey CP, Harb Z, et al. Diagnosis of glenoid labral tears using 3-tesla MRI vs. 3-tesla MRA: a systematic review and meta-analysis. Arch Orthop Trauma Surg 2018;138(5):699–709.

9. McGarvey C, Harb Z, Smith C, et al. Diagnosis of rotator cuff tears using 3-Tesla MRI versus 3-Tesla MRA: a systematic review and meta-analysis. Skeletal Radiol 2016;45(2):251–61.

10. Chhadia AM, Goldberg BA, Hutchinson MR. Abnormal translation in SLAP lesions on magnetic resonance imaging abducted externally rotated view. Arthroscopy 2010;26(1):19–25.

11. Borrero CG, Casagranda BU, Towers JD, et al. Magnetic resonance appearance of posterosuperior labral peel back during humeral abduction and external rotation. Skeletal Radiol 2010;39(1):19–26.

12. Modi CS, Karthikeyan S, Marks A, et al. Accuracy of abduction-external rotation MRA versus standard MRA in the diagnosis of intra-articular shoulder pathology. Orthopedics 2013;36(3):e337–42.

13. Polster JM, Schickendantz MS. Shoulder MRI: what do we miss? Am J Roentgenol 2010;195(3):577–84.

14. Subhas N, Conroy J, Koo J, et al. Cost-effectiveness of MR arthrography versus MRI for SLAP tears. Podium Presentation (Presented by Naveen Subhas) presented at the: Society of Skeletal Radiology 41st Annual Meeting. Austin, TX, March 25, 2018.

15. Woertler K, Waldt S. MR imaging in sports-related glenohumeral instability. Eur Radiol 2006;16(12):2622–36.

16. Dillman CJ, Fleisig GS, Andrews JR. Biomechanics of pitching with emphasis upon shoulder kinematics. J Orthop Sports Phys Ther 1993;18(2):402–8.

17. Chang I-YJ, Polster JM. Pathomechanics and magnetic resonance imaging of the thrower's shoulder. Radiol Clin North Am 2016;54(5):801–15.

18. Lintner D, Noonan TJ, Kibler WB. Injury patterns and biomechanics of the athlete's shoulder. Clin Sports Med 2008;27(4):527–51.

19. Lin DJ, Wong TT, Kazam JK. Shoulder injuries in the overhead-throwing athlete: epidemiology, mechanisms of injury, and imaging findings. Radiology 2018;286(2):370–87.

20. Burkhart SS, Morgan CD, Kibler WB. The disabled throwing shoulder: spectrum of pathology part II: evaluation and treatment of SLAP lesions in throwers. Arthroscopy 2003;19(5):531–9.

21. Jobe CM. Posterior superior glenoid impingement: expanded spectrum. Arthroscopy 1995;11(5):530–6.

22. Rassi J, Subhas N, Bullen J, et al. Characterization of glenoid bone remodeling in professional baseball pitchers. Skeletal Radiol 2019;48(7):1095–102.

23. Snyder SJ, Ferkel RD. SLAP lesions of the shoulder. Arthroscopy 1990;6(4):274–9.

24. Mohana-Borges AVR, Chung CB, Resnick D. Superior labral anteroposterior tear: classification and diagnosis on MRI and MR arthrography. Am J Roentgenol 2003;181(6):1449–62.

25. De Coninck T, Ngai SS, Tafur M, et al. Imaging the glenoid labrum and labral tears. Radiographics 2016;36(6):1628–47.

26. Burkhart SS, Morgan CD, Kibler WB. The disabled throwing shoulder: spectrum of pathology part I: pathoanatomy and biomechanics. Arthroscopy 2003;19(4):404–20.

27. Chang D, Mohana-Borges A, Borso M, et al. SLAP lesions: anatomy, clinical presentation, MR imaging diagnosis and characterization. Eur J Radiol 2008;68(1):72–87.

28. De Maeseneer M, Van Roy F, Lenchik L, et al. CT and MR arthrography of the normal and pathologic anterosuperior labrum and labral-bicipital complex. Radiographics 2000;20(suppl_1):S67–81.

29. Rajiah P, Holden D, Schils J, et al. Imaging of the sports injury: indications and findings. In: Miniaci A, editor. Disorders of the shoulder: diagnosis and management. Sports injuries, vol. 2. Philadelphia: Wolters Kluwer Health Adis (ESP); 2013. p. 31–60.

30. Waldt S, Burkart A, Lange P, et al. Diagnostic performance of MR arthrography in the assessment of superior labral anteroposterior lesions of the shoulder. Am J Roentgenol 2004;182(5):1271–8.

31. Popp D. Superior labral anterior posterior lesions of the shoulder: current diagnostic and therapeutic standards. World J Orthop 2015;6(9):660.

32. Schreinemachers SA, van der Hulst VPM, Willems WJ, et al. Detection of partial-thickness supraspinatus tendon tears: is a single direct MR arthrography series in ABER position as accurate as conventional MR arthrography? Skeletal Radiol 2009;38(10):967–75.

33. Herold T, Bachthaler M, Hamer OW, et al. Indirect MR arthrography of the shoulder: use of abduction and external rotation to detect full- and partial-thickness tears of the supraspinatus tendon. Radiology 2006;240(1):152–60.

34. Lesniak BP, Baraga MG, Jose J, et al. Glenohumeral findings on magnetic resonance imaging correlate with innings pitched in asymptomatic pitchers. Am J Sports Med 2013;41(9):2022–7.

35. Su B-Y, Yeh W-C, Lee Y-C, et al. Internal derangement of the shoulder joint in asymptomatic professional baseball players. Acad Radiol 2019. https://doi.org/10.1016/j.acra.2019.06.010. S1076633219303149.

36. Polster JM, Lynch TS, Bullen JA, et al. Throwing-related injuries of the subscapularis in professional baseball players. Skeletal Radiol 2016; 45(1):41–7.

37. Calcei JG, Boddapati V, Altchek DW, et al. Diagnosis and treatment of injuries to the biceps and superior labral complex in overhead athletes. Curr Rev Musculoskelet Med 2018;11(1):63–71.

38. Taylor SA, Newman AM, Nguyen J, et al. Magnetic resonance imaging currently fails to fully evaluate the biceps-labrum complex and bicipital tunnel. Arthroscopy 2016;32(2):238–44.

39. Polster JM, Bullen J, Obuchowski NA, et al. Relationship between humeral torsion and injury in professional baseball pitchers. Am J Sports Med 2013; 41(9):2015–21.

40. Kim JY, Rhee S-M, Rhee YG. Accuracy of MRI in diagnosing intra-articular pathology of the long head of the biceps tendon: results with a large cohort of patients. BMC Musculoskelet Disord 2019;20(1):270.

Capsular Injury and Inflammation

Jad S. Husseini, MD[a], Marc Levin, MD[b], Connie Y. Chang, MD[a],*

KEYWORDS

- Glenohumeral joint • Glenoid labrum • Glenohumeral capsule • Glenohumeral ligaments
- Adhesive capsulitis

KEY POINTS

- The capsular and ligamentous structures of the glenohumeral joint are important stabilizing structures that are best evaluated by conventional MR imaging and MR arthrography.
- Traumatic capsular injury, particularly involving the inferior glenohumeral ligament, can occur in the setting of instability or other trauma.
- Adhesive capsulitis has characteristic imaging features on MR imaging and should be considered in the appropriate clinical setting.

INTRODUCTION

The glenohumeral ligamentous and capsular structures are important for providing stability to the shoulder. As static stabilizers, these function primarily in the extremes of motion and work in concert with the glenohumeral joint articulation, the glenoid labrum, and the rotator cuff tendons.[1] Traumatic and inflammatory processes of these structures can result in decreased range of motion, pain, and instability. In this article, we discuss imaging of the capsular and ligamentous structures, normal and variant anatomy, and describe some of the traumatic injuries and inflammatory conditions that are encountered.

NORMAL ANATOMY AND IMAGING TECHNIQUE

Normal Anatomy

The glenohumeral joint is defined by multiple capsular ligaments, many of which fuse with rotator cuff muscle fascia or attach on the glenoid labrum. These ligaments are, from cranial to caudal, coracohumeral ligament (CHL), the superior glenohumeral ligament (SGHL), middle glenohumeral ligament (MGHL), and inferior glenohumeral ligament (IGHL).[1]

The CHL and SGHL are found in the rotator interval, the space between the anterior supraspinatus and cranial subscapularis created by the coracoid process as it protrudes between the two muscle bellies. The roof of the rotator interval is composed of a portion of the glenohumeral joint capsule that is not reinforced by the rotator cuff musculature. The intra-articular portion of the biceps tendon also courses through this space as it travels from its origin at the superior glenoid tubercle to its muscle belly in the anterior upper arm (**Fig. 1**).[1–4]

The CHL arises from the lateral aspect of the base of the coracoid process, outside of the glenohumeral joint. It broadens and merges with the rotator interval capsule and inserts on the lesser and greater tuberosities of the humerus. The CHL divides into two major functional bands, a larger lateral band and small medial band. The

a Division of Musculoskeletal Imaging and Intervention, Department of Radiology, Massachusetts General Hospital, 55 Fruit Street, Yawkey 6E, Boston, MA 02114, USA; b Department of Radiology, Mt. Auburn Hospital, 330 Mount Auburn Street, Cambridge, MA 02138, USA
* Corresponding author.
E-mail address: cychang@mgh.harvard.edu

Magn Reson Imaging Clin N Am 28 (2020) 257–267
https://doi.org/10.1016/j.mric.2019.12.008
1064-9689/20/© 2019 Elsevier Inc. All rights reserved.

lateral band surrounds the superior and lateral aspect of the intra-articular long head of the biceps tendon before inserting on the greater tuberosity of the humerus, at the anterior margin of the subscapularis tendon. The medial band (MCHL) blends with fibers of the SGHL to form a ligamentous complex (SGHL-MGHL) surrounding the medial and inferior aspects of the intra-articular portion of the long head of the biceps tendon before it inserts on the lesser tuberosity of the humerus and the rotator interval capsule along the superior fibers of the subscapularis tendon.[5] Together, the CHL and SGHL form the biceps pulley, a sling-like structure that stabilizes the biceps tendon, preventing anterior tendon subluxation or dislocation. When the arm is abducted and externally rotated, the pulley limits medial subluxation of the biceps tendon.[1–3]

The subcoracoid fat triangle is an anatomic structure bounded by the CHL superiorly, the coracoid anterosuperiorly, and the joint capsule posteroinferiorly (**Fig. 2**). Because of its close relationship with the CHL and joint capsule, the subcoracoid fat triangle is affected in adhesive capsulitis.[6–8]

The SGHL is a focal thickening of the glenohumeral joint capsule.[9] The origin is variable and may include the supraglenoid tubercle, superior labrum, long head of biceps tendon, MGHL, or a combination. The SGHL is anterior to the biceps tendon and maintains a close relationship along its course. It inserts on the fovea capitis of the humerus, a small depression above the lesser tuberosity, and contributes to the biceps pulley.[5]

The origin of the MGHL is also variable but is most commonly the labrum or glenoid neck. In approximately 40% of cases the MGHL and SGHL share a common origin. Distally, the MGHL fuses with the deep fascia of the subscapularis tendon over a distance of approximately 2.5 cm. MGHL has a cordlike variation (~18%) (**Fig. 3**A) and can also be hypertrophied in combination with an absent labrum, also called a Buford complex (1.2%) (**Fig. 3**B).[10,11]

The IGHL is the largest and most important component of the glenohumeral labroligamentous complex.[12] The anterior and posterior bands of the IGHL represent bandlike thickenings of the inferior joint capsule. In between these ligaments, the capsule is referred to as the "axillary pouch."[13] The anterior band is stronger and thicker and originates as high as 2 o'clock superiorly on the anterior glenoid rim and labrum and as low as 5 o'clock inferiorly and prevents anterior translation in abduction and external rotation. Because the most common shoulder injuries involve anterior subluxation and dislocation with the arm abducted

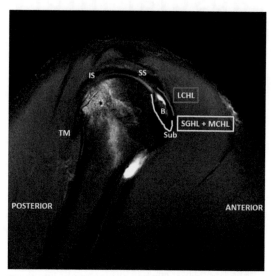

Fig. 1. Rotator interval anatomy on MR arthrogram. Bone marrow edema from the patient's recent shoulder dislocation and Hill-Sachs fracture (*asterisk*). B, biceps tendon; IS, infraspinatus; LCHL, lateral coracohumeral ligament; MCHL, medial coracohumeral ligament; SS, supraspinatus; Sub, subscapularis; TM, teres minor.

and externally rotated, injuries to the IGHL most frequently involve the anterior band. The posterior band extends from the 7-o'clock to 9-o'clock position and limits posterior translation in abduction

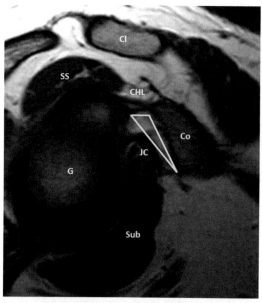

Fig. 2. The borders of the subcoracoid fat triangle (*yellow triangle*) are: Cl, clavicle; Co, coracoid; G, glenoid; JC, joint capsule; SS, supraspinatus; Sub, subscapularis.

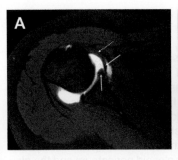
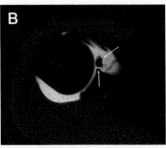

Fig. 3. MGHL normal variation. (*A*) The MGHL originates from the glenoid labrum or neck (*solid white arrow*) and inserts on the deep surface of the subscapularis (*dashed arrow*). This MGHL is thick and cord-like. The anterior labrum (*yellow arrow*) is present. (*B*) The MGHL is thickened (*white arrow*) and the anterior labrum is absent (*yellow arrow*). The combination of a thickened MGHL and an absent anterior labrum is called a Buford complex.

and internal rotation. As abduction of the shoulder increases, more support is derived from the IGHL with decreased support from the SGHL and MGHL.[14,15] The attachments of the IGHL at the glenoid and labrum strengthen with age and are therefore more likely injured in younger patients.[16] Laterally, IGHL inserts on the anatomic neck of the humerus in a collarlike or V-like configuration.[17,18] The insertion on the humerus is 1 to 3 cm wide, broader than focal SGHL/MCHL attachments (**Fig. 4**).

with arthroscopy.[19–22] Direct MR arthrography, or MR imaging following injection of intra-articular contrast, is likely more sensitive for detection of labroligamentous abnormalities.[20,23,24] As a result, direct MR imaging arthrography is often performed if there is concern for a labral pathology that may require surgical intervention. The capsule and ligaments, like the rotator interval and labrum, may be better outlined by the presence of intra-articular contrast, improving the sensitivity for detection of associated pathology.

Imaging Technique

MR imaging is the modality of choice for evaluation of the ligamentous and capsular structures of the shoulder. Studies using conventional MR imaging have produced mixed results in terms of identifying labral injury in the setting of instability, with sensitivities ranging from 44% to 93% compared

Intervention

Glenohumeral intra-articular steroid injection is diagnostic and therapeutic for adhesive capsulitis. In a 2019 study of 212 patients, MR imaging findings of adhesive capsulitis were associated with statistically significantly higher pain relief at 1 month after a glenohumeral joint injection.

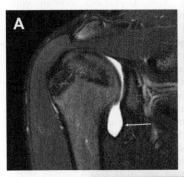
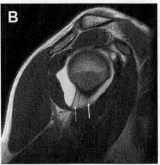
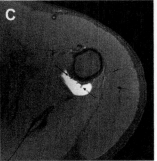

Fig. 4. A 29-year-old man with shoulder pain. (*A*) IGHL (*arrow*). The coronal T1 fat-suppressed sequence is useful for visualizing IGHL tears and inflammation. (*B*) Sagittal T1 fat-suppressed sequence is helpful for identifying the anterior (*solid arrow*) and posterior (*dashed arrow*) bands of the IGHL. (*C*) Axial T1 fat-suppressed sequence can show the anterior (*solid arrow*) and posterior (*dashed arrow*) bands of the IGHL.

Some groups have shown that glenohumeral joint hydrodilatation performed in conjunction with corticosteroid injection can decrease pain and improve range of motion, noting that there is no standardized injectate volume.[25] However, the value of hydrodilatation remains uncertain, as meta-analyses have suggested that it has only a small effect on the clinical course of adhesive capsulitis.[26,27]

IMAGING FINDINGS/PATHOLOGY
Capsular Trauma

Anterior shoulder dislocation can result a variety of injuries, including soft tissue Bankart, bony Bankart, Perthes (nondisplaced labral tear with intact periosteum), anterior labroligamentous periosteal sleeve avulsion (ALPSA), and humeral avulsion of the glenohumeral ligament (HAGL) lesions.[28] Only ALPSA and HAGL lesions are discussed in this article.

ALPSA injuries refer to a detached anterior inferior labroligamentous complex (including anterior inferior labrum and the anterior band of the IGHL). Like a Perthes lesion, the periosteum remains intact. In contrast to a Perthes lesion, the labroligamentous complex is medially displaced and inferiorly rotated (**Fig. 5**). Chronically, the complex can scar in this location, contributing to anterior instability (**Fig. 6**). ALPSA lesions are more common with repeated dislocations, and a soft tissue Bankart or Perthes lesion can progress to a ALPSA.[1,14,28–33]

On MR imaging, an ALPSA lesion can be missed when a joint effusion is not present. Medial and inferior shifting of the IGHL complex is the best clue to diagnose an ALPSA lesion. On MR arthrography, displaced labroligamentous tissue is best seen on axial and coronal T1 fat-saturated sequences.[34] Abduction and external rotation views may accentuate the undercutting of contrast between the anterior glenoid periosteum and the glenoid neck and make the ALPSA lesion more apparent (see **Fig. 5**).

The posterior labroligamentous periosteal sleeve avulsion was first described in 1998 as an avulsion of the glenohumeral capsule at its posterior attachment with associated stripping of the posterior glenoid periosteum.[35,36] This lesion is the posterior counterpart of the ALPSA lesion. As with ALPSA lesions, the posterior labroligamentous periosteal sleeve avulsion can be missed on conventional MR imaging when a joint effusion is not present. On MR arthrography, contrast undercutting the displaced posterior glenoid periosteum and the adjacent posterior glenoid neck is seen (**Fig. 7**).[37]

A humeral avulsion of the IGHL, or HAGL, can also occur in the setting of anterior dislocation (**Fig. 8**). On conventional MR imaging or MR arthrography, the anterior band of the IGHL humeral attachment is detached, producing a "J"-

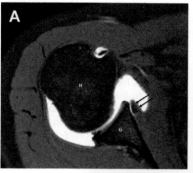
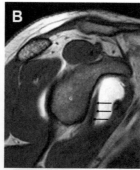
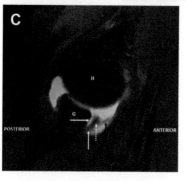

Fig. 5. A 32-year-old woman with chronic anterior shoulder instability. (*A*) Axial T1 fat-suppressed and (*B*) sagittal T1 images with intra-articular contrast demonstrate labroligamentous tissue displaced along the glenoid neck, consistent with an ALPSA (*arrows*). (*C*) T1 fat-suppressed image of the shoulder with intra-articular contrast in abduction and external rotation (ABER) demonstrates contrast (*solid white arrow*) undercutting displaced anterior labrum (*dashed white arrow*) and IGHL (*black arrow*) along the glenoid neck. The periosteum is intact (*yellow arrow*). G, glenoid; H, humerus.

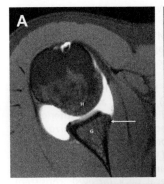
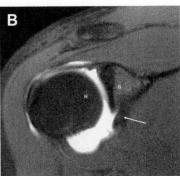
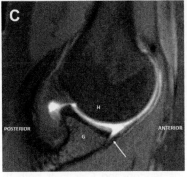

Fig. 6. A 21-year-old woman with approximately 20 dislocations in the past 6 years. (A) Axial, (B) coronal, and (C) ABER T1 fat-suppressed images with intra-articular contrast demonstrate medialization of the anterior inferior labroligamentous complex, which is scarred down on the anterior inferior glenoid neck (arrow). This finding is compatible with a chronic ALPSA. G, glenoid; H, humerus.

shaped IGHL on coronal images.[38] Glenohumeral joint fluid on conventional MR imaging or injected intra-articular contrast on MR arthrography may extend into the adjacent soft tissues through the capsular defect. In up to 20% of cases of HAGL, there is an avulsed bony fragment at the humeral attachment (Fig. 9).[39] If a fracture fragment is seen near the surgical neck of the humerus on

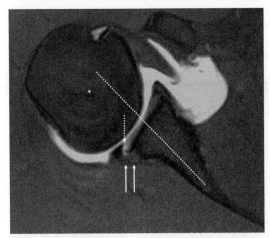

Fig. 7. A 17-year-old man with posterior shoulder pain after a fall while playing football 1 year ago. Axial T1 fat-suppressed image with intra-articular contrast demonstrates contrast undercutting the posterior labrum (white dashed arrow) with associated chronic periostitis and periosteal stripping (solid white arrows), consistent with a posterior labroligamentous periosteal sleeve avulsion. There is also posterior decentering of the humeral head with respect to the glenoid (dashed line should intersect with the asterisk, which is at the center of the humeral head).

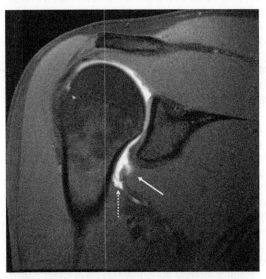

Fig. 8. A 54-year-old man with sudden onset of pain when reaching behind him in the car. Coronal T1 fat-suppressed image with intra-articular contrast demonstrates "J-shaped" inferior glenohumeral ligament (solid arrow) with extravasation of contrast along the humeral neck (dashed arrow), compatible with a HAGL.

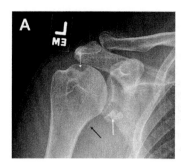
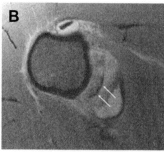

Fig. 9. A 46-year-old man with recent anterior inferior dislocation after fall while skiing. (*A*) Frontal radiograph demonstrates a thin curvilinear ossific fragment along the medial humeral neck, compatible with a bony avulsion of the IGHL (BHAGL) (*black arrow*). There is also a displaced anterior inferior glenoid fracture (*solid while arrow*) and a depressed Hill-Sachs fracture (*dashed white arrow*). (*B*) Axial T1 fat-suppressed image with intra-articular contrast demonstrates the curvilinear bony fragment at the humeral neck (*arrows*), consistent with a BHAGL.

radiographs, it should raise the suspicion for an IGHL injury, particularly in the setting of instability.

Tear of the anterior bands of the IGHL from the glenoid rim can also occur. This is referred to as a glenoid avulsion of the glenohumeral ligament. On MR imaging or MR arthrography, the anterior bands appear detached from the glenoid attachment and also produce a "J"-shaped IGHL on coronal images. The "J"-shape is in the opposite configuration as seen with a HAGL. Similarly, glenohumeral joint fluid on conventional MR imaging or injected intra-articular contrast on MR arthrography may extend into the adjacent soft tissues.[40]

Injuries to the posterior band of the IGHL can also occur. As with anterior band injuries, the tear may occur at the glenoid attachment (reverse glenoid avulsion of the glenohumeral ligament) or at the humeral attachment (reverse HAGL). The imaging findings are similar to anterior band IGHL injuries, with disruption of the ligament and extension of glenohumeral joint fluid or intra-articular injected contrast into the adjacent soft tissues.[41]

A potential pitfall in MR arthrography is iatrogenic contrast extravasation. Discontinuity of the anterior band is always a tear, and isolated involvement of the posterior band is 100% specific for iatrogenic extravasation.[42] True tears have thick, scarred ends, which may demonstrate a "reverse taper," where the end of the torn ligament is thicker than the ligament midsubstance. Contrast extravasation margins are thin and may have a "mop head" configuration (**Fig. 10**).[42]

Rotator interval abnormalities have been called "hidden" lesions and are one of the reasons for a failed arthroscopic glenohumeral repair for instability or biceps tendon instability and persistent pain after a rotator cuff repair.[43–48] Forty-seven percent of subscapularis tendon tears extend into the SGHL and mCHL.[49,50] Anterosuperior

tears of the rotator cuff (supraspinatus tendon) propagating through the rotator interval can result in lateral CHL injury (**Fig. 11**).[5] Even though the supraspinatus tendon is not a constituent of the biceps pulley, it is closely related to the rotator interval capsule and provides superolateral tension on the MCHL. Rupture of the lateral CHL and loss of normal tension of the MCHL allows subluxation of the biceps tendon, superficial to the subscapularis tendon and CHL.[51] If both the medial and lateral CHL are injured, the biceps tendon can freely dislocate into the joint or anteriorly.[51] In approximately 6% of cases, the CHL may be congenitally aplastic or hypoplastic, predisposing to traumatic injury.[52] Rotator interval defects can also occur in isolation in overhead throwing athletes or other professions and athletes with repetitive overhead motion.[49,53–55] Rotator interval defects are congenital or postsurgical.[56,57] These

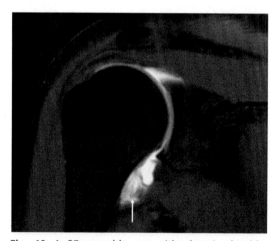

Fig. 10. A 35-year-old man with chronic shoulder pain. Coronal T1 fat-suppressed image with intra-articular contrast demonstrates the posterior band of the inferior glenohumeral ligament with thin wispy ends ("mop-like" configuration) (*arrow*), suggesting contrast extravasation rather than a tear.

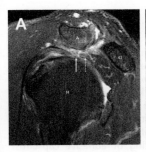
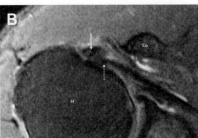

Fig. 11. A 61-year-old man with acute on chronic shoulder pain. (*A*) Sagittal T2 fat-suppressed image demonstrates a full-thickness anterior supraspinatus tear (*solid arrow*). The coracohumeral ligament is also torn (*dashed arrow*). (*B*) Axial T2 fat-suppressed image demonstrates subluxation of the biceps tendon (*solid arrow*) over the subscapularis tendon (*dashed arrow*). A, acromion; Cl, clavicle; Co, coracoid; H, humerus.

patients may be at risk for additional injury because of humeral head instability.[45]

Capsular Inflammation

Adhesive capsulitis is a condition characterized by inflammation of the glenohumeral joint capsule and synovium. Typical clinical features are progressive onset of pain and decreased range of motion with active and passive movement of the shoulder.[58] These inflammatory changes may be primary, occurring in the absence of preceding trauma or other insult, or secondary, occurring as a result of prior injury, surgery, or repetitive trauma.[59] Adhesive capsulitis has been linked with multiple comorbidities, including inflammatory arthropathy, Parkinson disease, diabetes mellitus, and other endocrine disorders.[60–63] Primary adhesive capsulitis is generally a self-limited process that lasts 18 to 24 months.[64] However, symptoms may persist and result in chronic disability.[65–67] Management is typically conservative and involves physical therapy and corticosteroid injection.[58,59]

Clinical and surgical literature describe four stages of adhesive capsulitis, originally outlined by Neviaser and since modified to incorporate associated arthroscopic findings.[64,68–70] Stage 1, the prefreezing stage, occurs within the first 3 months and is characterized by limited range

of motion and pain. Arthroscopy shows an erythematous synovium. Stage 2, the freezing stage, occurs within 3 to 9 months after symptom onset and is associated with severe restriction of range of motion. This is the most common time of presentation. On arthroscopy, the patients show a thickened, red synovial with contraction at the rotator interval and the axillary recess. Stage 3, the frozen stage, presents primarily with stiffness but minimal pain and is typically 9 to 15 months after symptom presentation. Arthroscopic findings are a pink synovium with contraction of the rotator interval and axillary recess. In stage 4, the thawing stage, range of motion improves and there is minimal pain. Arthroscopy shows contraction of the glenohumeral joint space but not synovitis.

Adhesive capsulitis is typically a clinical diagnosis made by a combination of history and physical examination. However, overlap between adhesive capsulitis and other causes of limited passive and active range of motion, such as rotator cuff pathology and osteoarthritis, means that additional imaging is often acquired.[55]

The primary role of plain radiographs in the assessment of adhesive capsulitis is to evaluate for other causes of shoulder pain. Radiographs showing substantial osteoarthritis of the glenohumeral joint, calcific rotator cuff tendinopathy or

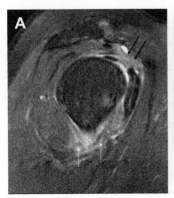
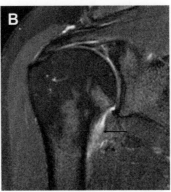

Fig. 12. A 51-year-old woman with severe shoulder pain for 5 months. (*A*) Sagittal T2 fat-suppressed imaging demonstrates thickened (6 mm) and edematous coracohumeral ligament (*arrows*). (*B*) Coronal T2 fat-suppressed image demonstrates thickened (8 mm) and edematous inferior glenohumeral ligament (*arrow*). These findings are seen in the setting of adhesive capsulitis.

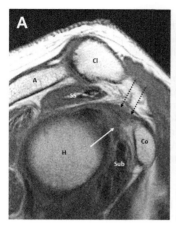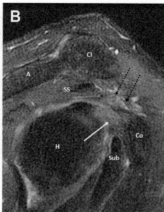

Fig. 13. A 65-year-old man with 6 months of shoulder pain. (*A*) Sagittal T1 and (*B*) sagittal T2 fat-suppressed images demonstrate partial obliteration of the subcoracoid fat triangle (*solid arrow*). The coracohumeral ligament is thick (3.5 mm) (*dashed arrows*). Other than a low-grade, chronic-appearing rotator cuff tear, the study was normal. These findings are seen in the setting of adhesive capsulitis. A, acromion; Cl, clavicle; Co, coracoid; H, humerus; SS, supraspinatus; Sub, subscapularis.

bursitis, and/or secondary findings of a chronic full-thickness rotator cuff tear may suggest an alternate diagnosis to adhesive capsulitis.

MR imaging findings of adhesive capsulitis are seen at the rotator interval/CHL, the axillary pouch, and the subcoracoid fat triangle. At the rotator interval, MR imaging shows soft tissue thickening of the CHL (**Fig. 12**A). This finding is best appreciated on sagittal oblique T2 fat-saturated images. Authors have proposed different values for abnormal thickening, with 3 mm of thickness of the CHL as seen on MR arthrography shown to be most accurate.[7,25,71]

At the axillary pouch, MR imaging shows thickening of the inferior joint capsule of greater than 4 mm and decreased volume of the axillary recess (**Fig. 12**B).[71,72] Capsular thickening is best measured on coronal oblique T2-weighted sequences with or without fat saturation. Measuring the area of the IGHL may decrease measurement variability and increase sensitivity for the detection of adhesive capsulitis.[73] The axillary pouch can show associated inflammatory changes, including intrasubstance and surrounding abnormal T2 hyperintense intrasubstance signal and signal of the surrounding soft tissues. If intravenous contrast is administered, the axillary pouch and surrounding soft tissues can show avid enhancement.

Capsular inflammation in adhesive capsulitis can obliterate the normal fat signal in the subcoracoid fat triangle, a finding that is best seen on sagittal oblique images (**Fig. 13**).[7,71,73] This finding is specific (100%) but not sensitive (32%) for adhesive capsulitis.[71]

Imaging findings may vary with the clinical stage of adhesive capsulitis. Edema of the IGHL and biceps tendon sheath effusion are present in almost all patients in stage 1, with decreasing prevalence as the patient progresses through stages 2 to 4. Conversely, obliteration of the subcoracoid triangle fat is more common in stages 3 and 4 than in stages 1 and 2. Anterior and posterior pericapsular edema is most common in stage 2 and is rarely present in stage 4.[25,74] The presence of three of the four findings of adhesive capsulitis-thickening of the CHL, thickening of the joint capsule at the rotator interval, obliteration of the subcoracoid fat triangle, and reduced volume of the axillary recess with edema of the joint capsule, in the absence of labral pathology is associated with a high level of pain decrease with intra-articular corticosteroid injection (**Box 1, Table 1**).[25,74]

PEARLS, PITFALLS, VARIANTS
Trauma

- Anterior shoulder dislocation can result in a variety of different lesions of the anteroinferior labroligamentous complex. In the setting of chronic dislocations, a soft tissue Bankart or Perthes can progress to an ALPSA.
- A chronic ALPSA scars along the medial glenoid neck.

Box 1
Diagnostic criteria

Adhesive capsulitis

  Thickening of CHL (>3 mm)

  Thickening of IGHL (>4 mm)

  Decreased volume of axillary recess

  Obliteration of fat signal in the subcoracoid fat triangle

Data from Refs.[7,25,68–70]

Table 1
Differential diagnosis

Diagnosis	Differential Diagnosis
ALPSA	Soft tissue Bankart Bony Bankart Perthes
Posterior labroligamentous periosteal sleeve avulsion	Reverse soft tissue Bankart Reverse bony Bankart
HAGL	Iatrogenic contrast extravasation (for MR arthrography) BAGL Glenoid avulsion of the glenohumeral ligament
Adhesive capsulitis	Normal variation

Abbreviation: BHAGL, bony humeral avulsion of the glenohumeral ligament.
Data from Refs.[28–39]

- HAGL typically involves the IGHL anterior band and can occur with or without a bony avulsion.
- If there is an isolated abnormality of the IGHL posterior band on MR arthrography, consider contrast extravasation.
- Anterior supraspinatus tears are associated with CHL tears and biceps subluxation.

Adhesive Capsulitis

- Most specific imaging finding is obliteration of the fat signal in the subcoracoid fat triangle.
- Clinical context is important.

What the Referring Physician Needs to Know

- In acute traumatic lesions of the labroligamentous complex, MR arthrography is likely more sensitive than conventional MR imaging.
- Adhesive capsulitis is a clinical diagnosis. Imaging findings are supportive and not diagnostic. In addition, MR imaging findings vary based on the stage of adhesive capsulitis.

SUMMARY

The capsular and ligamentous structures of the glenohumeral joint play an important role in the stability of the shoulder. These structures are best evaluated by MR arthrography. The IGHL is the largest and most important capsular structure and is commonly injured in the setting of instability or other trauma. Capsular injury may be associated with concomitant injuries to the glenoid labrum. Adhesive capsulitis, a common inflammatory condition of the glenohumeral joint capsule, may be difficult to distinguish from other causes of pain and instability by clinical examination. If no other cause for symptoms is identified, MR imaging findings are supportive but not diagnostic for this condition.

DISCLOSURE

The authors have no disclosures.

REFERENCES

1. Chung CB, Steinbach LS. MRI of the upper extremity: shoulder, elbow, wrist and hand. Philadelphia: Lippincott Williams & Wilkins; 2009.
2. Nakata W, Katou S, Fujita A, et al. Biceps pulley: normal anatomy and associated lesions at MR arthrography. Radiographics 2011;31(3):791–810.
3. Frank RM, Taylor D, Verma NN, et al. The rotator interval of the shoulder: implications in the treatment of shoulder instability. Orthop J Sports Med 2015; 3(12). 2325967115621494.
4. Gaskill TR, Braun S, Millett PJ. Multimedia article. The rotator interval: pathology and management. Arthroscopy 2011;27(4):556–67.
5. Petchprapa CN, Beltran LS, Jazrawi LM, et al. The rotator interval: a review of anatomy, function, and normal and abnormal MRI appearance. AJR Am J Roentgenol 2010;195(3):567–76.
6. Park S, Lee D-H, Yoon S-H, et al. Evaluation of adhesive capsulitis of the shoulder with fat-suppressed T2-weighted MRI: association between clinical features and MRI findings. AJR Am J Roentgenol 2016;207(1):135–41.
7. Lee S-Y, Park J, Song S-W. Correlation of MR arthrographic findings and range of shoulder motions in patients with frozen shoulder. AJR Am J Roentgenol 2012;198(1):173–9.
8. Zhao W, Zheng X, Liu Y, et al. An MRI study of symptomatic adhesive capsulitis. PLoS One 2012;7(10): e47277.
9. Massengill AD, Seeger LL, Yao L, et al. Labrocapsular ligamentous complex of the shoulder: normal anatomy, anatomic variation, and pitfalls of MR imaging and MR arthrography. Radiographics 1994; 14(6):1211–23.
10. Chahla J, Aman ZS, Godin JA, et al. Systematic review of the anatomic descriptions of the glenohumeral ligaments: a call for further quantitative studies. Arthroscopy 2019;35(6):1917–26.e2.
11. Williams MM, Snyder SJ, Buford D. The Buford complex: the "cord-like" middle glenohumeral ligament and absent anterosuperior labrum complex: a normal anatomic capsulolabral variant. Arthroscopy 1994;10(3):241–7.

12. Bencardino JT, Gyftopoulos S, Palmer WE. Imaging in anterior glenohumeral instability. Radiology 2013; 269(2):323–37.

13. Turkel SJ, Panio MW, Marshall JL, et al. Stabilizing mechanisms preventing anterior dislocation of the glenohumeral joint. J Bone Joint Surg Am 1981; 63(8):1208–17.

14. Ozbaydar M, Elhassan B, Diller D, et al. Results of arthroscopic capsulolabral repair: Bankart lesion versus anterior labroligamentous periosteal sleeve avulsion lesion. Arthroscopy 2008;24(11):1277–83.

15. Bigliani LU, Pollock RG, Soslowsky LJ, et al. Tensile properties of the inferior glenohumeral ligament. J Orthop Res 1992;10(2):187–97.

16. Rowe CR. Prognosis in dislocations of the shoulder. J Bone Joint Surg Am 1956;38-A(5):957–77.

17. O'Brien SJ, Neves MC, Arnoczky SP, et al. The anatomy and histology of the inferior glenohumeral ligament complex of the shoulder. Am J Sports Med 1990;18(5):449–56.

18. Ticker JB, Bigliani LU, Soslowsky LJ, et al. Inferior glenohumeral ligament: geometric and strain-rate dependent properties. J Shoulder Elbow Surg 1996;5(4):269–79.

19. Magee TH, Williams D. Sensitivity and specificity in detection of labral tears with 3.0-T MRI of the shoulder. AJR Am J Roentgenol 2006;187(6):1448–52.

20. Chandnani VP, Yeager TD, DeBerardino T, et al. Glenoid labral tears: prospective evaluation with MRI imaging, MR arthrography, and CT arthrography. AJR Am J Roentgenol 1993;161(6):1229–35.

21. Zlatkin MB, Hoffman C, Shellock FG. Assessment of the rotator cuff and glenoid labrum using an extremity MR system: MR results compared to surgical findings from a multi-center study. J Magn Reson Imaging 2004;19(5):623–31.

22. Gusmer PB, Potter HG, Schatz JA, et al. Labral injuries: accuracy of detection with unenhanced MR imaging of the shoulder. Radiology 1996;200(2): 519–24.

23. Palmer WE, Caslowitz PL. Anterior shoulder instability: diagnostic criteria determined from prospective analysis of 121 MR arthrograms. Radiology 1995;197(3):819–25.

24. Jee WH, McCauley TR, Katz LD, et al. Superior labral anterior posterior (SLAP) lesions of the glenoid labrum: reliability and accuracy of MR arthrography for diagnosis. Radiology 2001;218(1): 127–32.

25. Fritz B, Del Grande F, Sutter R, et al. Value of MR arthrography findings for pain relief after glenohumeral corticosteroid injections in the short term. Eur Radiol 2019. https://doi.org/10.1007/s00330-019-06237-1.

26. Buchbinder R, Green S, Youd JM, et al. Arthrographic distension for adhesive capsulitis (frozen shoulder). Cochrane Database Syst Rev 2008;(1): CD007005.

27. Saltychev M, Laimi K, Virolainen P, et al. Effectiveness of hydrodilatation in adhesive capsulitis of shoulder: a systematic review and meta-analysis. Scand J Surg 2018;107(4):285–93.

28. Saba L, De Filippo M. MR arthrography evaluation in patients with traumatic anterior shoulder instability. J Orthop 2017;14(1):73–6.

29. Neviaser TJ. The anterior labroligamentous periosteal sleeve avulsion lesion: a cause of anterior instability of the shoulder. Arthroscopy 1993;9(1):17–21.

30. Beltran J, Bencardino J, Mellado J, et al. MR arthrography of the shoulder: variants and pitfalls. Radiographics 1997;17(6):1403–12 [discussion: 1412–5].

31. Connell DA, Potter HG. Magnetic resonance evaluation of the labral capsular ligamentous complex: a pictorial review. Australas Radiol 1999;43(4):419–26.

32. McCauley TR. MR imaging of the glenoid labrum. Magn Reson Imaging Clin N Am 2004;12(1): 97–109, vi–vii.

33. Tischer T, Vogt S, Kreuz PC, et al. Arthroscopic anatomy, variants, and pathologic findings in shoulder instability. Arthroscopy 2011;27(10):1434–43.

34. Chloros GD, Haar PJ, Loughran TP, et al. Imaging of glenoid labrum lesions. Clin Sports Med 2013;32(3): 361–90.

35. Yu JS, Ashman CJ, Jones G. The POLPSA lesion: MR imaging findings with arthroscopic correlation in patients with posterior instability. Skeletal Radiol 2002;31(7):396–9.

36. Shah N, Tung GA. Imaging signs of posterior glenohumeral instability. AJR Am J Roentgenol 2009; 192(3):730–5.

37. De Coninck T, Ngai SS, Tafur M, et al. Imaging the glenoid labrum and labral tears. Radiographics 2016;36(6):1628–47.

38. Bui-Mansfield LT, Taylor DC, Uhorchak JM, et al. Humeral avulsions of the glenohumeral ligament: imaging features and a review of the literature. AJR Am J Roentgenol 2002;179(3):649–55.

39. Oberlander MA, Morgan BE, Visotsky JL. The BHAGL lesion: a new variant of anterior shoulder instability. Arthroscopy 1996;12(5):627–33.

40. Mannem R, DuBois M, Koeberl M, et al. Glenoid avulsion of the glenohumeral ligament (GAGL): a case report and review of the anatomy. Skeletal Radiol 2016;45(10):1443–8.

41. Chung CB, Sorenson S, Dwek JR, et al. Humeral avulsion of the posterior band of the inferior glenohumeral ligament: MR arthrography and clinical correlation in 17 patients. AJR Am J Roentgenol 2004; 183(2):355–9.

42. Wang W, Huang BK, Sharp M, et al. MR arthrogram features that can be used to distinguish between true inferior glenohumeral ligament complex tears and iatrogenic extravasation. AJR Am J Roentgenol 2019;212(2):411–7.

43. Morag Y, Jacobson JA, Shields G, et al. MR arthrography of rotator interval, long head of the biceps brachii, and biceps pulley of the shoulder. Radiology 2005;235(1):21–30.

44. Walch G, Nove-Josserand L, Levigne C, et al. Tears of the supraspinatus tendon associated with "hidden" lesions of the rotator interval. J Shoulder Elbow Surg 1994;3(6):353–60.

45. Field LD, Warren RF, O'Brien SJ, et al. Isolated closure of rotator interval defects for shoulder instability. Am J Sports Med 1995;23(5):557–63.

46. Sethi N, Wright R, Yamaguchi K. Disorders of the long head of the biceps tendon. J Shoulder Elbow Surg 1999;8(6):644–54.

47. Walch G, Nové-Josserand L, Boileau P, et al. Subluxations and dislocations of the tendon of the long head of the biceps. J Shoulder Elbow Surg 1998; 7(2):100–8.

48. Berlemann U, Bayley I. Tenodesis of the long head of biceps brachii in the painful shoulder: improving results in the long term. J Shoulder Elbow Surg 1995;4(6):429–35.

49. Bennett WF. Subscapularis, medial, and lateral head coracohumeral ligament insertion anatomy. Arthroscopic appearance and incidence of "hidden" rotator interval lesions. Arthroscopy 2001;17(2):173–80.

50. Le Huec JC, Schaeverbeke T, Moinard M, et al. Traumatic tear of the rotator interval. J Shoulder Elbow Surg 1996;5(1):41–6.

51. Bennett WF. Arthroscopic repair of anterosuperior (supraspinatus/subscapularis) rotator cuff tears: a prospective cohort with 2- to 4-year follow-up. Classification of biceps subluxation/instability. Arthroscopy 2003;19(1):21–33.

52. Neer CS, Satterlee CC, Dalsey RM, et al. The anatomy and potential effects of contracture of the coracohumeral ligament. Clin Orthop Relat Res 1992;(280):182–5.

53. O'Donoghue DH. Subluxing biceps tendon in the athlete. Clin Orthop Relat Res 1982;(164):26–9.

54. Zarins B, McMahon MS, Rowe CR. Diagnosis and treatment of traumatic anterior instability of the shoulder. Clin Orthop Relat Res 1993;(291):75–84.

55. Ho CP. MR imaging of rotator interval, long biceps, and associated injuries in the overhead-throwing athlete. Magn Reson Imaging Clin N Am 1999;7(1):23–37.

56. Karas SG. Arthroscopic rotator interval repair and anterior portal closure: an alternative technique. Arthroscopy 2002;18(4):436–9.

57. Cole BJ, Rodeo SA, O'Brien SJ, et al. The anatomy and histology of the rotator interval capsule of the shoulder. Clin Orthop Relat Res 2001;(390):129–37.

58. Andrews JR. Diagnosis and treatment of chronic painful shoulder: review of nonsurgical interventions. Arthroscopy 2005;21(3):333–47.

59. Hannafin JA, Chiaia TA. Adhesive capsulitis. A treatment approach. Clin Orthop Relat Res 2000;(372): 95–109.

60. Zreik NH, Malik RA, Charalambous CP. Adhesive capsulitis of the shoulder and diabetes: a meta-analysis of prevalence. Muscles Ligaments Tendons J 2016;6(1):26–34.

61. Riley D, Lang AE, Blair RD, et al. Frozen shoulder and other shoulder disturbances in Parkinson's disease. J Neurol Neurosurg Psychiatry 1989;52(1): 63–6.

62. Choy EH, Corkill MM, Gibson T, et al. Isolated ACTH deficiency presenting with bilateral frozen shoulder. Br J Rheumatol 1991;30(3):226–7.

63. Milgrom C, Novack V, Weil Y, et al. Risk factors for idiopathic frozen shoulder. Isr Med Assoc J 2008; 10(5):361–4.

64. Sofka CM, Ciavarra GA, Hannafin JA, et al. Magnetic resonance imaging of adhesive capsulitis: correlation with clinical staging. HSS J 2008;4(2):164–9.

65. Manske RC, Prohaska D. Diagnosis and management of adhesive capsulitis. Curr Rev Musculoskelet Med 2008;1(3–4):180–9.

66. Binder AI, Bulgen DY, Hazleman BL, et al. Frozen shoulder: a long-term prospective study. Ann Rheum Dis 1984;43(3):361–4.

67. Hand C, Clipsham K, Rees JL, et al. Long-term outcome of frozen shoulder. J Shoulder Elbow Surg 2008;17(2):231–6.

68. Neviaser JS. Adhesive capsulitis of the shoulder: a study of the pathological findings of periarthritis in the shoulder. J Bone Joint Surg 1945;(27):211–22.

69. Neviaser RJ. Painful conditions affecting the shoulder. Clin Orthop Relat Res 1983;(173):63–9.

70. Neviaser RJ, Neviaser TJ. The frozen shoulder. Diagnosis and management. Clin Orthop Relat Res 1987;223:59–64.

71. Mengiardi B, Pfirrmann CWA, Gerber C, et al. Frozen shoulder: MR arthrographic findings. Radiology 2004;233(2):486–92.

72. Emig EW, Schweitzer ME, Karasick D, et al. Adhesive capsulitis of the shoulder: MR diagnosis. AJR Am J Roentgenol 1995;164(6):1457–9.

73. Bang Y-S, Park J, Lee SY, et al. Value of anterior band of the inferior glenohumeral ligament area as a morphological parameter of adhesive capsulitis. Pain Res Manag 2019;2019:9301970.

74. Chellathurai A, Subbiah K, Elangovan A, et al. Adhesive capsulitis: MRI correlation with clinical stages and proposal of MRI staging. Indian J Radiol Imaging 2019;29(1):19–24.

Acromioclavicular Joint
What to Look for

Terence Patrick Farrell, MB BCh, BAO, MRCPI, FFRRCSI, FRCRUK[a],*, Adam Zoga, MD, MBA[b]

KEYWORDS

- Acromioclavicular joint • Shoulder girdle • Rockwood classification • MR imaging

KEY POINTS

- Shoulder girdle pathologies frequently coexist.
- Acromioclavicular joint (ACJ) pathologies are a common cause of shoulder girdle pain with significant overlap in clinical presentations.
- The role of MR imaging in evaluating ACJ pathologies is expanding, with dedicated sequences and imaging planes now available.
- MR imaging can accurately classify ACJ injuries, delineating injury patterns and acting as an important diagnostic tool in the treatment decision algorithm for ACJ injuries, especially in instances of clinical and radiographic uncertainty.
- ACJ pathology can be detected earlier on MR imaging, compared with radiographs, allowing for earlier intervention.

INTRODUCTION

The acromioclavicular joint (ACJ) is an important source of shoulder girdle pathology, which often is neglected in search of glenohumeral lesions and rotator cuff disease. Evaluation traditionally begins with clinical assessment and dedicated ACJ radiographs, including weight-bearing views in the setting of trauma. MR imaging is the most frequently used secondary imaging modality and typically performed as part of standard shoulder MR imaging protocols.

ACJ injuries dominate acute presentations. Previously, imaging of the ACJ has been dictated by surgical management, which has focused on achieving satisfactory reduction and alignment posttrauma. Developments in evidence-based treatment strategies for ACJ injuries with an emphasis on restoration of ligamentous ACJ stabilizers[1,2] as well as limitations in radiographic assessment of the ACJ have expanded the role for MR imaging in the evaluation of ACJ pathology. There is a growing recognition for the need for dedicated ACJ imaging planes and sequences. A knowledge of ACJ anatomy, biomechanics, and pathology is fundamental to accurately interpreting and providing a clinically relevant ACJ MR imaging report.

NORMAL ANATOMY AND IMAGING TECHNIQUES

The ACJ is a plane-type diarthrodial synovial joint between the medially and anteriorly orientated flat medial facet of the acromion and laterally and posteriorly orientated convex distal end of the clavicle.[3] The clavicle forms from 3 ossification centers and is the first bone to ossify. The acromial ossification centers appear in early adolescence and the 2 coracoid ossification centers begin to

[a] Department of Radiology, Thomas Jefferson University Hospitals, 132 South 10th Street, 10 Main, Philadelphia, PA 19107, USA; [b] Department of Radiology, Thomas Jefferson University Hospitals, Sidney Kimmel Medical Center, 132 South 10th Street, Suite 1096, Philadelphia, PA 19107, USA
* Corresponding author.
E-mail address: terence.farrell@jefferson.edu

Magn Reson Imaging Clin N Am 28 (2020) 269–283
https://doi.org/10.1016/j.mric.2019.12.009
1064-9689/20/© 2019 Elsevier Inc. All rights reserved.

ossify at 12 months to 18 months, with fusion occurring by 18 years to 20 years for both.[4,5]

The joint has an intra-articular synovium. The articular surfaces are covered in hyaline cartilage initially, which is later replaced by fibrocartilage in early adulthood. A fibrocartilaginous intra-articular disk usually is present and typically is meniscoid in morphology,[3,6] varies in thickness, and undergoes significant degeneration between the second and fourth decades.[6]

Blood supply is derived from branches of the suprascapular and thoracoacromial arteries, originating from the subclavian and axillary arteries, respectively. Innervation is provided by branches of multiple nerves, including suprascapular, lateral pectoral, and axillary nerves. ACJ pain can refer to the neck, shoulder, deltoids, and trapezius.

Acromioclavicular Joint Stabilizers

ACJ stabilization is achieved through static reinforcement by ligaments and dynamic reinforcement by muscles. The acromioclavicular (AC) and coracoclavicular (CC) ligaments are the primary stabilizers of the ACJ (**Fig. 1**). The ACJ is surrounded by a thin capsule, which is reinforced by 4 AC ligaments: anterior, posterior, superior, and inferior. The CC ligament complex consists of the conoid ligament, inserting into the conoid tubercle at the lateral posterior clavicle, and the trapezoid ligament, which inserts into the trapezoid ridge of the inferior lateral third of the clavicle.[7] The conoid ligament has an inverted cone shape with a broader thicker clavicular insertion.[8] The trapezoid

ligament also has a thick clavicular insertion. Horizontal stability is predominantly mediated by the AC ligaments,[9] with vertical stability provided by the CC ligaments.[9] The ACJ also is reinforced by fibers of the coracoacromial (CA) ligament, which blend with the capsule inferiorly.[10] The CA ligament is a triangular ligament with a broad coracoid base that inserts into the tip of the acromion anterior to the ACJ and predominantly functions to brace the acromion and coracoid process and protect the humerus from superior subluxation.

Muscular attachments further assist in dynamic joint stability. The anterior deltoid originates from the lateral clavicle and ACJ capsule, and the trapezius insertion spans the posterosuperior joint from medial acromion to posterosuperior clavicle blending with the superior ACJ ligament.

Functions and Biomechanics

The ACJ is an important component of the shoulder girdle and transmits motion and force between the appendicular and axial skeleton. Under normal conditions, gliding movements in the anteroposterior (AP) plane dominate motion at the ACJ.[11] During shoulder abduction, the clavicle rotates up to 9°.[12] These movements occur in tandem with movements at the glenohumeral and sternoclavicular joints.

The AC interval normally is 1 mm to 3 mm. A distance of greater than 6 mm or a difference of greater than 2 mm to 3 mm between the 2 sides is considered pathologic.[13] The normal CC interval is 11 mm to 13 mm. A difference of greater than 5 mm between the 2 sides is considered pathologic.[14]

MR Imaging Protocols

The ACJ is imaged most commonly as part of standard shoulder MR imaging protocols in the assessment of shoulder girdle pathology. This provides satisfactory morphologic evaluation for a majority of ACJ pathologies; however, dedicated sequences are required for the morphologic assessment of ACJ stabilizers. Imaging in the coronal oblique plane, parallel to the distal clavicle and perpendicular to the coracoid with non–fat-suppressed proton density (PD)-weighted fast spin-echo (FSE) imaging, provides the optimal technique to evaluate ACJ stabilizers owing to its in-plane orientation to the AC and CC ligaments.[14] This allows for the evaluation of both intact and disrupted ligaments. Utilization of fat suppression can make visualization of injury to the ligaments challenging in the subacute and chronic phase.

The MR pulse sequences utilized vary from institute to institute. The sequences acquired at the

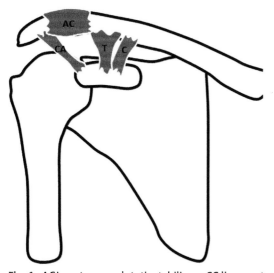

Fig. 1. ACJ anatomy and static stabilizers. CC ligament composed of trapezoid ligament (T) and conoid ligament (C), AC capsule and ligament (AC), and CA ligament.

Table 1
MR imaging shoulder protocol

Sequence	Field of View (cm)	Matrix/ Number of Excitations	Slice (mm)	Repetition Time (ms)	Echo Time (ms)	TI (Inversion time) ms	Echo Train Length	Bandwidth
Axial PD FSE, fat-suppressed	12–14	512 × 256 2	4/0.5	2000–3000	20–40	—	8	16
Cor oblique, short tau inverted recovery	16–18	256 × 192 2	4/0.5	>1500	20–40	—	8	16
Cor oblique, T1 spin-echo	16–18	256 × 256 1	4/.05	400–800	Minimum	3T: 180 1.5T: 150	—	16
Sag oblique, T2 FSE	14–16	256 × 192 1	4/1	>2000	90–110	—	8	16
aCor oblique, PD FSE	14–16	256 × 512 2	4/0.5	3000–3600	30–36	—	8	16

a Additional Cor oblique proton density, fast spin-echo sequence, for acromioclavicular joint stabilizer integrity.

authors' institute for a standard shoulder MR imaging are summarized in **Table 1**. An additional PD sequence in the described coronal oblique plane is performed when evaluation of ACJ stabilizer integrity is requested.

Differentiating complete and partial tears in the acute and subacute setting can be challenging on resting MR imaging. Similarly, resting MR imaging cannot assess functional capacity of a scarred CC ligament in chronic ACJ injuries. Combining resting and stress MR imaging has successfully demonstrated both ACJ stabilizer morphology and functionality. Although not widely available, this technique is promising for the evaluation of challenging acute and chronic ACJ injuries in terms of guiding appropriate therapy.[15]

IMAGING FINDINGS/PATHOLOGY
Trauma

ACJ injuries encompass a range of pathologies from sprains to physeal injuries and fractures. ACJ sprain or separation accounts for approximately 10% of all shoulder girdle injuries.[16] They occur most frequently in male athletes participating in contact and overhead sports.[17] The most common mechanism of injury is direct force to the acromion with the shoulder adducted. Indirect trauma from falling onto an outstretched hand is another, less common, cause. ACJ injuries are described most commonly on ACJ radiographs

using the Rockwood classification, which includes 6 grades of injury[18,19] (**Table 2**), and describes a sequential pattern of acute ACJ injury beginning with AC ligament disruption, followed by disruption of the CC ligament and subsequent deltotrapezial fascial disruption.

Clinical and radiographic evaluation, including weight-bearing views, typically are used to initially assess for instability and grade of injury. Accurate classification of injury is important for treatment planning. The Rockwood classification relies on radiographic measurements, including the AC interval and CC interval, to determine the likely extent of injury to the ACJ stabilizers. Limitations exist to this system, including difficulty differentiating between type II and type III injuries[20] as well as identifying type IV injuries with posterior subluxation on standard AP views. Nontraumatic ACJ widening can occur with normal aging, inflammatory arthropathies, infection, and other causes of distal clavicular osteolysis (DCO) and can further limit evaluation on radiographs.

MR imaging allows for direct assessment of the ACJ stabilizers as well as evaluation of joint congruency and displacement. Low-grade sprains as well as partial-thickness and full-thickness tears of the AC, CC, and CA ligaments can be visualized directly on PD FSE imaging. Thickening and hypointensity as well as calcification of the ligaments can be seen in chronic ACJ injuries.[14] Detachment of the deltoid and trapezius lateral clavicular

Table 2
Rockwood classification for acromioclavicular joint injuries

Grade	Acromiocla-vicular Ligament	Coracocla-vicular Ligament	Deltotra-pezial Fascia	Clavicular Displacement	Acromiocla-vicular Distance	Coracocla-vicular Distance
1	Intact/ partial tear	Intact	Intact	None	Normal	Normal
2	Ruptured	Incomplete tear	Intact to partial tear	50% superior	Widened	Slight increase
3	Ruptured	Ruptured	Partial tear	100% superior	Widened	Increase 25%–100%
4	Ruptured	Ruptured	Partial tear to detached	Posterior	Normal to widened	Normal to increased
5	Ruptured	Ruptured	Detached	>100% superior	Widened	Increased >100%
6	Ruptured	Intact to complete tear	Partial tear to detached	Inferior	Widened	Reduced

attachments, present in high-grade injuries, also can be seen with MR imaging.

MR imaging appearances of acromioclavicular joint injury by grade

Imaging has been dictated by surgical management of the ACJ, which has focused on achieving satisfactory reduction and alignment post-trauma.[14,21,22] Biomechanical tests have demonstrated superior outcomes with restoration of ligamentous ACJ stabilizers,[1,2] and MR imaging is becoming increasingly important in the preoperative evaluation and treatment planning.

Grade 1 injury Grade 1 injury typically demonstrates tearing of the superior AC ligament with surrounding soft tissue edema and hemorrhage as well as possible bone marrow edema (**Fig. 2**).

Grade 2 injury Grade 2 injury is associated with complete tears of the ACJ capsule and AC ligaments. The ACJ is widened and there may be a normal or mildly increased CC interval. MR imaging allows for assessment of extent of CC ligament disruption from low-grade sprain seen as ligament edema to partial tearing with hemorrhage and attenuation of the ligament. There is surrounding soft tissue edema and hemorrhage as well as possible bone marrow edema (**Fig. 3**).

Grade 3 injury There is complete disruption of the ACJ capsule and AC and CC ligaments, with edema and hemorrhage at the disrupted ligament interspaces. The ACJ is widened and CC interval is increased. The ACJ is incongruent with elevation

of the lateral clavicle (**Fig. 4**). A modification of this grading has been suggested with the introduction of grades IIIA and IIIB injuries signifying stable injuries likely to respond to nonsurgical management and unstable injuries likely requiring surgical intervention, respectively.[23]

Grade 4 injury In addition to the ligamentous findings seen in G3 injuries, there is posterior

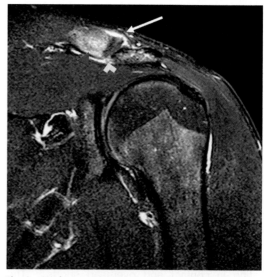

Fig. 2. Grade 1 ACJ injury. Coronal oblique STIR image of the left shoulder. Edematous and thickened superior AC ligament and AC capsule (*arrow*) with surrounding soft tissue edema (*yellow arrowhead*) and associated bone marrow edema (*red arrowhead*). Intact alignment.

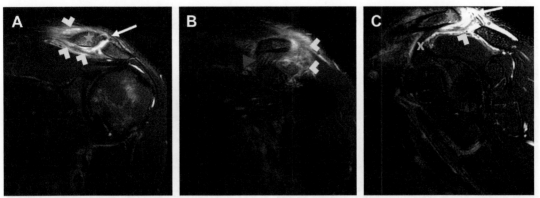

Fig. 3. Grade 2 ACJ injury. (*A*) Complete disruption of the AC capsule and ligament (*arrow*) with soft tissue (*yellow arrowheads*) and bone marrow edema (*star*). (*B, C*) Intact CC ligament (trapezoid ligament [*red arrowhead*] and conoid ligament [*X*]). Intact alignment. (*A*) Coronal oblique STIR (short tau inversion recovery), (*B*) Coronal oblique STIR and (*C*) Sagittal oblique T2 fat saturated images of the left shoulder.

displacement of the clavicle, with MR imaging demonstrating detachment of the deltoid and trapezius muscles insertions from the lateral clavicle (**Fig. 5**).

Grade 5 injury Grade 5 injury demonstrates the same ligamentous disruption as G3 injuries. As with grade 4 injuries, the deltoid and trapezius muscles are detached from the lateral clavicle; however, the clavicle is not displaced posteriorly; instead, the unopposed actions of sternocleidomastoid results in significant superior displacement of the lateral clavicle and marked increase in the CC interval (**Fig. 6**).

Grade 6 injury Grade 6 injury results from a downward force on the clavicle with inferior dislocation. MR imaging demonstrates disruption of the ACJ

capsule and AC ligaments with a typically intact CC ligament. The deltoid and trapezius clavicular attachments may be disrupted.

Indications for MR imaging in acromioclavicular joint injury

The Rockwood classification, determined by ACJ radiographs, has classically been utilized to guide management of ACJ injuries. Rockwood type I and type II usually are treated conservatively[24] whereas types IV to VI injuries are considered inherently unstable and typically managed with operative intervention using a variety of techniques. The management of grade III injuries remains controversial, with a growing trend toward nonoperative management.[25] This radiographic approach to ACJ injury grading is cost effective and accurate in identifying the grade of ACJ injury

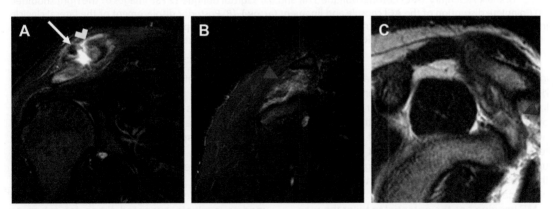

Fig. 4. Grade 3 ACJ injury. (*A*) Coronal oblique STIR, (*B*) Coronal oblique STIR and (*C*) Sagittal oblique T2 FSE images of the right shoulder. (*A*) Complete disruption of the ACJ capsule and ligament (*arrow*) and (*B, C*) complete disruption of the CC ligaments (*red arrowheads*) with edema at the ligament interspaces. The ACJ is widened and incongruent with elevation of the lateral clavicle (*yellow arrowhead*).

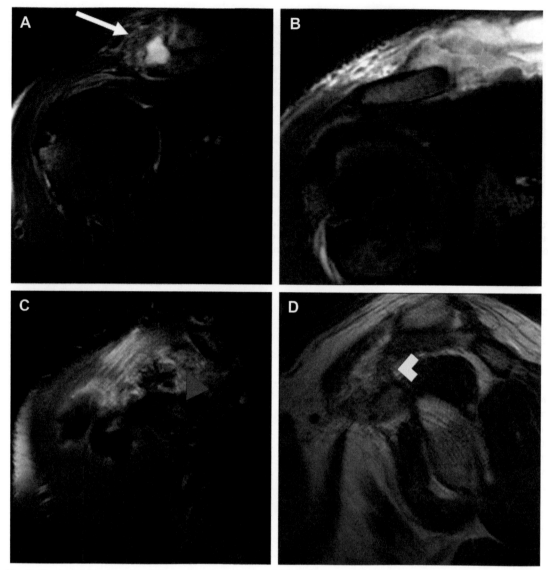

Fig. 5. Grade 4 ACJ injury. (*A-C*) Coronal oblique STIR and (*D*) Sagittal oblique T2 FSE images of the right shoulder. (*A*) Complete disruption of the ACJ capsule and ligament (*arrow*). (*B*) Posterior displacement of the lateral clavicle into the trapezius with associated intramuscular edema (*star*). (*C, D*) Disruption of the CC ligaments (trapezoid ligament [*red arrowhead*] and conoid ligament [*yellow arrowhead*]) with edema at the disrupted ligament interspaces.

in most cases.[26] MR imaging has the added benefit, however, of direct evaluation of ACJ stabilizers and can result in a significant reclassification of ACJ injuries when compared with radiographic evaluation. In 1 study, 47.8% of injuries were reclassified (36.4% downgraded and 11.4% upgraded) and 25% of cases had ligament injuries that were not predicted based on the Rockwood classification.[26]

MR imaging has the potential to tailor the management of ACJ injuries on a patient-by-patient basis, depending on the exact soft tissue injury and impact on joint stability, and may be of particular benefit in cases of clinical uncertainty, in particular in the differentiation of type II and type III injuries as well as in the evaluation of clinically and radiographically low-grade injuries that are not responding to conservative therapy. In high-grade injuries, MR imaging also can assist in operative planning and surgical technique.

In the overhead athlete, MR imaging can be used to evaluate expected times for return to play. MR imaging also is valuable in differentiating between normal variation and low-grade ACJ injuries and can exclude ACJ injury in

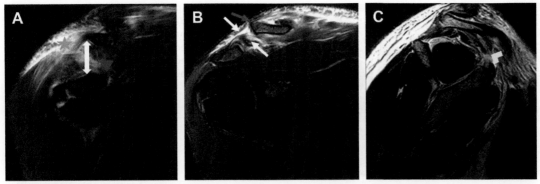

Fig. 6. Grade 5 ACJ injury. (*A, B*) Coronal oblique STIR and (*C*) Sagittal oblique T2 FSE images of the right shoulder. (*A, C*) Complete disruption of the AC ligament/capsule (*white arrows*) and CC ligament (trapezoid ligament [*red arrowhead*] and conoid ligament [*yellow arrowhead*]) with significant superior displacement of the lateral clavicle (*red arrow*) and marked increase in the CC interval (*double-headed arrow*). Tearing and edema of the deltoid ([*A*] *star*) and edema of the trapezius ([*B*] *X*).

settings of clinical uncertainty.[26] Concomitant injuries are common in cases of traumatic ACJ injury, in particular, SLAP tears (superior labral tear from anterior to posterior); MR imaging has the potential added benefit of excluding concomitant shoulder girdle pathology that cannot be evaluated with radiography.[27,28] The ACJ also can be injured as part of distal clavicular or acromion fractures (Neer classification).[29] These may occur concurrently with higher-grade ACJ injuries or occasionally occur independent to an ACJ injury.

Postoperative imaging findings

The overall goal of treating ACJ injuries is the return to activity with a pain free shoulder. Accurate diagnosis and classification are critical in determining the optimal treatment. There are a wide variety of surgical techniques available for the treatment of grades IV to VI ± grade III ACJ injuries with a lack of significant comparative data available on long-term outcomes and without a clear consensus on the optimum surgical approach to utilize.[23] These can be divided into anatomic and nonanatomic ACJ reconstruction with more anatomic reconstructions becoming increasingly

popular in recent years due to improved clinical and radiological outcomes.[30]

Anatomic reconstructions aim to stabilize the joint with tendon grafts (allograft or autograft) for the AC and/or CC ligaments (**Figs. 7** and **8**). Nonanatomic reconstructions aim to provide biomechanical stability, allowing the native ligaments to heal, and include ACJ fixation with metal hardware (K-wires or hook plate), CA ligament transfer (Weaver-Dunn procedure), and CC interval fixation with both rigid (Bosworth screw technique) and nonrigid implants (suspension devices with suture, flip buttons, and washers). Both open and arthroscopic approaches are available with an increasing tendency toward less invasive techniques.[31,32]

Complications are common with both nonanatomic and anatomic reconstructions,[33] with similar complication rates for open and arthroscopic procedures.[32] Depending on the type of repair, complications include loss of reduction, hardware and graft failure, coracoid and clavicle fracture, and pain.[33]

MR imaging has an evolving role in the postoperative assessment of ACJ reconstruction and can be used to assess ACJ reconstruction integrity,[30]

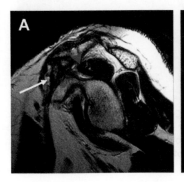
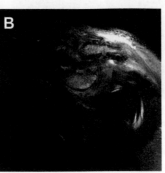

Fig. 7. (*A*) Sagittal oblique T2 FSE and (*B*) Coronal oblique STIR images of the left shoulder. Weaver-Dunn reconstruction. (*A*) CA ligament transfer to the lateral clavicle (*arrow*) and (*B*) reinforcement with sutures (*arrowheads*).

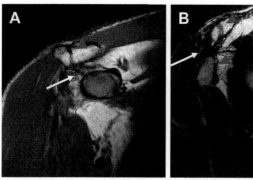
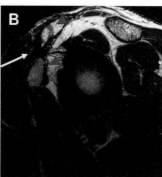

Fig. 8. (*A*) Coronal oblique T1 SE and (*B*) Sagittal oblique T2 FSE images of the right shoulder. Anatomic ACJ reconstruction. Autologous tendon reconstruction ([*A*] *arrows*) and suture reinforcement ([*A, B*] *arrowheads*).

postprocedural complications,[34] and CC ligament healing[35,36] after conservative and surgical intervention.

Distal Clavicular Osteolysis

DCO is a well-known cause of shoulder pain and can be traumatic and atraumatic in etiology. Clinical presentation can include pain, point tenderness, soft tissue swelling, and reduced function. DCO frequently also can mimic other shoulder pathologies, including rotator cuff tears. The diagnosis is dependent on clinical and radiological findings. Other causes of distal clavicular destruction must be excluded, including inflammatory disorders, for example, rheumatoid arthritis, hyperparathyroidism, scleroderma, infection, and lytic metastasis.

Atraumatic cases are associated strongly with chronic repetitive stress related to weightlifting[37] and overhead sports.[38] Traumatic cases are associated with an antecedent injury and may present weeks to months posttrauma.[39] Traumatic and atraumatic cases have similar imaging characteristics, including distal clavicular bone marrow

edema out of proportion to edema at the acromion, subchondral fractures, subchondral cystic changes, and distal clavicular periostitis in advanced cases[40,41] with sparing of the acromion articular surface (**Fig. 9**). Osteolysis with ACJ widening is a late finding.

MR imaging directly evaluates bone marrow edema and is more sensitive for the detection of early DCO. An MR imaging grading system has been proposed for DCO based on the extent of clavicular bone marrow and periostitis.[38] MR imaging grading is associated with interval development of ACJ osteoarthritis (OA) and ACJ widening.[38]

Osteoarthritis

OA is the most common disorder of the ACJ and may be primary or secondary to several entities, including posttraumatic, inflammatory, and postinfection. Joint incongruency, an incomplete or degenerated intra-articular disk, and/or high load forces transmitted across the joint all predispose to early OA, which typically presents in the fifth and sixth decades.[42,43] Although it can be a cause of debilitating

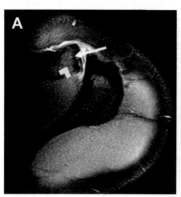
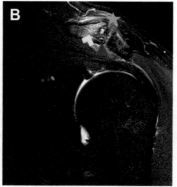
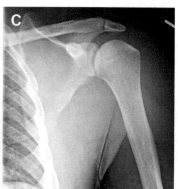

Fig. 9. DCO. (*A*) Axial oblique proton density (PD) FSE fat suppressed and (*B*) Coronal oblique STIR images of the left shoulder as well as (*C*) Left shoulder AP radiograph. (*A, B*) Distal clavicular subchondral fracture (*arrow*) with distal clavicular edema (*open arrowheads*) and sparing of the acromion, surrounding soft tissue edema (*star*) as well as early distal clavicular erosions/osteolysis (*red arrowhead*). (*C*) Findings of DCO, as described previously, not clearly visualized on concurrent AP radiograph of the shoulder.

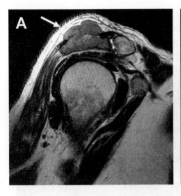
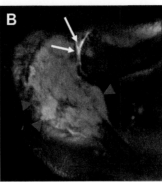

Fig. 10. (*A*) Sagittal oblique T2 FSE and (*B*) axial PD fat-saturated FSE of the left shoulder demonstrating a T2 hyperintense expansile and destructive lesion of the distal acromion extending into the ACJ (*arrows*) and surrounding soft tissues (*arrowheads*), consistent with a metastasis from lung carcinoma.

shoulder girdle pain, ACJ OA most often is asymptomatic.[44] When symptomatic, it often presents with poorly localized shoulder girdle and neck pain, making clinical and radiological diagnosis challenging.[45] MR imaging has been advocated in the evaluation of symptomatic ACJ OA.[46,47] The presence of bone marrow edema, of ACJ distention, and of impression on the supraspinatus muscle[46] as well as of superior joint capsule distention[47] all have been correlated with symptomatic ACJ OA. Superior joint capsule distention has been shown to predict pain relief after intra-articular steroid injection and can help in selecting patients likely to benefit from this treatment.[48] These findings also can be seen in asymptomatic patients[49] and should be interpreted in combination with the clinical history and focused physical examination.

Infection

Septic arthritis of the ACJ is uncommon; however, it must be considered in the setting of ACJ pain and clinical findings of infection. Affected patients typically are immunosuppressed or have a discontinuity of defense barriers.[50] Direct inoculation in the setting of intra-articular injections and prior surgery are additional risk factors.[51] It commonly occurs in the setting of a septic polyarthritis and typically is hematogenous in origin. As with other joints, staphylococcus aureus is the most common causative organism.[50] It can be rapidly destructive; early diagnosis is critical. MR imaging is sensitive for the detection of joint effusion and edema in the surrounding soft tissues as well as identifying bony changes of osteomyelitis (bone marrow edema and T1 fatty marrow signal replacement) before destructive changes develop on radiographs.[52]

Inflammatory/crystal Arthropathies

The ACJ commonly is involved in inflammatory arthropathies, in particular rheumatoid arthritis, with two-thirds of patients developing ACJ involvement with this arthropathy.[53] MR imaging is sensitive for

the early detection of joint involvement and demonstrates the typical features of inflammatory arthropathies, including synovitis, joint effusion, bone marrow and soft tissue edema, and joint erosions. Erosive changes can present as DCO. MR imaging can help identify inflammatory causes of DCO with bilateral joint involvement as well as pan-articular involvement, commonly seen in rheumatoid arthritis and other inflammatory arthropathies.

Crystal arthropathies, including calcium pyrophosphate deposition and gout, rarely involve the ACJ; however, they remain part of the differential in the evaluation of acute ACJ monoarthritis. The small number of reported cases of calcium pyrophosphate deposition demonstrates typical imaging findings on MR imaging, including chondrocalcinosis, joint effusion, and soft tissue edema.[54]

Neoplasia

Bone tumors involving the ACJ are exceedingly rare, which may be related to the poor vascularity and minimal red marrow.[55] Clavicular tumors most commonly involve the lateral third of the bone. Lesions of the clavicle and acromion can be subarticular in location or extend to involve the ACJ. Lesion type and frequency depend on patient age. In young patients, eosinophilic granuloma is the most common lesion of the clavicle, followed by aneurysmal bone cyst, Ewing sarcoma, and osteosarcoma.[56] In older patients, metastases (**Fig. 10**) are the most common lesion, followed by myeloma, osteosarcoma, and chondrosarcoma.[56] A similar distribution/frequency of lesions is noted in the acromion.[57] As with tumors of other bones, MR imaging is useful in the characterization of lesions involving the ACJ and in biopsy and treatment planning.[58]

PEARLS, PITFALLS, AND VARIANTS
Os acromiale

The acromion is formed from 4 ossification centers, with fusion occurring at varying ages from

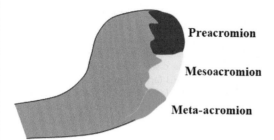

Fig. 11. Acromion ossification centers.

early adolescence to 20 years of age[59,60] (**Fig. 11**). An os acromiale results from the failure of fusion of 1 or more ossification centers and is bilateral in 60% of cases.[61] The junction of the mesoacromion and meta-acromion is involved most frequently (**Fig. 12**). An os acromiale frequently can be missed on AP and scapular Y views of the shoulder; an axial view is useful to make this diagnosis.

Os acromiale is increasingly recognized as a cause of shoulder pain in athletes.[62] Hypermobility of the unfused acromiale fragment, an unstable os

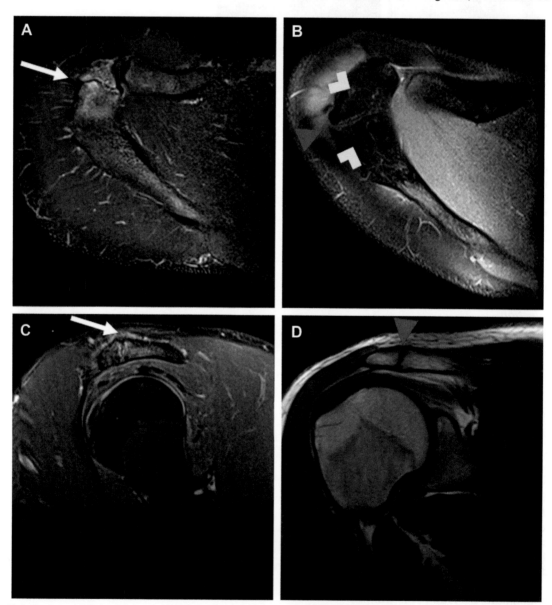

Fig. 12. Os acromiale. (A) Axial oblique PD FSE fat suppressed and (C) Sagittal oblique T2 fat saturated images of the right shoulder from patient 1. (B) Axial oblique PD FSE fat suppressed and (D) Coronal oblique T1 SE images of the right shoulder from patient 2. (A, C) Preacromion os acromiale with edema and early degenerative changes across the synchondrosis consistent with instability (*arrows*). (B, D) Mesoacromion os acromiale, stable with absence of edema (*yellow arrowheads*) or degenerative changes at the synchondrosis (*red arrowheads*).

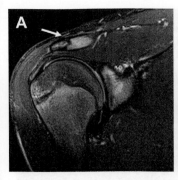 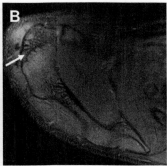

Fig. 13. Ossification center. (*A*) Coronal oblique STIR and (*B*) Axial oblique PD FSE fat saturated images of the right shoulder. (*A, B*) Skeletally immature patient with an acromiale ossification center, which demonstrates a lobulated margin with absence of edema (*white arrows*).

acromiale, is associated with pain secondary to degenerative changes at the synchondrosis[63] and through dynamic rotator cuff impingement.[63,64] MR imaging is useful in the differentiation of os acromiale from a developing unfused ossification center in adolescents.[65] Os acromiale demonstrates a transverse orientation with irregular margins and frequently demonstrates interface marrow edema and fluid signal (see **Fig. 12**). Unfused ossification centers typically demonstrate arched, lobulated interfaces, with an absence of interface marrow edema and fluid signal[65] (**Fig. 13**).

Coracoclavicular Joint

The CC joint is an uncommon anomalous synovial joint between the coracoid process of the scapula and the conoid tubercle of the clavicle (**Fig. 14**). Reported prevalence is 0.7% to 10%.[66,67] A majority of cases are identified incidentally and likely to be asymptomatic. The presence of a CC joint, however, has been implicated in shoulder pain, shoulder impingement, and thoracic outlet syndrome.[68] Static and dynamic MR imaging can help in the identification of a symptomatic CC joint, demonstrating strain with marrow edema across

the joint and in the surrounding soft tissues and early arthritis of the joint as well as evidence of neurovascular impingement on dynamic imaging.

Acromioclavicular Joint Cysts

ACJ cysts or ganglia occur most commonly in the setting of advanced rotator cuff disease (type 2 cyst). Cysts also can be seen with advanced ACJ OA (type 1 cyst) or a combination of these pathologies[69] (**Fig. 15**). In ACJ OA, synovial inflammation results in excess synovial fluid production. In type 2 cysts, cephalad migration of the humeral head results in irritation and tearing of the ACJ capsule, allowing glenohumeral fluid to extend into the ACJ, where it can become encysted. These cysts often extend through the superior ACJ capsule and into the subcutaneous tissues,[69] presenting as a clinically palpable lump. This finding has been described on arthrography and MR imaging as the geyser sign[70] and should prompt further evaluation with MR imaging of the shoulder and ACJ with particular attention to rotator cuff pathology. These lesions also can be seen as an iatrogenic finding post–subacromial decompression with injury to the ACJ capsule.[71] Diagnosis can be made on standard noncontrast shoulder MR

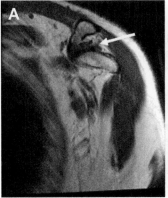 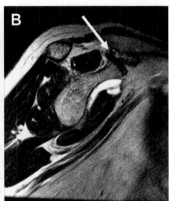

Fig. 14. (*A*) Coronal oblique T1 SE and (*B*) Sagittal oblique T2 FSE images. (*A, B*) Two cases of a CC joint: an accessory articulation between the coracoid process and clavicle with osteophytosis at the joint (*white arrows*).

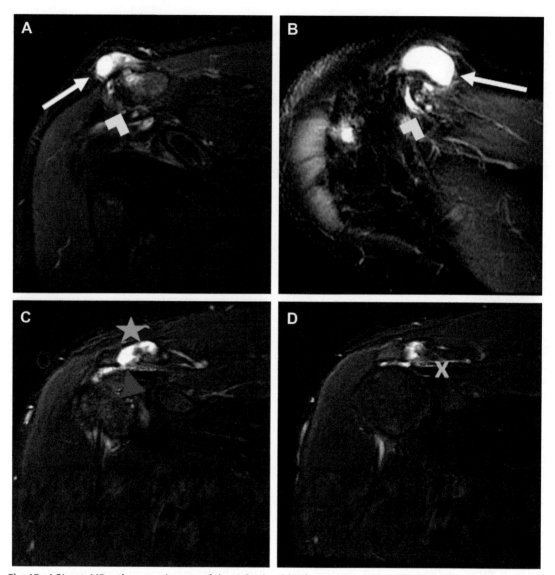

Fig. 15. ACJ cyst. MR arthrogram images of the right shoulder from patient 1 including (*A*) coronal oblique T1 fat suppressed and (*B*) axial oblique T1 fat suppressed images. (*C, D*) Coronal oblique T1 fat suppressed MR arthrogram images of the right shoulder from patient 2. (*A, B*) Patient 1: cyst superficial to and communicating with the ACJ (*arrows*) with moderate OA (*yellow arrowheads*). (*C, D*) Patient 2: full-thickness tear of supraspinatus with tendon retraction (*X*) and fluid extending from the subacromial/subdeltoid bursa into the ACJ (*star*) through a defect in the inferior ACJ capsule (*red arrowhead*) (geyser sign).

imaging, typically demonstrating a fluid signal lesion centered on the ACJ, which may extend superiorly into the subcutaneous soft tissues.

WHAT THE REFERRING PHYSICIAN NEEDS TO KNOW

1. Shoulder girdle pathologies frequently coexist.
2. ACJ pathologies are a common cause of shoulder girdle pain with significant overlap in clinical presentations.
3. The role of MR imaging in evaluating ACJ pathologies is expanding, with dedicated sequences and imaging planes now available.
4. MR imaging can accurately classify ACJ injuries and is an important secondary diagnostic tool in particular in cases of clinical and radiographic uncertainty.
5. ACJ pathology can be detected earlier on MR imaging compared with radiographs, allowing for earlier intervention.

SUMMARY

ACJ pathology is a common source of shoulder girdle pain, which frequently coexists with and shares overlapping clinical features of rotator cuff, labral, and glenohumeral joint disease. MR imaging of the ACJ is a powerful tool that can be used for the early diagnosis of ACJ pathology and in the accurate assessment of ACJ injuries, helping to resolve clinically challenging cases and allowing for individualized treatment planning.

DISLCOSURE

The authors have nothing to disclose.

REFERENCES

1. Abat F, Sarasquete J, Natera LG, et al. Biomechanical analysis of acromioclavicular joint dislocation repair using coracoclavicular suspension devices in two different configurations. J Orthop Traumatol 2015;16(3):215–9.
2. Mazzocca AD, Santangelo SA, Johnson ST, et al. A biomechanical evaluation of an anatomical coracoclavicular ligament reconstruction. Am J Sports Med 2006;34(2):236–46.
3. Renfree KJ, Wright TW. Anatomy and biomechanics of the acromioclavicular and sternoclavicular joints. Clin Sports Med 2003;22(2):219–37.
4. Roedl JB, Morrison WB, Ciccotti MG, et al. Acromial apophysiolysis: superior shoulder pain and acromial nonfusion in the young throwing athlete. Radiology 2015;274(1):201–9.
5. Todd TW, D'Errico J. The clavicular epiphyses. Am J Anat 1928;41(1):25–50.
6. Heers G, Götz J, Schubert T, et al. MR imaging of the intraarticular disk of the acromioclavicular joint: a comparison with anatomical, histological and in-vivo findings. Skeletal Radiol 2007;36(1):23–8.
7. Klassen JF, Morrey BF, An KN. Surgical anatomy and function of the acromioclavicular and coracoclavicular ligaments. Oper Techn Sport Med 1997;5(2):60–4.
8. Harris RI, Vu DH, Sonnabend DH, et al. Anatomic variance of the coracoclavicular ligaments. J Shoulder Elbow Surg 2001;10(6):585–8.
9. Dawson PA, Adamson GJ, Pink MM, et al. Relative contribution of acromioclavicular joint capsule and coracoclavicular ligaments to acromioclavicular stability. J Shoulder Elbow Surg 2009;18(2):237–44.
10. Zlatkin MB. MRI of the shoulder. 2nd edition. Philadelphia: Lippincott Williams and Wilkins; 2003. p. 306.
11. Wong M, Kiel J. Anatomy, shoulder and upper limb, acromioclavicular joint. In: StatPearls. Treasure Island, FL: StatPearls Publishing; 2019. Available at: http://www.ncbi.nlm.nih.gov/books/NBK499858/. Accessed August 21, 2019.
12. Eckenrode BJ, Kelley MJ. Clinical biomechanics of the shoulder complex. In: Andrews JR, Wilk KE, Reinold M, editors. The athlete's shoulder. 2nd edition. Philadelphia: Elsevier; 2009. p. 17–41. https://doi.org/10.1016/B978-044306701-3.50005-0.
13. Petersson CJ, Redlund-Johnell I. Radiographic joint space in normal acromioclavicular joints. Acta Orthop Scand 1983;54(3):431–3.
14. Alyas F, Curtis M, Speed C, et al. MR imaging appearances of acromioclavicular joint dislocation. Radiographics 2008;28(2):463–79.
15. Izadpanah K, Winterer J, Vicari M, et al. A stress MRI of the shoulder for evaluation of ligamentous stabilizers in acute and chronic acromioclavicular joint instabilities. J Magn Reson Imaging 2013;37(6):1486–92.
16. Melenevsky Y, Yablon CM, Ramappa A, et al. Clavicle and acromioclavicular joint injuries: a review of imaging, treatment, and complications. Skeletal Radiol 2011;40(7):831–42.
17. Pallis M, Cameron KL, Svoboda SJ, et al. Epidemiology of acromioclavicular joint injury in young athletes. Am J Sports Med 2012;40(9):2072–7.
18. Rockwood CA. Subluxation of the shoulder: the classification, diagnosis and treatment. Orthop Trans 1979;(4):306.
19. Rockwood CJ, Williams G, Young D. Disorders of the acromioclavicular joint. In: Rockwood CJ, Matsen III FA, editors. The shoulder. 2nd edition. Philadelphia: Saunders; 1998. p. 483–553.
20. Bossart PJ, Joyce SM, Manaster BJ, et al. Lack of efficacy of "weighted" radiographs in diagnosing acute acromioclavicular separation. Ann Emerg Med 1988;17(1):20–4.
21. Schaefer FK, Schaefer PJ, Brossmann J, et al. Experimental and clinical evaluation of acromioclavicular joint structures with new scan orientations in MRI. Eur Radiol 2006;16(7):1488–93.
22. Antonio GE, Cho JH, Chung CB, et al. Pictorial essay. MR imaging appearance and classification of acromioclavicular joint injury. AJR Am J Roentgenol 2003;180(4):1103–10.
23. Beitzel K, Mazzocca AD, Bak K, et al. ISAKOS upper extremity committee consensus statement on the need for diversification of the Rockwood classification for acromioclavicular joint injuries. Arthroscopy 2014;30(2):271–8.
24. Tamaoki MJS, Belloti JC, Lenza M, et al. Surgical versus conservative interventions for treating acromioclavicular dislocation of the shoulder in adults. Cochrane Database Syst Rev 2010;(8):CD007429.
25. Tang G, Zhang Y, Liu Y, et al. Comparison of surgical and conservative treatment of Rockwood type-III acromioclavicular dislocation: a meta-analysis. Medicine (Baltimore) 2018;97(4):e9690.

26. Nemec U, Oberleitner G, Nemec SF, et al. MRI versus radiography of acromioclavicular joint dislocation. AJR Am J Roentgenol 2011;197(4):968–73.

27. Tischer T, Salzmann GM, El-Azab H, et al. Incidence of associated injuries with acute acromioclavicular joint dislocations types III through V. Am J Sports Med 2009;37(1):136–9.

28. Arrigoni P, Brady PC, Zottarelli L, et al. Associated lesions requiring additional surgical treatment in grade 3 acromioclavicular joint dislocations. Arthroscopy 2014;30(1):6–10.

29. Neer CS. Fractures of the distal third of the clavicle. Clin Orthop Relat Res 1968;58:43–50.

30. Tauber M, Gordon K, Koller H, et al. Semitendinosus tendon graft versus a modified Weaver-Dunn procedure for acromioclavicular joint reconstruction in chronic cases: a prospective comparative study. Am J Sports Med 2009;37(1):181–90.

31. Woodmass JM, Esposito JG, Ono Y, et al. Complications following arthroscopic fixation of acromioclavicular separations: a systematic review of the literature. Open Access J Sports Med 2015;6:97–107.

32. Gowd AK, Liu JN, Cabarcas BC, et al. Current concepts in the operative management of acromioclavicular dislocations: a systematic review and meta-analysis of operative techniques. Am J Sports Med 2018. https://doi.org/10.1177/0363546518795147.036354651879514.

33. Martetschläger F, Horan MP, Warth RJ, et al. Complications after anatomic fixation and reconstruction of the coracoclavicular ligaments. Am J Sports Med 2013;41(12):2896–903.

34. Alentorn-Geli E, Santana F, Mingo F, et al. Distal clavicle osteolysis after modified Weaver-Dunn's procedure for chronic acromioclavicular dislocation: a case report and review of complications. Case Rep Orthop 2014;2014:1–5.

35. Di Francesco A, Zoccali C, Colafarina O, et al. The use of hook plate in type III and V acromio-clavicular Rockwood dislocations: clinical and radiological midterm results and MRI evaluation in 42 patients. Injury 2012;43(2):147–52.

36. Faria RSS, Ribeiro FR, Amin Bde O, et al. Acromio-clavicular dislocation: postoperative evaluation of the coracoclavicular ligaments using magnetic resonance. Rev Bras Ortop 2015;50(2):195–9.

37. Cahill BR. Osteolysis of the distal part of the clavicle in male athletes. J Bone Joint Surg Am 1982;64(7):1053–8.

38. Roedl JB, Nevalainen M, Gonzalez FM, et al. Frequency, imaging findings, risk factors, and long-term sequelae of distal clavicular osteolysis in young patients. Skeletal Radiol 2015;44(5):659–66.

39. Asano H, Mimori K, Shinomiya K. A case of post-traumatic osteolysis of the distal clavicle: histologic lesion of the acromion. J Shoulder Elbow Surg 2002;11(2):182–7.

40. de la Puente R, Boutin RD, Theodorou DJ, et al. Post-traumatic and stress-induced osteolysis of the distal clavicle: MR imaging findings in 17 patients. Skeletal Radiol 1999;28(4):202–8.

41. Kassarjian A, Llopis E, Palmer WE. Distal clavicular osteolysis: MR evidence for subchondral fracture. Skeletal Radiol 2007;36(1):17–22.

42. Petersson CJ. Degeneration of the acromioclavicular joint: a morphological study. Acta Orthop Scand 1983;54(3):434–8.

43. Buttaci CJ, Stitik TP, Yonclas PP, et al. Osteoarthritis of the acromioclavicular joint: a review of anatomy, biomechanics, diagnosis, and treatment. Am J Phys Med Rehabil 2004;83(10):791–7.

44. Mall NA, Foley E, Chalmers PN, et al. Degenerative joint disease of the acromioclavicular joint: a review. Am J Sports Med 2013;41(11):2684–92.

45. Menge TJ, Boykin RE, Bushnell BD, et al. Acromio-clavicular osteoarthritis: a common cause of shoulder pain. South Med J 2014;107(5):324–9.

46. Veen EJD, Donders CM, Westerbeek RE, et al. Predictive findings on magnetic resonance imaging in patients with symptomatic acromioclavicular osteoarthritis. J Shoulder Elbow Surg 2018;27(8):e252–8.

47. Choo HJ, Lee SJ, Kim JH, et al. Can symptomatic acromioclavicular joints be differentiated from asymptomatic acromioclavicular joints on 3-T MR imaging? Eur J Radiol 2013;82(4):e184–91.

48. Strobel K, Pfirrmann CWA, Zanetti M, et al. MRI features of the acromioclavicular joint that predict pain relief from intraarticular injection. Am J Roentgenol 2003;181(3):755–60.

49. Singh B, Gulihar A, Bilagi P, et al. Magnetic resonance imaging scans are not a reliable tool for predicting symptomatic acromioclavicular arthritis. Shoulder Elbow 2018;10(4):250–4.

50. Martínez-Morillo M, Mateo Soria L, Riveros Frutos A, et al. Septic arthritis of the acromioclavicular joint: an uncommon location. Reumatol Clin 2014;10(1):37–42.

51. Bossert M, Prati C, Bertolini E, et al. Septic arthritis of the acromioclavicular joint. Joint Bone Spine 2010;77(5):466–9.

52. Widman DS, Craig JG, van Holsbeeck MT. Sonographic detection, evaluation and aspiration of infected acromioclavicular joints. Skeletal Radiol 2001;30(7):388–92.

53. Lehtinen JT, Kaarela K, Belt EA, et al. Incidence of acromioclavicular joint involvement in rheumatoid arthritis: a 15 year endpoint study. J Rheumatol 1999;26(6):1239–41.

54. Hakozaki M, Kikuchi S, Otani K, et al. Pseudogout of the acromioclavicular joint: report of two cases and review of the literature. Mod Rheumatol 2011;21(4):440–3.

55. Pressney I, Saifuddin A. Percutaneous image-guided needle biopsy of clavicle lesions: a retrospective study of diagnostic yield with description of safe biopsy routes in 55 cases. Skeletal Radiol 2015;44(4):497–503.

56. Priemel MH, Stiel N, Zustin J, et al. Bone tumours of the clavicle: histopathological, anatomical and epidemiological analysis of 113 cases. J Bone Oncol 2019;16:100229.

57. Paramesparan K. A case series review: the rarity of acromion tumours. European Society of Musculoskeletal Radiology 2017. https://doi.org/10.1594/essr2017/p-0319.

58. Nascimento D, Suchard G, Hatem M, et al. The role of magnetic resonance imaging in the evaluation of bone tumours and tumour-like lesions. Insights Imaging 2014;5(4):419–40.

59. Ogata S, Uhthoff HK. The early development and ossification of the human clavicle–an embryologic study. Acta Orthop Scand 1990;61(4):330–4.

60. Kothary P, Rosenberg ZS. Skeletal developmental patterns in the acromial process and distal clavicle as observed by MRI. Skeletal Radiol 2015;44(2):207–15.

61. Sammarco VJ. Os acromiale: frequency, anatomy, and clinical implications. J Bone Joint Surg Am 2000;82(3):394–400.

62. Pagnani MJ, Mathis CE, Solman CG. Painful os acromiale (or unfused acromial apophysis) in athletes. J Shoulder Elbow Surg 2006;15(4):432–5.

63. Hasan SA, Shiu B, Jauregui JJ. Symptomatic, unstable Os acromiale. J Am Acad Orthop Surg 2018;26(22):789–97.

64. Spiegl UJ, Millett PJ, Josten C, et al. Optimal management of symptomatic os acromiale: current perspectives. Orthop Res Rev 2018;10:1–7.

65. Winfeld M, Rosenberg ZS, Wang A, et al. Differentiating os acromiale from normally developing acromial ossification centers using magnetic resonance imaging. Skeletal Radiol 2015;44(5):667–72.

66. Cockshott WP. The geography of coracoclavicular joints. Skeletal Radiol 1992;21(4):225–7.

67. Nehme A, Tricoire J-L, Giordano G, et al. Coracoclavicular joints. Reflections upon incidence, pathophysiology and etiology of the different forms. Surg Radiol Anat 2004;26(1):33–8.

68. Singh VK, Singh PK, Balakrishnan SK. Bilateral coracoclavicular joints as a rare cause of bilateral thoracic outlet syndrome and shoulder pain treated successfully by conservative means. Singapore Med J 2009;50(6):e214–7.

69. Hiller AD, Miller JD, Zeller JL. Acromioclavicular joint cyst formation. Clin Anat 2010;23(2):145–52.

70. Craig EV. The geyser sign and torn rotator cuff: clinical significance and pathomechanics. Clin Orthop 1984;191:213–5.

71. Mohana-Borges AVR, Chung CB, Resnick D. MR imaging and MR arthrography of the postoperative shoulder: spectrum of normal and abnormal findings. Radiographics 2004;24(1):69–85.

Nerve and Muscle Abnormalities

David A. Rubin, MD[a,b,c,*]

KEYWORDS

- Shoulder • MR imaging • Muscle • Nerve • Rotator cuff • Denervation

KEY POINTS

- The MR imaging findings of muscle atrophy include decreased muscle bulk and/or fatty infiltration.
- In shoulders with rotator cuff tendon tears, muscle atrophy is associated with decreased function, decreased reparability, increased retears after repair, and poorer outcomes after surgery.
- Other than labral cysts compressing the suprascapular nerve, most nerve entrapments around the shoulder are not caused by mass lesions and show no nerve findings on routine MR imaging sequences.
- The pattern of muscle denervation predicts the location of nerve dysfunction, informing the differential diagnosis and guiding management.

INTRODUCTION

Although most shoulder MR imaging examinations are requested to evaluate the rotator cuff and biceps tendons and/or the glenoid labrum, imaging abnormalities related to the muscles and peripheral nerves are commonly encountered. Potential interpretative difficulties arise because many muscle diseases can superficially appear similar on MR images, with intramuscular edema or fatty infiltration being the primary abnormality. Furthermore, even in patients with profound clinical neurologic findings, imaging abnormalities in the peripheral nerves may be subtle or absent.

RECOGNIZING AND QUANTIFYING MUSCLE ABNORMALITIES

Abnormal muscles in the shoulder girdle are typically either atrophied or edematous. These changes most commonly affect the four rotator cuff muscles; most research also investigates those muscles.

Muscle Atrophy

Atrophy refers to decreased muscle size (bulk), fatty infiltration/replacement, or a combination. Although decreased bulk and fatty infiltration often coexist, they differ somewhat in their prognostic importance. Thus, I note these two findings separately when I describe muscle atrophy.

Normal shoulder muscles contain minimal (less than 10%) visible macroscopic fat on cross-sectional imaging studies (Fig. 1). Goutallier and colleagues[1] proposed a grading scheme based on transverse computed tomography images to semiquantitatively describe increased fat based on visually estimating the fat-containing pixels compared with pixels of soft tissue attenuation within a given muscle as follows:

- Grade 0: normal
- Grade 1: minimally increased fat
- Grade 2: substantially increased fat content with more muscle than fat

a All Pro Orthopedic Imaging Consultants, LLC, St Louis, MO, USA; b Radsource, Brentwood, TN, USA; c NYU Langone Medical Center, New York, NY, USA
* 7733 Forsyth Blvd, Suite 1100, St Louis, MO 63105.
E-mail address: drubin001@gmail.com

Magn Reson Imaging Clin N Am 28 (2020) 285–300
https://doi.org/10.1016/j.mric.2019.12.010
1064-9689/20/© 2019 Elsevier Inc. All rights reserved.

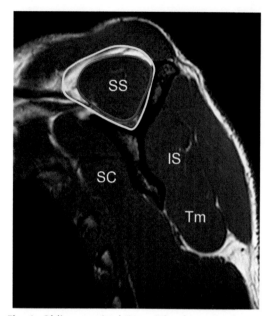

Fig. 1. Oblique sagittal T1-weighted image of a 25-year-old man shows normal rotator cuff muscles. Slice location is most lateral where scapular spine contacts scapular body. Minimal fatty streaks are present in the subscapularis (SC), supraspinatus (SS), infraspinatus (IS), and teres minor (Tm) muscles, which each have convex borders. IS and Tm muscles are inseparable. Note thickness of subtrapezial fat cranial to SS muscle is thicker than fat between other muscles. The occupancy ratio of the cross-section of the SS muscle (*red circle*) to its fossa (*yellow circle*) is greater than 75%.

- Grade 3: fat and muscle amounts approximately equal
- Grade 4: more fat than muscle tissue

Later authors applied the system to T1-weighted MR images[2] and others modified it for ultrasound, estimating the amount of hyperechoic tissue within each muscle.[3] More rigorous quantitative MR imaging methods for calculating intramuscular fat content using chemical shift imaging, MR spectroscopy, or segmentation software have also been published (**Table 1**).[4–6] Results of these methods correlate with Goutallier scoring,[4,7] but are impractical for routine use, and it is unclear how much precision is needed for clinical decision-making.

The largely subjective Goutallier method has drawbacks. It is unclear how best to handle muscles that are also decreased in size (eg, a muscle that has lost half of its volume where half of the remaining tissue is composed of fat is grade 3 even though the total amount of fat comprises <50% of the cross-section for a normal-size muscle). Studies examining the interobserver and

intraobserver agreement show mixed results,[8–10] although agreement is better when the number of grades is reduced from 5 to 3 (by combining grades 0 and 1, and then either combining grades 2 and 3 or grades 3 and 4).[2,11,12] Fatty replacement may occur because of aging or deconditioning (**Fig. 2**),[13,14] which can affect the assigned grade. Lastly, when applied to follow-up, the meaning of a change in one or two grades is inconsistent. For example, a muscle that is originally 40% fat (grade 2) that progresses to 60% (grade 4) changes by two Goutallier grades. But one that goes from 20% to 40% remains grade 2, although the muscle has again suffered a 20% increase in fat content.

For these reasons, my approach to interpreting clinical images is basic: I describe mild/moderate/severe fatty replacement based on prior experience and an overall impression (**Fig. 3**). I suspect that I use the term "mild" for muscle with approximately 10% to 25% fat content, moderate when I estimate 25% to 75% fatty replacement, and severe for the rest. Although I primarily rely on the oblique sagittal sequence, I also refer to the oblique coronal and transverse images, which often show more of the overall muscle bellies (**Fig. 4**).

Determining whether a muscle is smaller than normal requires an internal control; a young, healthy athlete and a geriatric patient are expected to have different size skeletal muscles (see **Figs. 1** and **2**).[13] Whole muscle volume determined by summing manually or automatically drawn cross-sections over the entire muscle length[19] is clinically impractical, so typically a single muscle cross-sectional area is a surrogate for muscle volume. The two-dimensional imaging slice specified is the most lateral oblique sagittal image where the scapular spine contacts the scapular body (see **Fig. 1**). At this location, the normal supraspinatus muscle should extend above a line connecting the cranial aspects of the scapular spine and coracoid (see **Fig. 2A**). If the muscle lies entirely caudal to this line, it is decreased in bulk, the so-called "tangent sign."[15] On the same image, an occupation ratio is calculated by manually tracing the outline of a muscle (typically the supraspinatus) and its bony fossa, and calculating the percentage of the fossa filled by the muscle (see **Fig. 1**).[15–17] Studies applying the occupation ratio for decision-making suggest a cutoff of approximately 40% as an indicator of clinically relevant supraspinatus atrophy.[16,20] Decreased muscle cross-section correlates with increased fatty content.[2,5,17]

These methods for evaluating muscle size have several limitations. In shoulders with large rotator cuff tears, myotendinous retraction shifts the

Table 1
Methods for assessing rotator cuff muscle atrophy

Modality	Technique	Details	References
Semiquantitative methods			
CT, later MR imaging, US	Goutallier	Visually estimate fat percentage within muscle cross-section	CT: Goutallier et al,[1] 1994 MR imaging: Fuchs et al,[2] 1999 US: Strobel et al,[3] 2005
MR imaging, later CT	Tangent sign	Assess SS muscle position relative to a reference line	MR imaging: Zanetti et al,[15] 1998 CT: Williams et al,[12] 2009
MR imaging, later CT, US	Occupation ratio	Calculate ratio of muscle cross-section to size of its fossa	MR imaging: Thomazeau et al,[16] 1996 CT: Tae et al,[17] 2011 US: Khoury et al,[18] 2008
Quantitative methods			
MR imaging	Spectroscopy	Calculate intramuscular lipid content	Pfirrmann et al,[4] 2004
MR imaging	Chemical shift	Calculate fat fraction with in/out phase sequences	Nozaki et al,[5] 2015
MR imaging	T1 quantification	Count fat pixels using segmentation software	Davis et al,[6] 2019
MR imaging	Muscle volume	Calculate muscle volumes by adding multiple cross-sectional areas	Tingart et al,[19] 2003

Abbreviations: CT, computed tomography; SS, supraspinatus; US, ultrasound.

muscle bulk medially, resulting in underestimation of the cross-sectional area on the typically used section (**Fig. 5**).[21] The techniques are difficult to apply to muscles other than the supraspinatus: there is no well-delineated fossa for the other cuff muscles, separating the infraspinatus from the teres minor muscle is often not possible (see **Fig. 1**), and no equivalent tangent line exists for the infraspinatus (although Warner and colleagues[22] proposed a line drawn from the medial coracoid to the inferior scapular tip for the subscapularis). Thus, similar to assessing fatty infiltration, my approach to evaluating muscle size on MR imaging studies is more Gestalt (see **Fig. 3**), applying

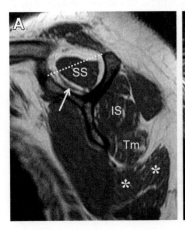
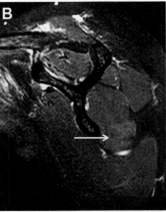

Fig. 2. Muscles in a 70-year-old woman on (*A*) oblique sagittal T1-weighted image are smaller and contain more fat compared with young man (compare with **Fig. 1**). Fatty content in infraspinatus (IS) approximates that in noncuff muscles (*asterisks*) and is likely normal for age. Supraspinatus (SS) muscle rises above tangent line (*dotted line*) connecting superior borders of coracoid and scapular spine. Note suprascapular nerve (*arrow*) in floor of supraspinatus fossa. Teres minor (Tm) muscle is abnormal with intramuscular fat greater than surrounding muscles, and mild edema on fat-suppressed T2-weighted image (*arrow, B*) representing subacute and chronic denervation.

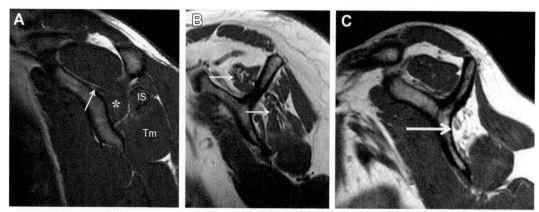

Fig. 3. Degrees of muscle atrophy in three different patients. (*A*) Infraspinatus (IS) shows mild fatty infiltration compared with other rotator cuff muscles, caused by subacute denervation from a labral cyst (*asterisk*) compressing suprascapular nerve (*arrow*). Muscle size is moderately decreased relative to teres minor (Tm). (*B*) Supraspinatus and infraspinatus show moderate fatty infiltration (*arrows*), and mildly decreased bulk compared with surrounding muscles, caused by a massive rotator cuff tendon tear. Note increased thickness of fat surrounding muscles indicating decreased bulk. (*C*) Infraspinatus muscle shows severe fatty replacement (*arrow*) and profoundly decreased size in patient with rotator cuff tear isolated to supraspinatus tendon.

these general rules when deciding whether a muscle is normal, or shows mild/moderate/severe decreased bulk:

- The width of fat between different muscle groups is usually constant (other than between the trapezius and supraspinatus, which is consistently thicker); increased fat between muscles indicates that one or both are small
- Normal muscles typically have convex outer margins where they are not against bone; concave borders suggest decreased muscle mass (see **Fig. 4**B)
- Normal muscles should not be hyperintense on T2-weighted images (see **Fig. 2**)
- Most importantly, overall muscle "bulkiness" is usually uniform throughout all the shoulder girdle muscles in each patient; a muscle that has decreased girth relative to other visible muscles is atrophic

Muscle Edema

Edema refers to muscle that is higher in signal intensity compared with adjacent muscles on water-sensitive MR imaging sequences. The finding is more conspicuous on fat-suppressed T2-weighted or STIR sequences. Edema may be easier to observe than atrophy but is more difficult to interpret correctly, with varied potential causes including mechanical injury, inflammation, infection, and neoplasm. A careful analysis of the pattern of the intramuscular edema, the specific muscles involved and spared, and associated imaging findings together with the clinical history narrows the diagnostic possibilities. In the shoulder, the two most important etiologies are trauma and denervation.

Edema centered around the myotendinous junction is characteristic of indirect muscle injury (strain or delayed-onset muscle soreness).[23]

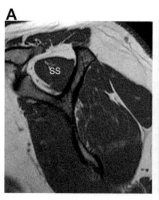

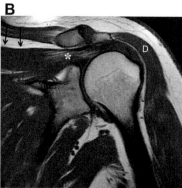

Fig. 4. In shoulder with a small rotator cuff tear, (*A*) oblique sagittal T1-weighted image underestimates supraspinatus (SS) muscle atrophy. (*B*) Oblique coronal T1-weighted image shows mild fatty infiltration (*asterisk*), and mildly concave superior contour (*arrows*) of more medial aspect of SS muscle, indicating mildly decreased muscle bulk. Normal deltoid (D) muscle lies lateral to humeral head and greater tuberosity.

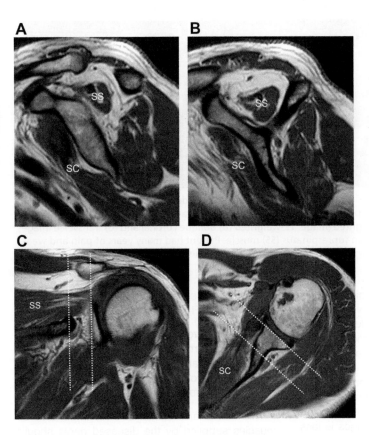

Fig. 5. (*A*) Oblique sagittal T1-weighted image through the glenoid face shows more apparent muscle atrophy of subscapularis (SC) and supraspinatus (SS) compared with (*B*) more medial section where the scapular spine contacts the scapular body. However, both images overestimate muscle atrophy because of muscle retraction. (*C*) Oblique coronal and (*D*) transverse images show bulk of SS and SC muscles lying medial to location of acquired sagittal images (*dotted lines*).

Isolated strains are rare in the rotator cuff[24] because few activities result in eccentric loading of these muscles, but they can occur in the other major muscle groups (**Fig. 6**). Acute shoulder dislocations, with stretching of the muscles surrounding the glenohumeral joint, can also result in the indirect injury pattern. Muscle edema coexists with atrophy in some "acute-on-chronic" rotator cuff tears (**Fig. 7**), corresponding to the common history of sudden exacerbation of long-standing pain, which the patient relates to a specific injury accompanied by a "pop." In these cases, I alert the clinician because some surgeons believe that torn cuffs with an acute component may be easier to mobilize and may want to operate on these shoulders sooner.

Intramuscular edema that varies in different parts of a muscle but is not centered at the myotendinous junction is common after direct trauma.[23] Muscle contusions from external blunt force trauma predominate in the more superficial muscles (**Fig. 8**). Penetrating injury, which may be iatrogenic, can produce the same pattern in deeper muscles (**Fig. 9**).

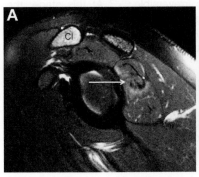
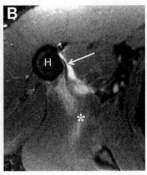

Fig. 6. Muscle strains. Muscle edema on oblique sagittal, fat-suppressed T2-weighted image surrounding a central tendon in infraspinatus (*A, arrow*) represents muscle strain; arm was violently pulled by machine while patient was resisting. Edema in distal clavicle (Cl) was caused by separate injury. (*B*) Transverse fat-suppressed T2-weighted image in second patient shows strain of latissimus dorsi between tendon (*arrow*) and muscle belly (*asterisk*) sustained in a college basketball game. H, humerus.

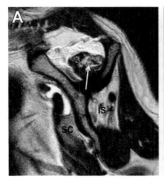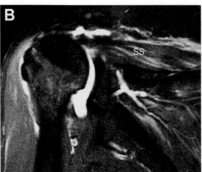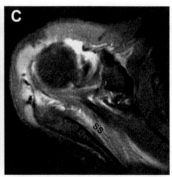

Fig. 7. Acute-on-chronic rotator cuff tear. (*A*) Oblique sagittal image shows decreased size of subscapularis (SC) and infraspinatus (IS) muscles. High signal intensity in supraspinatus (*arrow*) can be caused by fatty infiltration or edema on this non-fat-suppressed T2-weighted image. T2-weighted (*B*) oblique coronal and (*C*) transverse images with fat suppression clearly show edema in supraspinatus (SS) muscle. Patient had many years of pain and weakness but experienced a recent acute injury, felt a "pop," and pain intensified.

Denervation indicates the pathologic changes that a muscle undergoes when its nerve supply is compromised. Approximately 2 weeks following abrupt, complete disruption of a motor nerve axon (eg, after a nerve laceration), the muscles supplied by the nerve show increased water content manifest as edema, especially on STIR images.[25,26] However, most causes of nerve injury occur insidiously and more gradually so defining an exact time frame for imaging changes is less certain. Nevertheless, the pattern of muscle edema caused by subacute denervation differs

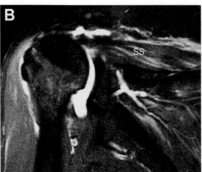

Fig. 8. Muscle contusion. Transverse fat-suppressed, T2-weighted image shows extensive muscle contusion in the deltoid muscle (*asterisks*) in a patient who fell from a bicycle onto lateral shoulder.

from other causes[27] and is characterized by the following (see **Fig. 2**B; **Fig. 10**):

- Uniform involvement of the entire muscle
- Lack of surrounding fascial edema (common with traumatic and inflammatory causes)
- Muscle involvement conforming to a specific nerve distribution

This last characteristic is most important: all muscles supplied by the diseased nerve should be affected and those outside of the distribution should be spared. Recognize that "nerve distribution" does not necessarily mean a single motor neuron. Insults located more proximally in the neuroaxis (anywhere from the cervical nerve roots through the brachial plexus) affect muscles supplied by multiple downstream peripheral nerves. The opposite is also true: injury to a nerve that branches to supply several muscles only affects those muscles located distal to the lesion (**Fig. 11**).

If the cause of nerve dysfunction is self-limited, or is recognized and treated, muscle signal intensity returns to normal. However, if the issue persists (typically for 6 months or longer), the affected muscles eventually become infiltrated by fat, which is irreversible.[26,28] At this stage, the key to recognizing chronic denervation is again noting that the atrophied muscles conform to a nerve distribution (**Fig. 12**).

MUSCLE ABNORMALITIES IN SHOULDERS WITH ROTATOR CUFF TENDON TEARS

Muscle atrophy (fatty infiltration and decreased size) is a sequala of chronic rotator cuff tendon tears; the degree of atrophy correlates to the size of the tear[13,29,30] and the duration of symptoms.[31,32] Isolated infraspinatus muscle atrophy

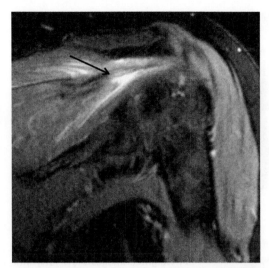

Fig. 9. Iatrogenic muscle injury. Oblique coronal fat-suppressed, T2-weighted image demonstrates focal infraspinatus muscle edema (*arrow*) in patient who had needle electromyography 2 days previously.

can occur with large tendon tears that involve the supraspinatus tendon, with or without the subscapularis (see **Fig. 3**C).[1,33] Theories to explain this observation include changes in force vectors and muscle fiber pennation angles following supraspinatus tendon tears, stretching of the suprascapular nerve, and renewed understanding of the overlap and intermingling of infraspinatus and supraspinatus tendon fibers at the insertional footprint.[34–36] Of course, massive cuff tears are associated with atrophy of multiple cuff muscles.

Unsurprisingly, muscle atrophy is associated with decreased shoulder function in patients with rotator cuff tears.[7,37] But the importance of recognizing muscle atrophy is that it prognosticates tear reparability and surgical outcomes. Diminished supraspinatus muscle size, defined by the tangent sign or an occupancy ratio of 40% or less, is associated with inability to completely cover the greater

tuberosity footprint during attempted cuff repair.[20,38] In a recent study, less than 15% of massive rotator cuff tears could be repaired when Goutallier grade 3 or higher infraspinatus fatty infiltration was present (compared with 77% with less severe fatty atrophy).[39] Diminished supraspinatus muscle size is also a predictor of recurrent tendon tears after repair,[40] whereas increased intramuscular fat (especially for the infraspinatus) is associated with poorer postoperative functional results[41] and retears.[42,43] A recent systemic review of 11 published studies (925 shoulders) found a 59% retear rate for shoulders with preoperative Goutallier grade 2 to 4 fatty infiltration compared with 25% in those with grade 0 to 1 muscles.[44] Even in patients with successful (intact) repairs of massive rotator cuff tears, preoperative subscapularis and infraspinatus fatty infiltration (Goutallier grade 2 and higher) is associated with worse clinical outcomes.[45]

Muscle fat may progress postoperatively in shoulders with failed cuff repairs[46]; with an intact repair fatty infiltration usually does not progress, and may partly improve long-term.[43,47,48] Supraspinatus muscle bulk can increase after a successful cuff repair, but the improvement is usually slight (11%–14%),[47] and better for smaller tendon tears.[48] Note that apparent postoperative improvement in muscle volume may be artifactual and caused by retracted muscle being moved laterally (into the oblique sagittal slice used for analysis) during cuff repair, rather than an actual increase in muscle volume.[49,50] Rotator cuff retears may lead to further decreases in muscle size.[51]

Deltoid muscle tears are a rare but frequently overlooked finding in shoulder MR imaging examinations. Injuries begin on the deep surface of the muscle belly and can progress to full-thickness tears with associated muscle atrophy (**Fig. 13**), or the muscle can dehisce from its acromial attachment, similar to what may occur following open acromioplasty.[52,53] Most cases of deltoid muscle

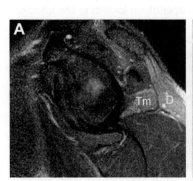
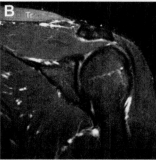

Fig. 10. Subacute muscle denervation. (*A*) Oblique sagittal fat-suppressed, T2-weighted image shows homogeneous muscle edema throughout teres minor (Tm) and deltoid (D) muscles without surrounding fascial edema. Distribution indicates axillary nerve insult within quadrilateral space. (*B*) Oblique coronal fat-suppressed T2-weighted image in second patient with presumed viral neuritis shows same pattern of edema in trapezius (Tr) muscle, corresponding to accessory spinal nerve (cranial nerve XI) distribution.

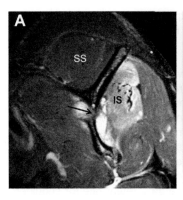
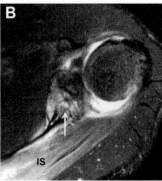

Fig. 11. Subacute denervation. (*A*) Oblique sagittal and (*B*) transverse fat-suppressed, T2-weighted images in shoulder with scapular fracture (*arrow*) demonstrate edema isolated to infraspinatus (IS) muscle, innervated by distal branches of suprascapular nerve. Supraspinatus (SS) is spared because fracture injures nerve distal to branches supplying SS.

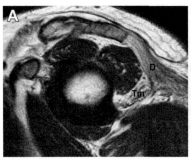
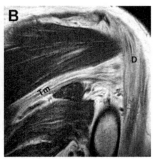

Fig. 12. Chronic denervation. (*A*) Oblique sagittal and (*B*) oblique coronal T1-weighted images show fatty infiltration uniformly throughout teres minor (Tm) and deltoid (D) muscles. Distribution is same as patient in **Fig. 10A**, but fatty infiltration instead of muscle edema indicates that denervation has reached chronic stage. No space-occupying lesion is present in the quadrilateral space.

failure have associated chronic, massive rotator cuff tears (see **Fig. 13**) with superior humeral subluxation and impingement by the greater tuberosity suggested as contributing factors.[52,54] Although a torn deltoid muscle is usually not repaired during rotator cuff surgery, deltoid atrophy negatively affects outcomes in reverse total shoulder arthroplasties performed for irreparable cuff lesions.[55]

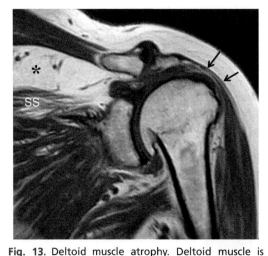

Fig. 13. Deltoid muscle atrophy. Deltoid muscle is chronically torn and severely atrophied (*arrows*, compare with **Fig. 4B**) on oblique coronal T1-weighted image in shoulder with massive chronic cuff tear and secondary cuff tear arthropathy. Supraspinatus (SS) muscle shows severe atrophy with hypertrophy of subtrapezial fat (*asterisk*).

MUSCLE ABNORMALITIES RELATED TO NERVE DISORDERS

Neuritis is often not suspected clinically: shoulder pain and weakness is attributed to an internal derangement so imaging findings of muscle denervation may be the first indication of a neurologic condition. Alternatively, when clinical neuropathy is present, imaging is useful to show alternative or additional pathology. Management of neuropathy depends on localizing the affected site. However, diagnostic electrical testing and the imaging appearance of the affected nerves can be nonspecific (or normal). Thus, the pattern of muscle involvement becomes a powerful tool predicting disease location within the neuroaxis.[56] Recognizing these patterns requires an understanding of the peripheral nerve anatomy.

Relevant Nerve Anatomy

The nerves most frequently implicated in shoulder symptoms are the suprascapular and axillary. Each nerve has muscular and sensory branches.

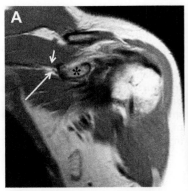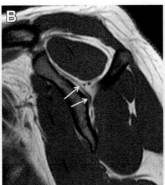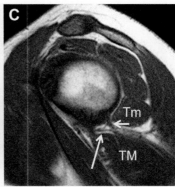

Fig. 14. Normal nerves and landmarks. Oblique coronal T1-weighted image shows suprascapular ligament (*short arrow, A*) emanating from medial border of coracoid (*asterisk*) with suprascapular nerve (*long arrow*) below. (*B*) In a second shoulder, oblique sagittal T1-weighted image demonstrates suprascapular nerve (*arrows*) passing through spinoglenoid notch. Spinoglenoid ligament is not visible. (*C*) Oblique sagittal T1-weighted image in third shoulder shows branching axillary nerve (*long arrow*) within quadrilateral space. *Short arrow* = long head triceps tendon; Tm, teres minor; TM, teres major.

Both originate primarily from the C5 and C6 nerve roots and arise from the brachial plexus.[57,58]

The suprascapular nerve extends from the upper trunk of the plexus, through the posterior triangle of the neck, and then passes through the suprascapular notch of the scapula.[59] The suprascapular (superior transverse scapular) ligament forms the roof of the notch and is often visible along the medial edge of the coracoid base on oblique coronal images (**Fig. 14**A).[60] The nerve next courses along the floor of the supraspinatus fossa (see **Fig. 2**A) where it innervates the supraspinatus muscle. From there it travels through the spinoglenoid notch (**Fig. 14**B), which is bounded by the spinoglenoid (inferior transverse scapular) ligament.[61] Terminal branches then supply the infraspinatus muscle.

The axillary nerve arises from the posterior cord of the brachial plexus, coursing under the coracoid and along the anterior surface of the subscapularis muscle. It then enters the quadrilateral space (**Fig. 14**C), an area bounded by the teres minor and major muscles, the long head of the triceps, and the humeral surgical neck.[62] The nerve divides into anterior and posterior limbs, with the anterior branch innervating most of the deltoid, and the posterior branch running along the inferior glenoid, sending variable branches to the teres minor muscle.[63,64]

Table 2 summarizes the usual locations of nerve injury together with the affected muscles and most common etiologies. Importantly, other than labral cysts producing suprascapular nerve compression, most nerve entrapments show no mass or mass-effect, and normal or nonspecific findings in the nerves on routine MR imaging sequences, meaning that findings of muscle denervation alone are typically the only imaging clue to a focal neuritis.[65,66]

Table 2
Shoulder nerve insults by location

Location	Muscles Involved	Common Etiologies
Suprascapular nerve		
Suprascapular notch	Supraspinatus Infraspinatus	Clavicle fracture Entrapment under suprascapular ligament Iatrogenic injury Parsonage-Turner syndrome (mimic)
Spinoglenoid notch	Infraspinatus	Labral cyst Scapular fracture Iatrogenic injury Traction/overuse in overhead athletes
Axillary nerve		
Quadrilateral space	Deltoid Teres minor	Glenohumeral dislocation Proximal humeral fracture Iatrogenic injury Fibrous bands
Postero-inferior glenoid	Teres minor	Idiopathic/ unknown Glenohumeral osteoarthritis Labral cyst

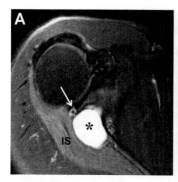
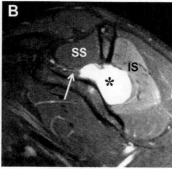

Fig. 15. Labral cyst compressing suprascapular nerve. (*A*) Transverse and (*B*) oblique sagittal fat-suppressed, T2-weighted images show cyst (*asterisk*), arising from posterior labral tear (*arrow* in *A*). Infraspinatus (IS) muscle demonstrates denervation edema, whereas supraspinatus (SS) is spared. Note relation of cyst to suprascapular nerve (*arrow* in *B*).

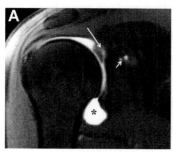
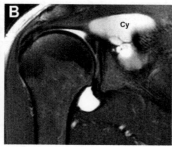

Fig. 16. Labral tear and cyst on MR arthrogram. (*A*) Oblique coronal, fat-suppressed T1-weighted image after intra-articular injection of dilute gadolinium shows high signal intensity contrast in joint (*asterisk*) and labral tear (*long arrow*), but minimal contrast communicating with labral cyst (*short arrow*). (*B*) T2-weighted image shows full extent of labral cyst (Cy).

Specific Suprascapular Nerve Disorders

Infraspinatus muscle denervation with sparing of the supraspinatus muscle indicates nerve injury around the spinoglenoid notch, distal to the branches supplying the supraspinatus (see **Table 2**). Entrapment caused by a compressing

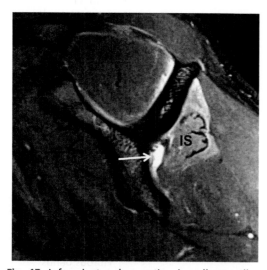

Fig. 17. Infraspinatus denervation in college volleyball player. Infraspinatus muscle (IS) is edematous and decreased in size (note concave margins) on oblique sagittal, fat-suppressed T2-weighted image. Vessels in suprascapular notch are mildly dilated (*arrow*), a nonspecific finding.

cyst (see **Fig. 3**A; **Fig. 15**) has a better prognosis compared with other causes. A cyst in the spinoglenoid notch virtually always originates from a tear of the posterosuperior glenoid labrum, even though 21% of the time, the labral tear is not visible on a conventional MR imaging examination.[67] Although MR arthrography is more sensitive for showing labral tears compared with conventional MR imaging,[68,69] most labral cysts do not freely communicate with their labral tear. Thus, when performing MR arthrography, T2-weighted images are needed in addition to the T1-weighted images that best depict the injected contrast (**Fig. 16**).[70] Although labral cysts may be aspirated percutaneously with imaging guidance, they tend to recur if the underlying labral tear is not also treated. Cysts typically resolve after arthroscopic repair of the labral tear.[67,71]

Other causes of suprascapular nerve dysfunction localized to the spinoglenoid notch include acute trauma (see **Fig. 11**), iatrogenic injuries,[72,73] and overuse or traction in overhead athletes.[59,74] Approximately one-third of high-level volleyball players (**Fig. 17**) and 4% of major league baseball pitchers demonstrate isolated infraspinatus denervation, which usually does not negatively affect performance.[58,75,76] Dilated veins in the spinoglenoid notch may be seen in patients with neuritis (see **Fig. 17**),[77] although I suspect that the enlarged vessels may simply reflect increased local pressure in this location (unlike for the

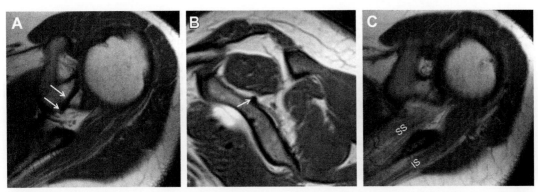

Fig. 18. Iatrogenic suprascapular nerve injury. (*A*) Transverse and (*B*) oblique sagittal T1-weighted images show suture anchor from prior superior labral repair abutting suprascapular nerve (*arrows*) proximal to spinoglenoid notch. Six months later, (*C*) transverse image shows progressive supraspinatus (SS) and infraspinatus (IS) atrophy indicating chronic denervation.

suprascapular ligament, the vessels travel under the spinoglenoid ligament, together with the nerve[57,61]) rather than a cause of nerve compression. First-line treatment of suprascapular neuritis localized to the spinoglenoid notch is nonoperative,[78] with operative release of the spinoglenoid ligament reserve for refractory cases.[57,79]

Denervation involving the supraspinatus and infraspinatus muscles suggests an injury to the suprascapular nerve at or proximal to the suprascapular notch. Etiologies here include trauma (eg, midclavicle fractures,[80] and chronic stretching and traction); iatrogenic injuries, including

mobilization during rotator cuff repair[74] and malpositioned implants (**Fig. 18**); and entrapment or friction under the suprascapular ligament (**Fig. 19**).[59] Approximately 10% of patients with massive rotator cuff tears may have enough muscle retraction to stretch the suprascapular nerve,[81,82] leading some researchers to postulate that chronic denervation contributes to the muscle

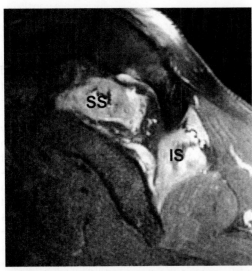

Fig. 19. Nerve entrapment in suprascapular notch. Subacute supraspinatus (SS) and infraspinatus (IS) denervation on oblique sagittal, fat-suppressed T2-weighted image. At surgery, suprascapular nerve was entrapped by thickened suprascapular ligament, which was released. Parsonage-Turner syndrome could present with same findings.

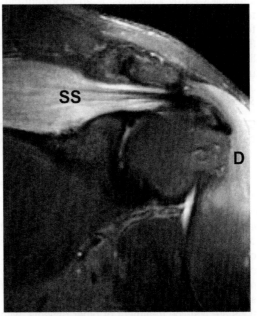

Fig. 20. Parsonage-Turner syndrome. Subacute supraspinatus (SS) denervation alone on oblique coronal, fat-suppressed T2-weighted image would be difficult to differentiate from suprascapular nerve entrapment (compare **Fig. 19**). Involvement of deltoid (D) is clue to localization more proximally in brachial plexus. Clinical symptoms and imaging findings resolved spontaneously approximately 8 months later.

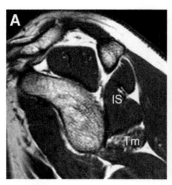 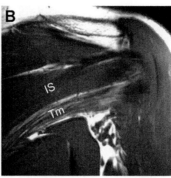

Fig. 21. Isolated teres minor denervation. Teres minor (Tm) muscle is decreased in size and partly replaced with fat compared with infraspinatus (IS) on (*A*) oblique sagittal and (*B*) oblique coronal T1-weighted images. Finding was incidental and asymptomatic.

atrophy seen in association with rotator cuff tears.[34,83,84] Regardless of cause, initial treatment is nonoperative[78]; surgical release of the suprascapular ligament is reserved for patients with progressive chronic denervation.[79,85]

Parsonage-Turner syndrome is a neuritis of unknown cause involving the upper trunk of the brachial plexus, most often (97%) the suprascapular nerve with or without other nerves.[28,86] In approximately 50% of cases, only the supraspinatus and infraspinatus muscle are denervated mimicking suprascapular neuropathy (see **Fig. 19**).[86] The characteristic history (acute onset pain, sometimes preceded by a viral infection, later followed by weakness) is an important clue to the correct diagnosis. The diagnosis is easier to recognize when other muscles are involved (**Fig. 20**).[87] Parsonage-Turner syndrome is self-limited (although complete recovery make take up to 2 years) and managed conservatively.[88]

Specific Axillary Nerve Disorders

Classic quadrilateral space syndrome affects the deltoid and teres minor muscles (see **Figs. 10**A and **12**). Approximately half the patients with proximal humeral fractures and anterior shoulder dislocations have electromyography evidence of nerve injury, most commonly axonal loss involving the axillary nerve.[58,89,90] Iatrogenic injury in the quadrilateral space can also occur after open rotator cuff or instability surgery.[58] Nontraumatic cases are often attributed to fibrous bands resulting in nerve compression or friction.[62] Most patients with axillary nerve compression caused by acute trauma recover spontaneously[89,90]; physical therapy and medications are first-line treatment of other patients, with surgery (neurolysis, resection of fibrous bands) reserved for refractory cases or the rare instances where a space-occupying lesion is present.[62]

Isolated subacute or chronic teres minor denervation with sparing of the deltoid muscle is observed in 3% of shoulder MR imaging examinations performed for any reason (see **Fig. 2**; **Fig. 21**).[91]

Radiologists may erroneously attribute this finding to quadrilateral space syndrome, but it is a distinct entity and virtually never caused by a compressing mass lesion.[64,92] Rarely a large labral cyst can cause denervation of the infraspinatus and teres minor muscles, although in these shoulders a branch of the suprascapular nerve supplying the teres minor (a normal variant), may be responsible.[67,70] A subset of shoulders with glenohumeral osteoarthritis demonstrate chronic teres minor atrophy, possibly caused by irritation by inferior humeral head osteophytes.[93] Although the denervation is not specifically treated in these patients, it may have prognostic significance because teres minor muscle atrophy negatively affects outcomes following reverse total shoulder arthroplasty.[94]

SUMMARY

The presence of muscle atrophy (decreased bulk and/or fatty replacement) in shoulders with rotator cuff tendon tears is a negative prognosticator, associated with decreased function, decreased reparability, increased retears after repair, and poorer outcomes after surgery. Muscle edema or atrophy within a neurologic distribution characterizes denervation. Because most nerve entrapments around the shoulder are not caused by mass lesions and show no nerve findings on routine MR imaging sequences, the pattern of muscle denervation is often the best clue to predicting the location of nerve dysfunction, which in turn narrows the differential diagnosis and guides clinical management. The exception is suprascapular nerve compression in the spinoglenoid notch, which can be caused by a compressing cyst. These cysts originate from labral tears, which are treated arthroscopically.

DISCLOSURE

The author has no commercial or financial conflicts of interest and has not received funding from any source.

REFERENCES

1. Goutallier D, Postel JM, Bernageau J, et al. Fatty muscle degeneration in cuff ruptures. Pre- and post-operative evaluation by CT scan. Clin Orthop Relat Res 1994;304:78–83.

2. Fuchs B, Weishaupt D, Zanetti M, et al. Fatty degeneration of the muscles of the rotator cuff: assessment by computed tomography versus magnetic resonance imaging. J Shoulder Elbow Surg 1999;8(6):599–605.

3. Strobel K, Hodler J, Meyer DC, et al. Fatty atrophy of supraspinatus and infraspinatus muscles: accuracy of US. Radiology 2005;237(2):584–9.

4. Pfirrmann CW, Schmid MR, Zanetti M, et al. Assessment of fat content in supraspinatus muscle with proton MR spectroscopy in asymptomatic volunteers and patients with supraspinatus tendon lesions. Radiology 2004;232(3):709–15.

5. Nozaki T, Tasaki A, Horiuchi S, et al. Quantification of fatty degeneration within the supraspinatus muscle by using a 2-point Dixon method on 3-T MRI. AJR Am J Roentgenol 2015;205(1):116–22.

6. Davis DL, Kesler T, Gilotra MN, et al. Quantification of shoulder muscle intramuscular fatty infiltration on T1-weighted MRI: a viable alternative to the Goutallier classification system. Skeletal Radiol 2019; 48(4):535–41.

7. Nardo L, Karampinos DC, Lansdown DA, et al. Quantitative assessment of fat infiltration in the rotator cuff muscles using water-fat MRI. J Magn Reson Imaging 2014;39(5):1178–85.

8. Oh JH, Kim SH, Choi JA, et al. Reliability of the grading system for fatty degeneration of rotator cuff muscles. Clin Orthop Relat Res 2010;468(6):1558–64.

9. Lippe J, Spang JT, Leger RR, et al. Inter-rater agreement of the Goutallier, Patte, and Warner classification scores using preoperative magnetic resonance imaging in patients with rotator cuff tears. Arthroscopy 2012;28(2):154–9.

10. Schiefer M, Mendonca R, Magnanini MM, et al. Intraobserver and interobserver agreement of Goutallier classification applied to magnetic resonance images. J Shoulder Elbow Surg 2015;24(8):1314–21.

11. Slabaugh MA, Friel NA, Karas V, et al. Interobserver and intraobserver reliability of the Goutallier classification using magnetic resonance imaging: proposal of a simplified classification system to increase reliability. Am J Sports Med 2012;40(8):1728–34.

12. Williams MD, Ladermann A, Melis B, et al. Fatty infiltration of the supraspinatus: a reliability study. J Shoulder Elbow Surg 2009;18(4):581–7.

13. Barry JJ, Lansdown DA, Cheung S, et al. The relationship between tear severity, fatty infiltration, and muscle atrophy in the supraspinatus. J Shoulder Elbow Surg 2013;22(1):18–25.

14. Dow DF, Mehta K, Xu Y, et al. The relationship between body mass index and fatty infiltration in the shoulder musculature. J Comput Assist Tomogr 2018;42(2):323–9.

15. Zanetti M, Gerber C, Hodler J. Quantitative assessment of the muscles of the rotator cuff with magnetic resonance imaging. Invest Radiol 1998;33(3): 163–70.

16. Thomazeau H, Rolland Y, Lucas C, et al. Atrophy of the supraspinatus belly. Assessment by MRI in 55 patients with rotator cuff pathology. Acta Orthop Scand 1996;67(3):264–8.

17. Tae SK, Oh JH, Kim SH, et al. Evaluation of fatty degeneration of the supraspinatus muscle using a new measuring tool and its correlation between multidetector computed tomography and magnetic resonance imaging. Am J Sports Med 2011;39(3): 599–606.

18. Khoury V, Cardinal E, Brassard P. Atrophy and fatty infiltration of the supraspinatus muscle: sonography versus MRI. AJR Am J Roentgenol 2008;190(4): 1105–11.

19. Tingart MJ, Apreleva M, Lehtinen JT, et al. Magnetic resonance imaging in quantitative analysis of rotator cuff muscle volume. Clin Orthop Relat Res 2003; 415:104–10.

20. Jeong JY, Chung PK, Lee SM, et al. Supraspinatus muscle occupation ratio predicts rotator cuff reparability. J Shoulder Elbow Surg 2017;26(6):960–6.

21. Fukuta S, Tsutsui T, Amari R, et al. Tendon retraction with rotator cuff tear causes a decrease in cross-sectional area of the supraspinatus muscle on magnetic resonance imaging. J Shoulder Elbow Surg 2016;25(7):1069–75.

22. Warner JJ, Higgins L, Parsons IMT, et al. Diagnosis and treatment of anterosuperior rotator cuff tears. J Shoulder Elbow Surg 2001;10(1):37–46.

23. Flores DV, Mejia Gomez C, Estrada-Castrillon M, et al. MR imaging of muscle trauma: anatomy, biomechanics, pathophysiology, and imaging appearance. Radiographics 2018;38(1):124–48.

24. Taneja AK, Kattapuram SV, Chang CY, et al. MRI findings of rotator cuff myotendinous junction injury. AJR Am J Roentgenol 2014;203(2):406–11.

25. Fleckenstein JL, Watumull D, Conner KE, et al. Denervated human skeletal muscle: MR imaging evaluation. Radiology 1993;187(1):213–8.

26. Polak JF, Jolesz FA, Adams DF. Magnetic resonance imaging of skeletal muscle. Prolongation of T1 and T2 subsequent to denervation. Invest Radiol 1988; 23(5):365–9.

27. Sallomi D, Janzen DL, Munk PL, et al. Muscle denervation patterns in upper limb nerve injuries: MR imaging findings and anatomic basis. AJR Am J Roentgenol 1998;171(3):779–84.

28. Blum A, Lecocq S, Louis M, et al. The nerves around the shoulder. Eur J Radiol 2013;82(1):2–16.

29. Lee S, Lucas RM, Lansdown DA, et al. Magnetic resonance rotator cuff fat fraction and its relationship

with tendon tear severity and subject characteristics. J Shoulder Elbow Surg 2015;24(9):1442–51.

30. Bureau NJ, Deslauriers M, Lepage-Saucier M, et al. Rotator cuff tear morphologic parameters at magnetic resonance imaging: relationship with muscle atrophy and fatty infiltration and patient-reported function and health-related quality of life. J Comput Assist Tomogr 2018;42(5):784–91.

31. Melis B, Wall B, Walch G. Natural history of infraspinatus fatty infiltration in rotator cuff tears. J Shoulder Elbow Surg 2010;19(5):757–63.

32. Melis B, DeFranco MJ, Chuinard C, et al. Natural history of fatty infiltration and atrophy of the supraspinatus muscle in rotator cuff tears. Clin Orthop Relat Res 2010;468(6):1498–505.

33. Yao L, Mehta U. Infraspinatus muscle atrophy: implications? Radiology 2003;226(1):161–4.

34. Laron D, Samagh SP, Liu X, et al. Muscle degeneration in rotator cuff tears. J Shoulder Elbow Surg 2012;21(2):164–74.

35. Cheung S, Dillon E, Tham SC, et al. The presence of fatty infiltration in the infraspinatus: its relation with the condition of the supraspinatus tendon. Arthroscopy 2011;27(4):463–70.

36. Mochizuki T, Sugaya H, Uomizu M, et al. Humeral insertion of the supraspinatus and infraspinatus. New anatomical findings regarding the footprint of the rotator cuff. J Bone Joint Surg Am 2008;90(5): 962–9.

37. Yoon JP, Jung JW, Lee CH, et al. Fatty degeneration of the rotator cuff reflects shoulder strength deficits in patients with rotator cuff tears. Orthopedics 2018;41(1):e15–21.

38. Kissenberth MJ, Rulewicz GJ, Hamilton SC, et al. A positive tangent sign predicts the repairability of rotator cuff tears. J Shoulder Elbow Surg 2014; 23(7):1023–7.

39. Kim JY, Park JS, Rhee YG. Can preoperative magnetic resonance imaging predict the reparability of massive rotator cuff tears? Am J Sports Med 2017; 45(7):1654–63.

40. Thomazeau H, Boukobza E, Morcet N, et al. Prediction of rotator cuff repair results by magnetic resonance imaging. Clin Orthop Relat Res 1997;344: 275–83.

41. Gladstone JN, Bishop JY, Lo IK, et al. Fatty infiltration and atrophy of the rotator cuff do not improve after rotator cuff repair and correlate with poor functional outcome. Am J Sports Med 2007;35(5): 719–28.

42. Goutallier D, Postel JM, Gleyze P, et al. Influence of cuff muscle fatty degeneration on anatomic and functional outcomes after simple suture of full-thickness tears. J Shoulder Elbow Surg 2003;12(6):550–4.

43. Nozaki T, Tasaki A, Horiuchi S, et al. Predicting retear after repair of full-thickness rotator cuff tear: two-point Dixon MR imaging quantification of fatty

muscle degeneration-initial experience with 1-year follow-up. Radiology 2016;280(2):500–9.

44. Khair MM, Lehman J, Tsouris N, et al. A systematic review of preoperative fatty infiltration and rotator cuff outcomes. HSS J 2016;12(2):170–6.

45. Ohzono H, Gotoh M, Nakamura H, et al. Effect of preoperative fatty degeneration of the rotator cuff muscles on the clinical outcome of patients with intact tendons after arthroscopic rotator cuff repair of large/massive cuff tears. Am J Sports Med 2017;45(13):2975–81.

46. Deniz G, Kose O, Tugay A, et al. Fatty degeneration and atrophy of the rotator cuff muscles after arthroscopic repair: does it improve, halt or deteriorate? Arch Orthop Trauma Surg 2014;134(7):985–90.

47. Park YB, Ryu HY, Hong JH, et al. Reversibility of supraspinatus muscle atrophy in tendon-bone healing after arthroscopic rotator cuff repair. Am J Sports Med 2016;44(4):981–8.

48. Hamano N, Yamamoto A, Shitara H, et al. Does successful rotator cuff repair improve muscle atrophy and fatty infiltration of the rotator cuff? A retrospective magnetic resonance imaging study performed shortly after surgery as a reference. J Shoulder Elbow Surg 2017;26(6):967–74.

49. Chung SW, Oh KS, Moon SG, et al. Serial changes in 3-dimensional supraspinatus muscle volume after rotator cuff repair. Am J Sports Med 2017;45(10): 2345–54.

50. Lhee SH, Singh AK, Lee DY. Does magnetic resonance imaging appearance of supraspinatus muscle atrophy change after repairing rotator cuff tears? J Shoulder Elbow Surg 2017;26(3):416–23.

51. Jo CH, Shin JS. Cross-sectional area of the supraspinatus muscle after rotator cuff repair: an anatomic measure of outcome. J Bone Joint Surg Am 2013;95(19):1785–91.

52. Ilaslan H, Iannotti JP, Recht MP. Deltoid muscle and tendon tears in patients with chronic rotator cuff tears. Skeletal Radiol 2007;36(6):503–7.

53. Moser T, Lecours J, Michaud J, et al. The deltoid, a forgotten muscle of the shoulder. Skeletal Radiol 2013;42(10):1361–75.

54. Blazar PE, Williams GR, Iannotti JP. Spontaneous detachment of the deltoid muscle origin. J Shoulder Elbow Surg 1998;7(4):389–92.

55. Yoon JP, Seo A, Kim JJ, et al. Deltoid muscle volume affects clinical outcome of reverse total shoulder arthroplasty in patients with cuff tear arthropathy or irreparable cuff tears. PLoS One 2017;12(3): e0174361.

56. Moen TC, Babatunde OM, Hsu SH, et al. Suprascapular neuropathy: what does the literature show? J Shoulder Elbow Surg 2012;21(6):835–46.

57. Post M. Diagnosis and treatment of suprascapular nerve entrapment. Clin Orthop Relat Res 1999;368: 92–100.

58. Safran MR. Nerve injury about the shoulder in athletes, part 1: suprascapular nerve and axillary nerve. Am J Sports Med 2004;32(3):803–19.

59. Cummins CA, Messer TM, Nuber GW. Suprascapular nerve entrapment. J Bone Joint Surg Am 2000; 82(3):415–24.

60. Simeone FJ, Bredella MA, Chang CY, et al. MRI appearance of the superior transverse scapular ligament. Skeletal Radiol 2015;44(11):1663–9.

61. Plancher KD, Peterson RK, Johnston JC, et al. The spinoglenoid ligament. Anatomy, morphology, and histological findings. J Bone Joint Surg Am 2005; 87(2):361–5.

62. Flynn LS, Wright TW, King JJ. Quadrilateral space syndrome: a review. J Shoulder Elbow Surg 2018; 27(5):950–6.

63. Ball CM, Steger T, Galatz LM, et al. The posterior branch of the axillary nerve: an anatomic study. J Bone Joint Surg Am 2003;85(8):1497–501.

64. Friend J, Francis S, McCulloch J, et al. Teres minor innervation in the context of isolated muscle atrophy. Surg Radiol Anat 2010;32(3):243–9.

65. Bencardino JT, Rosenberg ZS. Entrapment neuropathies of the shoulder and elbow in the athlete. Clin Sports Med 2006;25(3):465–87. vi-vii.

66. Yanny S, Toms AP. MR patterns of denervation around the shoulder. AJR Am J Roentgenol 2010; 195(2):W157–63.

67. Schroder CP, Lundgreen K, Kvakestad R. Paralabral cysts of the shoulder treated with isolated labral repair: effect on pain and radiologic findings. J Shoulder Elbow Surg 2018;27(7): 1283–9.

68. Major NM, Browne J, Domzalski T, et al. Evaluation of the glenoid labrum with 3-T MRI: is intraarticular contrast necessary? AJR Am J Roentgenol 2011; 196(5):1139–44.

69. Symanski JS, Subhas N, Babb J, et al. Diagnosis of superior labrum anterior-to-posterior tears by using MR imaging and MR arthrography: a systematic review and meta-analysis. Radiology 2017;285(1): 101–13.

70. Tung GA, Entzian D, Stern JB, et al. MR imaging and MR arthrography of paraglenoid labral cysts. AJR Am J Roentgenol 2000;174(6):1707–15.

71. Youm T, Matthews PV, El Attrache NS. Treatment of patients with spinoglenoid cysts associated with superior labral tears without cyst aspiration, debridement, or excision. Arthroscopy 2006;22(5): 548–52.

72. Yoo JC, Lee YS, Ahn JH, et al. Isolated suprascapular nerve injury below the spinoglenoid notch after SLAP repair. J Shoulder Elbow Surg 2009;18(4): e27–9.

73. Kim SH, Koh YG, Sung CH, et al. Iatrogenic suprascapular nerve injury after repair of type II SLAP lesion. Arthroscopy 2010;26(7):1005–8.

74. Ahlawat S, Wadhwa V, Belzberg AJ, et al. Spectrum of suprascapular nerve lesions: normal and abnormal neuromuscular imaging appearances on 3-T MR neurography. AJR Am J Roentgenol 2015; 204(3):589–601.

75. Cummins CA, Messer TM, Schafer MF. Infraspinatus muscle atrophy in professional baseball players. Am J Sports Med 2004;32(1):116–20.

76. Lajtai G, Pfirrmann CW, Aitzetmuller G, et al. The shoulders of professional beach volleyball players: high prevalence of infraspinatus muscle atrophy. Am J Sports Med 2009;37(7):1375–83.

77. Carroll KW, Helms CA, Otte MT, et al. Enlarged spinoglenoid notch veins causing suprascapular nerve compression. Skeletal Radiol 2003;32(2):72–7.

78. Boykin RE, Friedman DJ, Higgins LD, et al. Suprascapular neuropathy. J Bone Joint Surg Am 2010; 92(13):2348–64.

79. Antoniou J, Tae SK, Williams GR, et al. Suprascapular neuropathy. Variability in the diagnosis, treatment, and outcome. Clin Orthop Relat Res 2001; 386:131–8.

80. Yu JS, Fischer RA. Denervation atrophy caused by suprascapular nerve injury: MR findings. J Comput Assist Tomogr 1997;21(2):302–3.

81. Shah AA, Butler RB, Sung SY, et al. Clinical outcomes of suprascapular nerve decompression. J Shoulder Elbow Surg 2011;20(6):975–82.

82. Albritton MJ, Graham RD, Richards RS 2nd, et al. An anatomic study of the effects on the suprascapular nerve due to retraction of the supraspinatus muscle after a rotator cuff tear. J Shoulder Elbow Surg 2003; 12(5):497–500.

83. Gerber C, Meyer DC, Fluck M, et al. Muscle degeneration associated with rotator cuff tendon release and/or denervation in sheep. Am J Sports Med 2017;45(3):651–8.

84. Shi LL, Freehill MT, Yannopoulos P, et al. Suprascapular nerve: is it important in cuff pathology? Adv Orthop 2012;2012:516985.

85. Mall NA, Hammond JE, Lenart BA, et al. Suprascapular nerve entrapment isolated to the spinoglenoid notch: surgical technique and results of open decompression. J Shoulder Elbow Surg 2013; 22(11):e1–8.

86. Gaskin CM, Helms CA. Parsonage-Turner syndrome: MR imaging findings and clinical information of 27 patients. Radiology 2006;240(2):501–7.

87. Scalf RE, Wenger DE, Frick MA, et al. MRI findings of 26 patients with Parsonage-Turner syndrome. AJR Am J Roentgenol 2007;189(1):W39–44.

88. Tsairis P, Dyck PJ, Mulder DW. Natural history of brachial plexus neuropathy. Report on 99 patients. Arch Neurol 1972;27(2):109–17.

89. Visser CP, Coene LN, Brand R, et al. The incidence of nerve injury in anterior dislocation of the shoulder and its influence on functional recovery. A

prospective clinical and EMG study. J Bone Joint Surg Br 1999;81(4):679–85.

90. de Laat EA, Visser CP, Coene LN, et al. Nerve lesions in primary shoulder dislocations and humeral neck fractures. A prospective clinical and EMG study. J Bone Joint Surg Br 1994;76(3):381–3.

91. Sofka CM, Lin J, Feinberg J, et al. Teres minor denervation on routine magnetic resonance imaging of the shoulder. Skeletal Radiol 2004;33(9):514–8.

92. Wilson L, Sundaram M, Piraino DW, et al. Isolated teres minor atrophy: manifestation of quadrilateral space syndrome or traction injury to the axillary nerve? Orthopedics 2006;29(5):447–50.

93. Millett PJ, Schoenahl JY, Allen MJ, et al. An association between the inferior humeral head osteophyte and teres minor fatty infiltration: evidence for axillary nerve entrapment in glenohumeral osteoarthritis. J Shoulder Elbow Surg 2013;22(2):215–21.

94. Simovitch RW, Helmy N, Zumstein MA, et al. Impact of fatty infiltration of the teres minor muscle on the outcome of reverse total shoulder arthroplasty. J Bone Joint Surg Am 2007;89(5):934–9.

Shoulder Tumor/Tumor-Like Lesions: What to Look for

James Thomas Patrick Decourcy Hallinan, MBChB[a,b,*], Brady K. Huang, MD[c]

KEYWORDS

• Shoulder • Tumors • Tumor-like lesions • Elastofibroma • Osteosarcoma • Chondrosarcoma
• Amyloid arthropathy • Synovial sarcoma

KEY POINTS

• Bone tumors at the shoulder rank second in incidence to those at the knee and include benign and malignant entities.
• MR imaging is critical for staging of malignant bone lesions and detection of skip lesions.
• Shoulder soft tissue tumors are overwhelmingly benign in nature, with lipomas predominating.
• Ultrasound often is used for soft tissue lesion screening, with MR imaging providing further characterization of indeterminate lesions.
• Tumor-like lesions may arise from the shoulder joints or bursae due to arthropathies (eg, amyloid).

INTRODUCTION

Tumor and tumor-like lesions are common at the shoulder and may arise from the bones, soft tissues, or underlying joints or bursae. Osseous tumors include benign osteochondromas and enchondromas or malignant lesions, including osteosarcoma and metastases.[1,2] Soft tissue tumors are overwhelmingly benign in nature, with lipomas predominating.[3,4] Numerous tumor-like lesions may arise from the joints or bursae, due either to an underlying degenerative process or inflammatory arthropathy or may be related to other conditions, including tenosynovial giant cell tumor (TGCT). This article discusses the role of imaging for the most common shoulder lesions.

NORMAL ANATOMY AND IMAGING TECHNIQUES

Initial assessment of shoulder tumor and tumor-like lesions should include radiographs to assess for fracture, joint degeneration, erosions, and soft tissue mineralization.[5] Radiographs remain vital in the work-up of bone tumor matrix characterization and identifying aggressive cortical destruction. Ultrasound is useful for the diagnosis of soft tissue lesions and can guide biopsy of indeterminate lesions. Computed tomography (CT) can assess for matrix mineralization and guide bone tumor biopsy. For a majority of bone tumors and large complex soft tissue lesions, MR imaging provides superior anatomic and morphologic characterization.[2]

MR imaging must be optimized to assess the lesion in detail (small field of view [FOV]) and the surrounding region for any satellite lesions, for example, skip lesions in osteosarcoma. The patient is imaged supine with the affected shoulder positioned within a dedicated coil close to the magnet isocenter. MR imaging protocols vary among institutions, although most include standard T1-weighted and short tau inversion recovery (STIR) or T2-weighted fat-suppressed sequences. Common additional sequences include gradient-echo or gadolinium-enhanced, fat-suppressed T1-weighted sequences.

[a] Department of Diagnostic Imaging, National University Health System, 1E Kent Ridge Road, Singapore 119074, Singapore; [b] Yong Loo Lin School of Medicine, National University of Singapore, Block MD11, 10 Medical Drive, Singapore 119074, Singapore; [c] Department of Radiology, University of California San Diego, School of Medicine, UCSD Teleradiology and Education Center, 408 Dickinson Street, Mail Code #8226, San Diego, CA 92103-8226, USA
* Corresponding author. Department of Diagnostic Imaging, National University Health System, 1E Kent Ridge Road, Singapore 119074, Singapore.
E-mail address: jim.hallinan@gmail.com

Magn Reson Imaging Clin N Am 28 (2020) 301–316
https://doi.org/10.1016/j.mric.2019.12.011
1064-9689/20/© 2019 Elsevier Inc. All rights reserved.

Table 1
Suggested shoulder tumor MR imaging protocol

Axial	Sagittal	Coronal	Additional Sequences
T1-weighted or gradient echo	T1-weighted	T1-weighted	1. Axial, coronal, and sagittal T1-weighted fat-suppressed postcontrast sequences with or without dynamic postcontrast for indeterminate lesion characterization and post-treatment assessment
Proton density or T2- weighted fat-suppressed	Proton density or T2- weighted fat-suppressed	T2-weighted, fat-suppressed, or STIR	2. Diffusion-weighted images with apparent diffusion coefficient maps can help differentiate benign from malignant lesions and assess treatment response (higher apparent diffusion coefficient values post-treatment are favorable).
			3. Chemical-shift fat-water separation techniques (eg, Dixon) may aid lesion characterization and marrow assessment.

Gradient-echo can identify blooming artifact arising from hemosiderin deposition (eg, TGCT) or metallic foreign bodies. Postcontrast sequences are deployed to differentiate between cystic and solid masses, necrosis, and increase lesion conspicuity.[2,5] A suggested imaging protocol for shoulder tumor and tumor-like lesions is summarized in **Table 1**.

BONE TUMOR AND TUMOR-LIKE LESIONS

Several benign and malignant bone tumors occur at the shoulder (**Box 1**) along with pseudolesions. A majority of bone tumors occur at the proximal humerus (70%). Benign bone tumors include osteochondromas, enchondromas, and giant cell tumors. Most malignant bone lesions are metastases or myeloma. Other primary malignant bone tumors include osteosarcoma and chondrosarcoma. Tumor-like lesions also predominate in the proximal humerus, with simple bone cysts the most common (90% of cases).[1,2,6]

BENIGN BONE TUMOR
Cartilaginous

Osteochondroma accounts for more than half of all benign bone tumors at the shoulder. The distinctive imaging feature is continuity of the lesion and medullary cavity of the bone (**Fig. 1**). Although benign, there is a risk of sarcomatous transformation at the cartilage cap, which is suspected if there is an enlarging or painful lesion. Cartilage cap measurements greater than 2 cm on CT/MR

imaging should raise concern for malignant transformation in the mature skeleton.[7,8]

Enchondroma is another common benign bony tumor at the shoulder accounting for 15% of lesions. Most occur at the proximal humerus and demonstrate ring and arc chondroid calcifications on radiographs and CT. On MR imaging, the chondroid calcification appears as low-signal septations between lobules of T2 hyperintense cartilage. Postcontrast imaging typically demonstrates mild septal enhancement with no soft tissue extension, which is more suggestive of chondrosarcoma.[2,9]

Box 1
Major shoulder bone tumors

Benign

  Osteochondroma

  Osteoid osteoma and osteoblastoma

  Chondroid lesions: chondroblastoma, enchondroma, and periosteal chondroma

  Giant cell tumor

  Fibrous dysplasia

Malignant

  Myeloma, metastases and lymphoma (multiplicity of lesions is key)

  Osteosarcoma

  Chondrosarcoma

  Ewing sarcoma

  Fibrous: pleomorphic undifferentiated sarcoma and fibrosarcoma

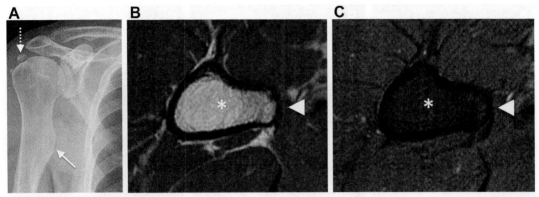

Fig. 1. Sessile osteochondroma at the medial proximal humerus in a 57-year-old man. (*A*) Frontal radiograph shows a sessile bony lesion (*arrow*) with additional rotator cuff calcific tendon deposits (*dashed arrow*). (*B*) Axial T1-weighted and (*C*) T2-weighted fat-suppressed MR images demonstrate continuity between the lesion (*arrowheads*) and medullary cavity (*asterisks*). No discernible cartilage cap, adjacent edema, or bursal formation is seen.

Osseous

Osteoid osteomas account for approximately 4% of shoulder bone tumors and consist of a small hypervascular nidus with a rind of surrounding reactive bone. MR imaging characteristics depend on the extent of nidal mineralization; nonmineralized nidi demonstrate homogeneous postcontrast enhancement and hyperintense T2 signal, whereas mineralized nidi may show low signal on all sequences. Most osteoid osteomas are associated with extensive surrounding inflammatory marrow edema, which can be misinterpreted as an underlying traumatic or infectious process.[2,10] These lesions can be treated with CT-guided radiofrequency ablation.

Other Benign Bone Tumors

Giant cell tumor is a benign but locally aggressive lesion with a predilection for the humeral head, typically in the closed epiphysis of young adults. On radiographs, the lesion is classically subarticular, expansile, and well defined with a nonsclerotic border. MR imaging typically shows heterogeneous low T2 tumor signal and enhancement. Secondary aneurysmal bone cyst formation can coexist.[11]

Fibrous dysplasia occurs in monostotic and polyostotic forms and involves the shoulder in approximately 3% of monostotic cases. Radiographs typically demonstrate ground-glass matrix with well-defined borders (**Fig. 2**). MR imaging can be challenging to interpret due to varying degrees of cellularity and mineralized components leading to heterogeneous low to intermediate T1 and T2 signals and varying enhancement.[12]

MALIGNANT BONE TUMORS

Metastases, myeloma, and secondary lymphoma are the most common malignant tumors of bone around the shoulder. Radiographs and MR imaging typically show aggressive lesions with nonspecific imaging features. More characteristic primary bone tumors include osteosarcoma and chondrosarcoma.

Osteosarcoma

After myeloma, the most common primary shoulder bone tumor is osteosarcoma, accounting for a third of cases. The most common subtype is the conventional, high-grade variant, with the surface and telangiectatic subtypes occurring less commonly. The conventional subtype is most common in the second decade of life, with secondary lesions occurring in older patients with preexisting bone lesions, for example, Paget's disease. Conventional osteosarcoma is typically located in the central humeral metaphysis, with osteoid matrix, soft tissue extension, and aggressive periosteal reaction.[13]

MR imaging shows tumor heterogeneity with hyperintense T2 signal and enhancing soft tissue adjacent to necrotic areas. Osteoid matrix can be seen as low-signal foci on all images. MR imaging should be optimized to assess the primary tumor with an additional large FOV to assess for skip lesions (**Fig. 3**).[14]

Chondrosarcoma

Chondrosarcoma accounts for approximately a third of primary malignant bone tumors of the shoulder, with 10% occurring at the proximal humerus and 5% at the scapula. Chondrosarcoma is the most common primary malignant bone lesion at the scapula.

Radiographs typically show a lytic lesion with a permeative appearance and aggressive periosteal

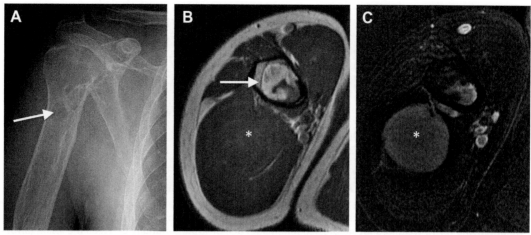

Fig. 2. Mazabraud syndrome in a 60-year-old man. (*A*) Frontal radiograph shows a lobulated mixed lytic and sclerotic lesion along the proximal humerus with areas of ground-glass matrix (*arrow*) and no cortical breach or periosteal reaction. (*B*) Axial T1-weighted and (*C*) T2-weighted fat-suppressed images show mixed signal abnormality in the humeral diaphysis with well-defined sclerotic margins (*arrow*) and no soft tissue extension. A well-defined, fairly homogeneous T2-weighted hyperintense lesion is seen separately in the triceps posteriorly (*asterisks*). Together these features were compatible with polyostotic fibrous dysplasia (other skeletal sites not shown) and a soft tissue myxoma.

reaction. Intralesional matrix calcifications are seen in up to 70% of chondrosarcoma, with CT revealing calcification in up to 94%. MR imaging demonstrates lobulated hyperintense T2 signal similar to enchondroma, although features favoring chondrosarcoma include deep endosteal scalloping (>2/3 thickness), bone expansion, cortical destruction, and soft tissue extension (**Fig. 4**).[15]

Tumor-Like Bone Lesions

Simple bone cysts account for 90% of non-neoplastic tumor-like lesions in the proximal humerus and typically are seen in the first to second decades. They appear as well-defined, geographic lesions at the central proximal humeral metaphysis (**Fig. 5**). They commonly present with a pathologic fracture leading to the characteristic fallen fragment sign. MR imaging typically reveals fluid signal characteristics with less common findings, including septations or fluid-fluid levels.[16] The latter typically occurs in aneurysmal bone cysts, which are another common non-neoplastic lesion at the proximal humerus. Up to a third of aneurysmal bone

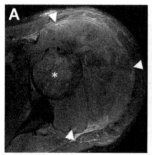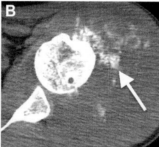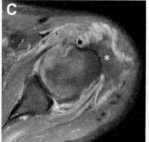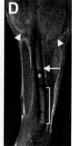

Fig. 3. Osteosarcoma of the proximal humerus in a 20-year-old man. (*A*) Axial T1-weighted fat-suppressed postcontrast MR image and (*B*) axial CT show a destructive bony lesion (*asterisk*) with enhancing soft tissue extension (*arrowheads*) and internal cloud-like osteoid (*arrow*), which is leading to anterior glenohumeral subluxation. (*C*) Axial T1-weighted fat-suppressed postcontrast MR image after neoadjuvant chemotherapy reveals marked reduction in the enhancing soft tissue, internal nonenhancing necrosis (*asterisk*), and resolution of the glenohumeral subluxation. (*D*) Sagittal T1-weighted fat-suppressed postcontrast, pretreatment MR image shows the primary tumor (*arrowheads*) and distal osseous margin (*arrow*). An enhancing skip lesion is seen in the distal humerus (*bracket*) with intervening normal marrow signal (*asterisk*). It is important to include a large FOV image of the entire humerus to detect skip lesions.

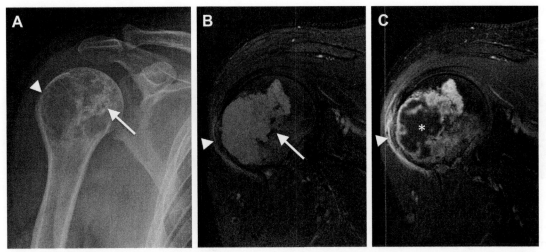

Fig. 4. Chondrosarcoma at the proximal humerus in a 48-year-old man. (*A*) Frontal radiograph shows a lucent lesion at the humeral head with characteristic chondroid ring and arc calcification (*arrow*). Deep endosteal scalloping is seen laterally at the greater tuberosity with suspicion of cortical breach (*arrowhead*). (*B*) Coronal T2-weighted fat-suppressed and (*C*) T1-weighted fat-suppressed postcontrast images show a lobulated T2 hyperintense lesion with nodular peripheral enhancement and central nonenhancing areas (*asterisk*). The low-signal chondroid calcification is noted (*arrow*) with cortical disruption and soft tissue extension laterally (*arrowheads*). These aggressive features make chondrosarcoma more likely than enchondroma.

cysts are secondary to an underlying lesion, for example, chondroblastoma, giant cell tumor, or even osteosarcoma.[2,17]

Bone Pseudolesions

A few pseudolesions occur at the shoulder, which could provoke unnecessary work-up. A proximal humeral cyst-like rarefaction due to a physiologic decrease in the trabeculae and increased marrow fat has been described. This radiolucency occurs at the superolateral head and can be misdiagnosed as a lytic lesion (**Fig. 6**). MR imaging typically is diagnostic, with clear demonstration of marrow fat signal.[18,19] Cortical and periosteal thickening at

the deltoid tuberosity of the humerus also can mimic a neoplasm.[20]

BENIGN SOFT TISSUE LESIONS

Box 2 lists the main types of benign soft tissue lesions at the shoulder. Lipomatous and neurogenic tumors are the most common and are discussed further.

Benign Lipomatous Lesions

Lipomas account for approximately 35% of benign soft tissue lesions around the shoulder and can be assessed on ultrasound if superficial (**Box 3**). Ultrasound can show variable echogenicity, although isoechogenicity or hyperechogenicity to

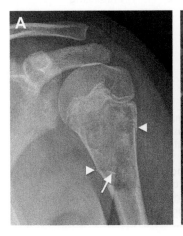
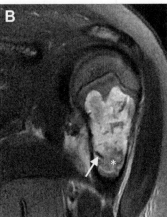

Fig. 5. Unicameral bone cyst and fallen fragment sign in a 15-year-old boy. (*A*) Frontal radiograph shows a predominantly lucent lesion in the left proximal humeral metaphysis with thinning of the endosteal cortex. There is a pathologic fracture (*arrowheads*) with a fallen fragment of bone present within the dependent portion of the lesion (*arrow*). (*B*) Coronal proton density MR image shows a high-signal intensity lesion with a low-signal fallen fragment (*arrow*) and intermediate signal likely due to posttraumatic hemorrhage (*asterisk*).

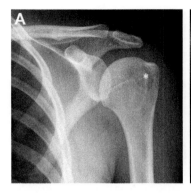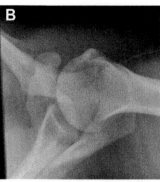

Fig. 6. Humeral head pseudolesion in a 17-year-old man with shoulder pain and reduced motion due to a football injury. (*A*) Frontal shoulder radiograph shows a nonaggressive lucency at the greater tuberosity (*asterisk*) with no periosteal reaction, cortical breach, or corresponding abnormality on the axial view (*B*). This was reported as a likely pseudolesion due to fatty marrow replacement.

the surrounding subcutaneous fat is most common. MR imaging is the most accurate imaging modality and demonstrates signal similar to subcutaneous fat with homogeneous fat-suppression Thin, enhancing internal septations can also occur (**Fig. 7**).[21] A more complex benign lipomatous lesion is the hibernoma, which is an uncommon tumor of brown fat with a predilection for the shoulder girdle. At MR imaging, these lesions typically demonstrate T1 signal slightly less than subcutaneous fat, with incomplete fat-suppression and internal enhancement due to prominent vascularity (**Fig. 8**).[22]

Elastofibroma is another benign fat-containing, fibroelastic tumor with a predilection for the infrascapular chest wall. This lesion is bilateral in 60% of cases and is found in up to 2% of thoracic CT studies. On CT, the characteristic finding is an infrascapular mass with internal fat striations. Similarly, on MR imaging, a streaky pattern of hyper and hypointense T1/T2 signal represents bands of lipomatous and fibroelastic tissue (**Fig. 9**). Ultrasound can also suggest the diagnosis, with the lesion appearing predominantly echogenic with streaks of hypoechoic fat.[2,23,24]

Box 2
Major shoulder soft tissue tumors

Benign

   Lipoma

   Fibrous lesions: benign fibrous histiocytoma, nodular fasciitis, and desmoid-type fibromatosis

   Elastofibroma

   Peripheral nerve sheath tumors: neurofibroma and schwannomas

   Vascular lesions: hemangioma or vascular malformations

Malignant

   Liposarcoma

   Fibrous lesions: myxofibrosarcoma, pleomorphic undifferentiated sarcoma, and dermatofibrosarcoma protuberans

   Synovial sarcoma

   Leiomyosarcoma

   MPNSTs

   Young children: rhabdomyosarcoma, hemangiosarcoma, and fibrosarcoma

---

Box 3
Differential diagnosis of lipomatous lesions

Lipoma (Benign)	*Liposarcoma*
Typically rounded or oval with a well-defined capsule	Lobulated with irregular margins
Subcutaneous, <5 cm in size	Deep intramuscular location, >5 cm in size
Smooth, thin, septal enhancement; no nodular enhancement	Nodular or thickened enhancing septations (>2 mm); enhancing, non–fat-containing nodules (dedifferentiated subtype)

Variants
Benign: hibernomas typically show inhomogeneous fat-suppression and more marked internal enhancement compared with lipomas.
Malignant: pleomorphic liposarcomas may have no internal fat on MR imaging and display nonspecific, aggressive features, including internal haemorrhage and necrosis.

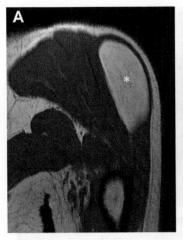
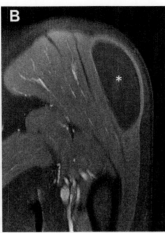

Fig. 7. Intramuscular lipoma at the deltoid in a 63-year-old woman. (A) Coronal T1-weighted and (B) T2-weighted fat-suppressed MR images show a well-defined T1-weighted hyperintense lesion in the deltoid (*asterisk*) with complete suppression of fat signal. No large nonlipomatous components or thickened septations are seen to suggest a liposarcoma.

Benign Neurogenic Tumors

Neurogenic tumors account for approximately 6% of benign shoulder tumors. On both ultrasound and MR imaging, a well-differentiated fusiform or rounded lesion along the course of a nerve should suggest the diagnosis. Schwannomas and neurofibromas are the main histologically distinct tumors with overlapping imaging signs. MR imaging typically shows hyperintense T2 signal, isointense to mildly hyperintense T1 signal, and avid contrast enhancement. MR imaging also can demonstrate a target sign, more commonly in neurofibromas, with central T2 hypointense fibrous tissue and peripheral T2 hyperintense myxoid tissue. Other imaging features more commonly seen in schwannomas include a fascicular sign on ultrasound or MR imaging, cystic change, and hemorrhage.[25]

MALIGNANT SOFT TISSUE TUMORS

Malignant soft tissue tumors are up to 100 times less common than benign tumors and comprise a wide variety of tumors that vary according to age (see **Box 2**).[26] The main role of the radiologist is to provide a categorization of soft tissue lesions into either benign or indeterminate lesions.[27] Patients with indeterminate lesions should be referred to specialist musculoskeletal oncology centers for biopsy and tissue diagnosis.[28] Ultrasound may be used for initial screening of these lesions with aggressive features, such as necrosis and prominent Doppler flow, triggering further evaluation with MR imaging.

A full discussion of the various subtypes of malignant soft tissue tumors is beyond the scope of this article and the most common lesions are discussed. A majority of malignant soft tissue lesions are seen in middle-aged adults and the elderly, with the most prevalent lesions being liposarcoma and myxofibrosarcoma (**Fig. 10**). MR imaging can suggest these diagnoses with macroscopic fat identified in liposarcoma and hyperintense T2/STIR myxoid signal in myxofibrosarcoma and myxoid liposarcoma. A

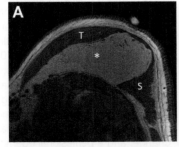
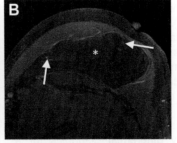

Fig. 8. Hibernoma in a 27-year-old man. (A) Sagittal T1-weighted and (B) T1-weighted postcontrast fat-suppressed MR images show a large lipomatous lesion (*asterisks*) interposed between the trapezius (T) and supraspinatus (S) muscles. The lesion shows T1-weighted hyperintensity and near complete fat-suppression, although there are prominent vessels (*arrows*) and subtle enhancement within. These features along with the size (>5 cm) were suspicious for an atypical lipomatous tumor or hibernoma. Resection and histology confirmed a hibernoma. The lesion was also negative for MDM2 amplification, which is more commonly positive in liposarcoma.

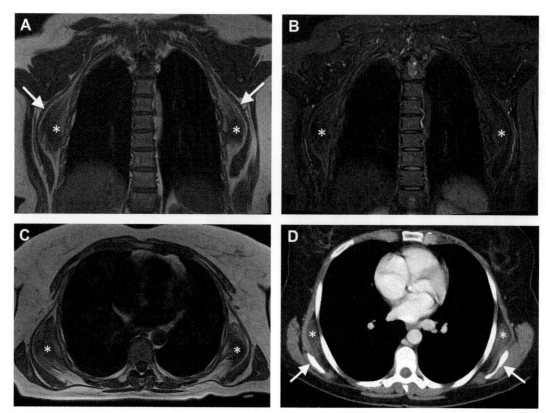

Fig. 9. Bilateral elastofibroma dorsi in a 49-year-old woman. (*A*) Coronal T1-weighted and (*B*) T2-weighted fat-suppressed MR images show bilateral lesions (*asterisks*) underlying the serratus anterior muscles (*arrows*). The lesions show internal fat signal (T1 hyperintensity with fat-suppression) with low-signal fibroelastic tissue. (*C*) Axial T1-weighted MR image and (*D*) CT demonstrate the fat-containing lesions (*asterisks*) underlying the scapulae (*arrows*). The location and internal fat signal are characteristic for elastofibromas.

majority of other malignant lesions show nonspecific, aggressive features on MR imaging, including intralesional hemorrhage, prominent vascularity and nonenhancing necrosis.[29]

Up to half of liposarcomas are of the well-differentiated/low-grade subtype, which can express MDM2 or CDK4. These lesions appear similar to lipomas on MR imaging, although suspicious features include size (>5 cm), deep intramuscular location, and thick enhancing septations (>2 mm). The higher-grade dedifferentiated liposarcoma can show intralesional enhancing nodules (>1 cm). Pleomorphic liposarcoma is an uncommon variant that may have a dearth of macroscopic fat on MR imaging, with additional internal hemorrhage and necrosis (see **Box 3**).[30]

In young adults and adolescents, synovial sarcoma is a key differential diagnosis for a juxta-articular soft tissue lesion (**Fig. 11**). On radiographs, the lesion may show internal calcifications (30%). MR imaging appearances depend on the size, with small lesions appearing more homogeneous and larger lesions typically

showing a triple sign on fluid-sensitive sequences due to low-signal calcifications/fibrosis, isointense cellular components, and hyperintense necrosis. Internal hemorrhage is also common with fluid-fluid levels, termed the *bowl of grapes sign*, seen in up to 25% of cases.[31]

Other malignant lesions include soft tissue metastases (typically multiple), leiomyosarcoma, dermatofibrosarcoma protuberans, and malignant peripheral nerve sheath tumors (MPNSTs). MPNSTs occur most commonly from pre-existing neurofibromas in neurofibromatosis type 1 (70%). Therefore, a rapidly enlarging or painful lesion in this subset of patients is concerning for malignant transformation. MR imaging can suggest a diagnosis of MPNST, usually showing internal hemorrhage and mineralization, peripheral enhancement, cystic change, and a perilesional edema-like zone.[32,33]

SOFT TISSUE TUMOR-LIKE LESIONS

Several benign cystic lesions occur commonly around the shoulder (**Box 4**). A characteristic cystic lesion (geyser) may arise superior to the

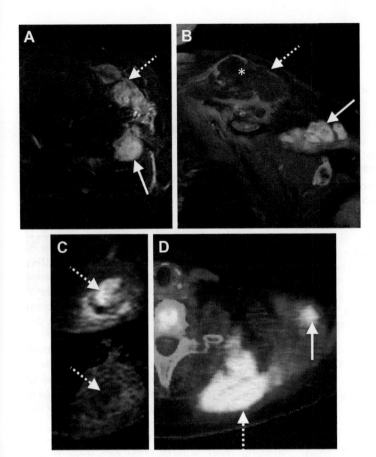

Fig. 10. Myxofibrosarcoma of the shoulder in a 78-year-old woman. (A) Sagittal T2-weighted fat-suppressed and (B) coronal T1-weighted fat-suppressed postcontrast MR images show a lobulated, T2-weighted hyperintense lesion with central necrosis (asterisk) involving the trapezius muscle (dashed arrows). A satellite nodule is seen in the deltoid (solid arrows). (C) Axial diffusion-weighted image (superior) and the ADC map (inferior) show restricted diffusion in the trapezius lesion (dashed arrows) suggestive of a hypercellular, likely malignant neoplasm. (D) Fluorodeoxyglucose-PET/CT demonstrates marked fluorodeoxyglucose uptake within the trapezius lesion (dashed arrow) with a hypermetabolic satellite nodule (solid arrow) and pulmonary metastases (not shown). Imaging features were compatible with a metastatic sarcoma and biopsy confirmed a myxofibrosarcoma.

acromioclavicular joint due to a chronic rotator cuff tear, humeral head instability, and degradation of the joint capsule. This is well demonstrated on ultrasound and MR imaging, with depiction of the rotator cuff tearing and T2 hyperintense cystic lesion (**Fig. 12**).[34]

Muscle and soft tissue trauma are common around the shoulder and can produce several

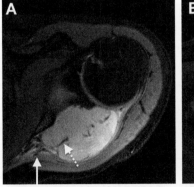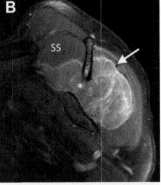

Fig. 11. Periscapular synovial sarcoma in a 34-year-old woman. (A) Axial T2-weighted fat-suppressed and (B) sagittal T1-weighted fat-suppressed postcontrast MR images show a lobulated, T2 hyperintense lesion with heterogeneous internal enhancement in the periscapular region extending through the spinoglenoid notch (asterisk). The lesion is inseparable and exerts mass effect on the rotator cuff musculature, especially the supraspinatus (SS) and infraspinatus (arrows) muscles. Internal low-signal foci could relate to fibrous tissue (dashed arrow). No calcifications were seen on the radiographs and CT (not shown).

Box 4
Tumor-like lesions: pearls, pitfalls, and variants

Bones

Pearls: fallen fragment sign is characteristic of a simple bone cyst.

Pitfalls:

- Fluid-fluid levels can be seen in benign aneurysmal bone cysts but also in malignant telangiectatic osteosarcomas.
- Deltoid tuberosity can mimic a bone lesion but has a characteristic location at the lateral midhumerus.

Soft tissue

Pearls: elastofibroma is a benign fat-containing, fibroelastic tumor with a characteristic location at the infrascapular chest wall.

Pitfalls: benign neurogenic lesions and MPNSTs overlap on imaging. A rapidly enlarging or painful lesion along with aggressive MR imaging findings, including internal hemorrhage, can suggest MPNSTs.

Variants: accessory muscles can present as a clinically apparent mass, for example, the axillary arch muscle of Langer.

Joint and bursal location

Pearls: MR imaging can show characteristic blooming on gradient-echo images in TGCT or fatty frond-like synovial proliferation in lipoma arborescens.

Pitfalls: fibrinous rice bodies are not unique to RA and occur in other inflammatory and infective arthropathies, for example, tuberculosis.

---

tumor-like lesions, such as myositis ossificans. Imaging of myositis ossificans typically shows a zonal ossification pattern proceeding from peripheral to central, which is best seen on radiographs and CT. At an early preossification phase, the imaging features are nonspecific, with MR imaging showing prominent enhancement and signal heterogeneity, which can be misleading for malignancy.[35]

Other tumor-like conditions include hematomas, infections (eg, abscesses), muscle tears, or contractures. Muscle contractures occur most commonly at the deltoid and are usually a consequence of repeated intramuscular injections. Fibrotic cords in the deltoid lead to fixed abduction and scapular winging, which can be seen on radiographs. Ultrasound shows mixed hypoechoic and hyperechoic

fibrotic cords at the deltoid, which typically appear hypointense on all MR imaging sequences (**Fig. 13**).[36,37]

Accessory muscles around the shoulder can present as a clinically apparent mass or mimic a mass on imaging. These variants include an accessory biceps brachii, an accessory pectoralis minor, and the axillary arch muscle of Langer (**Fig. 14**).[38,39]

ARTICULAR AND PERIARTICULAR LESIONS

TGCT is a benign tumor-like disorder of hypertrophic synovium and hemosiderin deposition that may affect joints (focally or diffusely), bursae, or tendon sheaths. The diffuse intra-articular subtype occurs most commonly at the knee (70%), hip, ankle, and shoulder in decreasing frequency.[40] TGCT in bursae or tendon sheaths can present as a focal shoulder mass, whereas intra-articular involvement can present as a glenohumeral joint effusion with bony erosions on radiographs.[41] Ultrasound findings are nonspecific, with intra-articular or bursal TGCT appearing as mixed hyperechoic villonodular lesions with increased vascularity on Doppler imaging. CT may show slightly hyperdense intra-articular lesions without calcification, which aids differentiation from synovial osteochondromatosis. MR imaging features have been well documented, with hemosiderin deposition typically exerting a paramagnetic effect that results in low to intermediate signal on all sequences, and prominent blooming artifact on gradient-echo sequences (**Fig. 15**).[42]

Other synovial tumor-like processes presenting with joint or bursal distension include a range of infectious/inflammatory, crystal, and metabolic arthropathies.

Rheumatoid arthritis (RA) and psoriatic arthritis are the most common inflammatory arthropathies and can initially present with enhancing synovial pannus and effusions. At a later stage, bony erosions occur (eg, circumferential humeral neck erosions with RA), along with joint rupture and rice bodies (**Fig. 16**).[5] Fibrinous rice bodies can mimic synovial osteochondromatosis in the joint or subacromial-subdeltoid bursa but do not show mineralization on radiographs or CT (**Fig. 17**). Infectious arthropathies, such as tuberculosis, may also produce rice bodies with similar overlapping imaging features.[43,44]

Crystalline arthropathies are a common cause of tumor-like lesions and include calcium hydroxyapatite deposition disease (HADD), gout, and pseudogout. HADD most commonly presents as a calcific deposit within the

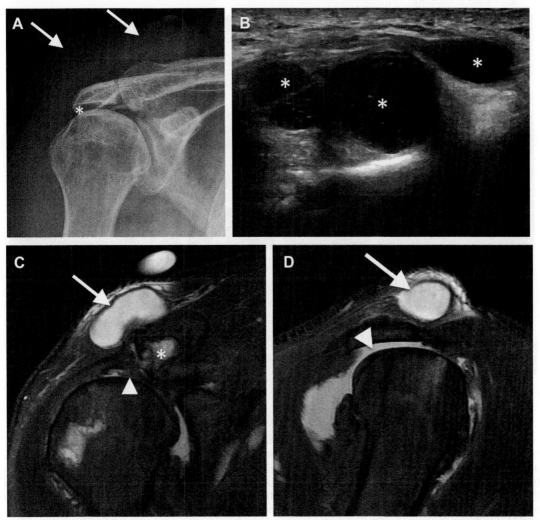

Fig. 12. Acromioclavicular joint (ACJ) geyser cyst in a 77-year-old man. (*A*) Frontal radiograph shows lobulated soft tissue masses superior to the ACJ (*arrows*). There is also loss of the acromiohumeral distance (*asterisk*) and superior humeral head subluxation suspicious for superior rotator cuff tearing. (*B*) Ultrasound shows lobulated cystic lesions superior to the ACJ (*asterisks*). (*C*) Coronal and (*D*) sagittal proton density fat-suppressed MR images confirm the cystic lesions arising superiorly from the ACJ (*arrows*). The cyst exhibits a geyser phenomenon, extending from the glenohumeral joint through a massive superior cuff tear (*arrowheads*), into a degenerative ACJ (subchondral cyst at the distal clavicle [*asterisk*]), and into the superior soft tissues.

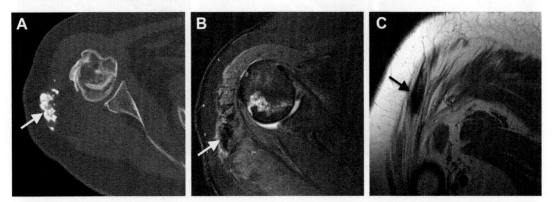

Fig. 13. Deltoid contracture in a 71-year-old woman with a history of humeral fracture complicated by avascular necrosis. (*A*) Axial CT with bone windowing and (*B*) axial proton density fat-suppressed MR image show calcification at the posterolateral deltoid and low signal on MR imaging (*arrows*). (*C*) Coronal T1-weighted MR image shows the characteristic elongated fibrous cord oriented along the fibers of the deltoid muscle (*arrow*).

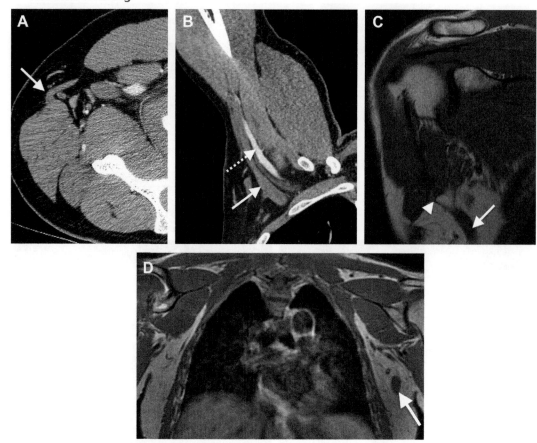

Fig. 14. Axillary arch muscle of Langer. (*A*) Axial CT and (*B*) coronal CT in a 37-year-old man with arms raised show the accessory muscle (*solid arrows*) crossing the axilla in close relation to the neurovascular structures (axillary artery [*dashed arrow* (*B*)]). (*C*) Coronal T1-weighted MR image in a 48-year-old woman shows the accessory muscle (*solid arrow*) crossing the axilla with no compression of the underlying brachial plexus. The muscle has a variety of insertions and in this case appears to blend with the coracobrachialis muscle and fascia (*arrowhead*). (*D*) Coronal T1-weighted MR image in a 59 year old for investigation of a palpable axillary mass shows the lesion to be a unilateral axillary arch muscle (*solid arrow*). As well as mimicking a soft tissue mass on examination, the accessory muscle may also obscure axillary lymph node enlargement. Note the absence of the accessory muscle in the contralateral axilla.

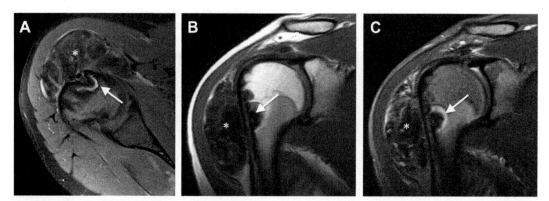

Fig. 15. TGCT in the subacromial-subdeltoid (SASD) bursa in a 30-year-old woman. (*A*) Axial proton density fat-suppressed, (*B*) coronal T1- weighted, and (*C*) proton density fat-suppressed MR images show a lobulated mass within the SASD bursa (*asterisks*). This shows mainly low signal and susceptibility on all sequences with erosions at the lateral humeral head and neck (*arrows*). Additional gradient-echo MR imaging can show blooming artifact in these lesions, although the current images were sufficient for diagnosis. Ultrasound-guided biopsy was performed with TGCT confirmed on histology.

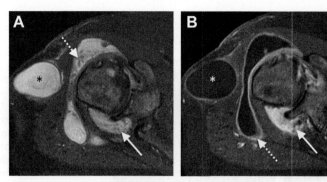

Fig. 16. Tumor-like lesion at the lateral shoulder in a 71-year-old woman with RA. (*A*) Axial proton density fat-suppressed and (*B*) T1-weighted postcontrast fat-suppressed MR images show a lateral subcutaneous cystic lesion (*asterisks*) extending through a mid-deltoid muscle defect (not shown) due to dehiscence of the subacromial-subdeltoid (SASD) bursa. Marked fluid, debris, and enhancing synovium are seen throughout the glenohumeral joint (*solid arrows*) and SASD bursa (*dashed arrows*) due to the underlying inflammatory arthropathy.

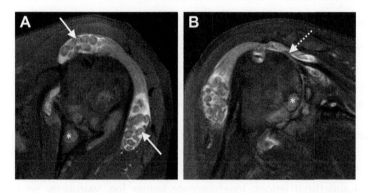

Fig. 17. Fibrinous rice bodies in RA of the shoulder. (*A*) Axial and (*B*) coronal proton density fat-suppressed MR images show fluid distension of the glenohumeral joint and subacromial-subdeltoid bursa (SASD). Internal fibrinous rice bodies are seen due to chronic synovial inflammation (*solid arrows*) with severe erosive glenohumeral arthropathy noted (*asterisks*). The glenohumeral joint and SASD bursa freely communicate through a retracted, full-thickness supraspinatus tendon tear (*dashed arrow*).

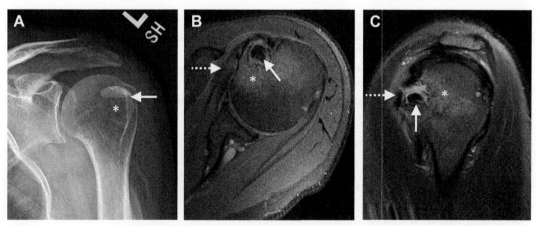

Fig. 18. Active calcium HADD at the subscapularis tendon insertion of a 53-year-old woman. (*A*) Frontal radiograph shows globular calcification (*solid arrow*) projected over the humeral head with surrounding lucency (*asterisk*). (*B*) Axial and (*C*) sagittal T2-weighted fat-suppressed MR images show low-signal intraosseous calcification (*solid arrows*) at the humeral insertion of the subscapularis tendon (*dashed arrows*). There is surrounding soft tissue and intraosseous edema (*asterisks*).

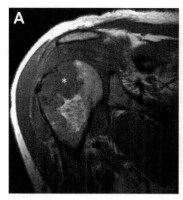 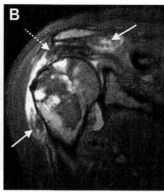

Fig. 19. Amyloid arthropathy. (*A*) Coronal T1-weighted and (*B*) proton density fat-suppressed MR images show an intraosseous lesion within the humeral head and greater tuberosity (*asterisks*). This displays isointense to low T1 signal with mixed T2 signal. There is adjacent bursal and joint fluid with nodular, mainly low-signal synovitis (*solid arrows*). Additional thickening of the supraspinatus tendon is noted (*dashed arrow*) with full-thickness tearing distally.

Box 5
Tumor/tumor-like lesions: what the referring physician needs to know

Suggested diagnostic imaging pathway

Bone lesions

- Radiographs (with or without CT) vital for matrix characterization, for example, chondroid or osteoid
- MR imaging for further characterization and staging of malignant lesions: skip lesions, soft tissue, and joint extension
- CT chest, abdomen, and pelvis or whole-body PET/CT for evaluation of metastases. CT for biopsy and tissue diagnosis of metastases

Soft tissues

- Ultrasound for initial screening of superficial lesions; indeterminate lesions (eg, vascularity on Doppler) or those with deep extent proceed to MR imaging
- MR imaging can visualize fat in lipomatous lesions but is most useful for lesion extent and margins
- Radiographs (with or without CT) useful for detection of calcifications, for example, synovial sarcoma (30% may show calcifications)

Joint and bursal location

- Ultrasound or MR imaging performed for a palpable soft tissue mass can confirm the location in the joint or bursa and readily identify cystic lesions
- MR imaging to assess for associated pathology, for example, rotator cuff tearing and a high-riding humerus in the superior acromioclavicular cyst geyser phenomenon
- Radiographs can demonstrate osteoarthritis or bony erosions in inflammatory arthropathies

What the radiologist needs to know

Accurate history is vital for diagnosis

- A soft tissue lesion after trauma makes myositis ossificans a key differential; otherwise, imaging and histologic appearances can mimic a malignant process. Radiographic follow-up in 2 to 4 weeks demonstrates characteristic peripheral ossification preventing biopsy
- Known arthropathy, dialysis (eg, amyloid), and family history (eg, tumoral calcinosis) are useful in diagnosing articular and periarticular tumor-like lesions

Treatment and management

    Suspected malignant bone and soft tissue tumors are best managed in specialist musculoskeletal oncology centers for biopsy and treatment planning

supraspinatus tendon but can rupture into the joint/bursae with potential osseous and joint destruction, termed *Milwaukee shoulder*. Radiographs can demonstrate HADD deposits as globular calcifications in the rotator cuff or deltoid tendons (see **Fig. 1; Fig. 18**), bursae, or joint capsule.[5,45]

Amyloid arthropathy is a metabolic arthropathy with a propensity for shoulder involvement. The condition is typically secondary to long-standing dialysis and can lead to a destructive arthropathy with large osteolytic lesions (amyloidomas) and sclerotic-rimmed erosions.[46] MR imaging can demonstrate amyloid infiltration as hypointense T1 and variable, mainly hypointense T2 signal soft tissue along the synovium with extension into the bony erosions, bursae, and periarticular soft tissues **(Fig. 19)**. These findings can overlap with those of a hemophilic arthropathy or TGCT, although amyloid does not show blooming on gradient-echo images.[47]

SUMMARY

The shoulder is a common location for tumors and tumor-like lesions arising in the bones, soft tissues, joints, and overlying bursae. Understanding of these common and uncommon lesions can allow accurate diagnosis and appropriate management **(Box 5)**.

CONFLICTS OF INTEREST STATEMENT

None of the authors have conflicts of interest to declare.

REFERENCES

1. Unni KK. Dahlin's bone tumors: general aspects and data on 10,165 cases. 6th edition. Philadelphia: Lippincott Williams & Wilkins; 2009.
2. Ritchie DA, Davies AM. MR imaging of tumors and tumor-like lesions of the shoulder girdle. Magn Reson Imaging Clin N Am 2004;12:125–41.
3. Kransdorf MJ. Benign soft-tissue tumors in a large referral population: distribution of diagnoses by age, sex, and location. AJR Am J Roentgenol 1995;164:395–402.
4. Kransdorf MJ. Malignant soft-tissue tumors in a large referral population: distribution of diagnoses by age, sex, and location. AJR Am J Roentgenol 1995;164:129–34.
5. Anderson SE, Johnston JO, Steinbach LS. Pseudotumors of the shoulder invited review. Eur J Radiol 2008;68:147–58.
6. Campanacci M. Bone and soft tissue tumours: clinical features, imaging, pathology and treatment. 2nd edition. New York: Springer; 1999.
7. Murphey MD, Choi JJ, Kransdorf MJ, et al. Imaging of osteochondroma: variants and complications with radiologic-pathologic correlation. Radiographics 2000;20:1407–34.
8. Mir BA, Wani MM, Halwai MA. Giant osteochondroma of proximal fibula in a skeletally mature patient. Musculoskelet Surg 2011;95:41–4.
9. Murphey MD, Walker EA, Wilson AJ, et al. From the archives of the AFIP: imaging of primary chondrosarcoma: radiologic-pathologic correlation. Radiographics 2003;23:1245–78.
10. Davies M, Cassar-Pullicino VN, Davies AM, et al. The diagnostic accuracy of MR imaging in osteoid osteoma. Skeletal Radiol 2002;31:559–69.
11. Murphey MD, Nomikos GC, Flemming DJ, et al. From the archives of AFIP. Imaging of giant cell tumor and giant cell reparative granuloma of bone: radiologic-pathologic correlation. Radiographics 2001;21:1283–309.
12. Kelle B, Polat Kelle A, Eren Erdoğan K, et al. A rare cause of shoulder pain: monostotic fibrous dysplasia. Arch Rheumatol 2016;31:184–7.
13. Murphey MD, Robbin MR, McRae GA, et al. The many faces of osteosarcoma. Radiographics 1997; 17:1205–31.
14. Rajiah P, Ilaslan H, Sundaram M. Imaging of primary malignant bone tumors (nonhematological). Radiol Clin North Am 2011;49:1135–61.
15. Murphey MD, Flemming DJ, Boyea SR, et al. Enchondroma versus chondrosarcoma in the appendicular skeleton: differentiating features. Radiographics 1998;18:1213–37.
16. Killeen KL. The fallen fragment sign. Radiology 1998;207:261–2.
17. Kransdorf MJ, Sweet DE. Aneurysmal bone cyst: concept, controversy, clinical presentation, and imaging. AJR Am J Roentgenol 1995;164: 573–80.
18. Resnick D, Cone RO 3rd. The nature of humeral pseudocysts. Radiology 1984;150:27–8.
19. Mhuircheartaigh JN, Lin YC, Wu JS. Bone tumor mimickers: a pictorial essay. Indian J Radiol Imaging 2014;24:225–36.
20. Berko NS, Kurian J, Taragin BH, et al. Imaging appearances of musculoskeletal developmental variants in the pediatric population. Curr Probl Diagn Radiol 2015;44:88–104.
21. Inampudi P, Jacobson JA, Fessell DP, et al. Soft-tissue lipomas: accuracy of sonography in diagnosis with pathologic correlation. Radiology 2004;233: 763–7.
22. Gupta P, Potti TA, Wuertzer SD, et al. Spectrum of fat-containing soft-tissue masses at MR imaging: the common, the uncommon, the characteristic,

and the sometimes confusing. Radiographics 2016; 36:753–66.

23. Naylor MF, Nascimento AG, Sherrick AD, et al. Elastofibroma dorsi: radiologic findings in 12 patients. AJR Am J Roentgenol 1996;167:683–7.

24. Burt AM, Huang BK. Imaging review of lipomatous musculoskeletal lesions. SICOT J 2017;3:34.

25. Beggs I. Pictorial review: imaging of peripheral nerve tumours. Clin Radiol 1997;52:8–17.

26. Walker EA, Fenton ME, Salesky JS, et al. Magnetic resonance imaging of benign soft tissue neoplasms in adults. Radiol Clin North Am 2011;49:1197–217.

27. Wu JS, Hochman MG. Soft-tissue tumors and tumor-like lesions: a systematic imaging approach. Radiology 2009;253:297–316.

28. Vanhoenacker FM, Van Looveren K, Trap K, et al. Grading and characterization of soft tissue tumors on magnetic resonance imaging: the value of an expert second opinion report. Insights Imaging 2012;3:131–8.

29. Vanhoenacker FM, Verstraete KL. Soft tissue tumors about the shoulder. Semin Musculoskelet Radiol 2015;19:284–99.

30. Murphey MD, Arcara LK, Fanburg-Smith J. From the archives of the AFIP: imaging of musculoskeletal liposarcoma with radiologic-pathologic correlation. Radiographics 2005;25:1371–95.

31. Murphey MD, Gibson MS, Jennings BT, et al. From the archives of the AFIP: imaging of synovial sarcoma with radiologic-pathologic correlation. Radiographics 2006;26:1543–65.

32. Wasa J, Nishida Y, Tsukushi S, et al. MRI features in the differentiation of malignant peripheral nerve sheath tumors and neurofibromas. AJR Am J Roentgenol 2010;194:1568–74.

33. Murphey MD, Smith WS, Smith SE, et al. From the archives of the AFIP. Imaging of musculoskeletal neurogenic tumors: radiologic-pathologic correlation. Radiographics 1999;19:1253–80.

34. Hiller AD, Miller JD, Zeller JL. Acromioclavicular joint cyst formation. Clin Anat 2010;23:145–52.

35. Lacout A, Jarraya M, Marcy PY, et al. Myositis ossificans imaging: keys to successful diagnosis. Indian J Radiol Imaging 2012;22:35–9.

36. Moser T, Lecours J, Michaud J, et al. The deltoid, a forgotten muscle of the shoulder. Skeletal Radiol 2013;42:1361–75.

37. Huang CC, Ko SF, Ko JY, et al. Contracture of the deltoid muscle: sonographic evaluation with MRI correlation. AJR Am J Roentgenol 2005;185:364–70.

38. Gheno R, Zoner CS, Buck FM, et al. Accessory head of biceps brachii muscle: anatomy, histology, and MRI in cadavers. AJR Am J Roentgenol 2010;194:W80–3.

39. Guy MS, Sandhu SK, Gowdy JM, et al. MRI of the axillary arch muscle: prevalence, anatomic relations, and potential consequences. AJR Am J Roentgenol 2011;196:W52–7.

40. Murphey MD, Rhee JH, Lewis RB, et al. Pigmented villonodular synovitis: radiologic-pathologic correlation. Radiographics 2008;28:1493–518.

41. Serra TQ, Morais J, Gonçalves Z, et al. An unusual case of diffuse pigmented villonodular synovitis of the shoulder: a multidisciplinary approach with arthroscopic synovectomy and adjuvant radiotherapy. Eur J Rheumatol 2017;4:142–4.

42. Masih S, Antebi A. Imaging of pigmented villonodular synovitis. Semin Musculoskelet Radiol 2003;7:205–16.

43. Choi JA, Koh SH, Hong SH, et al. Rheumatoid arthritis and tuberculous arthritis: differentiating MRI features. AJR Am J Roentgenol 2009;193:1347–53.

44. Hermann KG, Backhaus M, Schneider U, et al. Rheumatoid arthritis of the shoulder joint: comparison of conventional radiography, ultrasound, and dynamic contrast-enhanced magnetic resonance imaging. Arthritis Rheum 2003;48:3338–49.

45. Garcia GM, McCord GC, Kumar R. Hydroxyapatite crystal deposition disease. Semin Musculoskelet Radiol 2003;7:187–93.

46. Ross LV, Ross GJ, Mesgarzadeh M, et al. Hemodialysis-related amyloidomas of bone. Radiology 1991; 178:263–5.

47. Kiss E, Keusch G, Zanetti M, et al. Dialysis-related amyloidosis revisited. AJR Am J Roentgenol 2005; 185:1460–7.

Shoulder MR Imaging Versus Ultrasound
How to Choose

David C. Gimarc, MD[a],*, Kenneth S. Lee, MD[b]

KEYWORDS

• Ultrasound • MR imaging • Shoulder • Imaging • Algorithm • Appropriateness

KEY POINTS

• Imaging evaluation of the shoulder is performed using multiple modalities, including ultrasound and MR imaging.
• Ultrasound and MR imaging offer similar diagnostic information in regards to rotator cuff pathology and other soft tissues, although they differ in their technique, indications, and interpretation.
• A thorough understanding of these differences is imperative to appropriately use these modalities in clinical practice, including the unique interventional opportunities available with US.

INTRODUCTION

Shoulder pain accounts for a substantial proportion of patient visits to primary care providers and orthopedic and sports medicine specialists,[1] affecting up to 20% of the general population[2] and more commonly in women.[3] The initial evaluation of acute or chronic shoulder pain follows a similar approach to other musculoskeletal complaints, beginning with a focused history and physical examination. Clinicians are often able to create a differential diagnosis of the causes of shoulder pain and dysfunction based on their clinical assessment. The next step often leads to radiographs followed by the possibility of further advanced imaging if necessary.

Nonspecific shoulder pain most commonly is related to rotator cuff disease in nearly two-thirds of patients, although can also be attributed to other etiologies, such as labral tear, tendinosis, osteoarthritis, adhesive capsulitis, and referred pain from the neck.[4] Certain entities are more common in specific age groups; for example, degeneration of the rotator cuff and cartilage are more prevalent in older patients.[5] Although traumatic injuries can affect patients of all ages, the degenerated soft tissues are more prone to rotator cuff injury with less healing potential.

This article reviews ultrasound (US) and MR imaging evaluation of the shoulder, with a focus on the differences in technique, indications, and interpretation. In addition, we discuss the advantages of US, specifically dynamic evaluation of soft tissue structures and interventional procedures.

SHOULDER PATHOLOGY

The glenohumeral articulation is one of the least constrained articulations in the body,[6] thus requiring a unique balance of the stabilizing fibrocartilaginous labrum, rotator cuff muscles, and surrounding ligamentous and capsular attachments. A weakness or injury to any one of these components places increased strain on other components leading to a rapid progression of degeneration and instability.[7]

[a] Department of Radiology, University of Colorado School of Medicine, 12401 E. 17th Avenue, Mail Stop L954, Aurora, CO 80045, USA; [b] Department of Radiology, University of Wisconsin School of Medicine and Public Health, 600 Highland Avenue, E3/342, Madison, WI 53792, USA
* Corresponding author.
E-mail address: david.gimarc@cuanschutz.edu

Magn Reson Imaging Clin N Am 28 (2020) 317–330
https://doi.org/10.1016/j.mric.2019.12.012
1064-9689/20/© 2019 Elsevier Inc. All rights reserved.

The tendon unit is created by parallel collagen fibers, which are imaged and evaluated by either MR imaging or US. In younger patients, the tendon is strong, and patients generally suffer injuries as a result of acute trauma placing abnormal stress on otherwise healthy structures, such as the labrum.[8]

The normal fibrillar tendon architecture begins to degenerate with age, leading to tendon thickening and fiber disorganization, or tendinosis. Tendinosis may be painful and weakens the tendon, and if exposed to increased mechanical forces, the degenerated tendon is prone to rupture.

The fibrocartilage labrum deepens the glenoid articular surface to help increase stability of the glenohumeral articulation.[9] Although the posterior labrum is visualized by US, it remains limited in its ability to reliably visualize labral tears and cartilage degeneration.[10] However, US may show secondary signs of a labral tear, such as a paralabral cyst within the spinoglenoid notch (**Fig. 1**). MR arthrography is the gold standard for the diagnosis of labral tears, and should remain the optimal modality for labral tear evaluation.[11,12]

IMAGING MODALITIES
Radiographs

Radiography is an important initial imaging evaluation that is inexpensive, fast, and provides an important evaluation of osseous structures and alignment. In addition to osseous pathology, secondary signs of soft tissue pathology are seen on radiographs leading to a suspected diagnosis, such as calcific tendinosis or a chronic rotator cuff tear resulting in a decreased acromiohumeral distance.[13] Based on the clinical scenario, and in combination with patient symptoms and physical examination findings, clinicians often choose to pursue further imaging to evaluate soft tissue pathology of the shoulder.

Ultrasound

US evaluation of the shoulder was introduced in 1977,[14] and has increased in utility in the past few years, although it still represents a minority of advanced shoulder imaging.[15] US provides excellent spatial resolution of soft tissues, such as tendons and muscles, but poor visualization of bone because of its high attenuation coefficient,[16] and intra-articular structures, such as the labrum and articular cartilage. The fibrillar composition of myotendinous units and their superficial location within the body make for exceptional imaging quality and spatial resolution with US, to a higher degree than can currently be performed with MR imaging.[17] US is also well-suited for looking for the presence of fluid within and surrounding a joint, such as an effusion or bursitis.[18] Another advantage of US is its dynamic capability to evaluate for subacromial impingement, biceps tendon subluxation, and AC joint separation. The real-time capability of US also enables US-guided procedures for the skilled radiologist. Patient satisfaction is often increased when a clinically indicated US-guided injection is performed on the same day as a diagnostic US examination.

MR Imaging

MR imaging is largely considered to be the gold standard for noninvasive evaluation of the shoulder for its superior soft tissue contrast and large field of view to adequately evaluate soft tissues, such as the tendons, muscles, and labrum. Unlike US, MR imaging is superior at visualizing osseous structures, bone marrow, and overlying cartilage. Orthopedic surgeons also often prefer MR imaging over US for the evaluation of the shoulder.

SHOULDER IMAGING ALGORITHM

In 2011, the Society of Radiologists in Ultrasound created a consensus committee document outlining a proposed algorithm for the use of advanced imaging techniques in the clinical evaluation of shoulder pathology, specifically in the setting of suspected rotator cuff disease.[19] The panel included experts from various medical subspecialties, and categorized recommendations

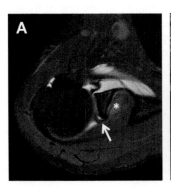
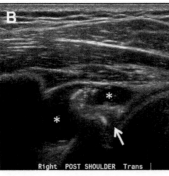

Fig. 1. Paralabral cyst in a 48-year-old man. (*A*) MR imaging axial T1 fat-saturated sequence after intra-articular gadolinium injection, and (*B*) transverse US of the posterior shoulder on the same patient demonstrate a paralabral cyst within the spinoglenoid notch (*asterisks*) denoting a posterior labral tear (*arrows*), although the tear is not well-visualized on the US. Note the cyst does not fill with intra-articular contrast.

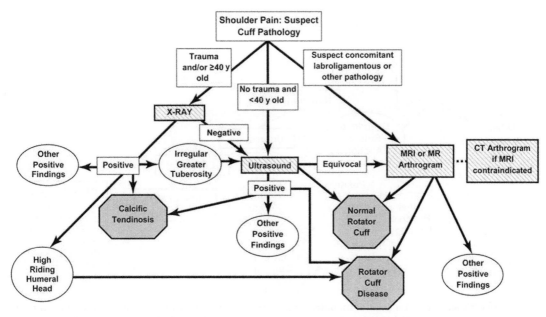

Fig. 2. Diagnostic algorithm for painful native shoulders suspected of having rotator cuff pathology. CT, computed tomography. (*From* Nazarian LN, Jacobson JA, Benson CB, et al. Imaging algorithms for evaluating suspected rotator cuff disease: Society of Radiologists in Ultrasound consensus conference statement. Radiology 2013;267(2):592; with permission.)

into patients with native shoulders, those who have undergone rotator cuff repair, and those with prosthetic glenohumeral joints. The subsequent report was created with respect to the American College of Radiology Appropriateness Criteria to help providers decide between ordering MR imaging or US of the shoulder for their patients.[20]

Shoulder Pain with Suspected Rotator Cuff Pathology

The algorithm for native (no history of prior surgery) shoulder divides shoulder pain in the setting of suspected rotator cuff pathology into post-traumatic and older patients (greater than 40 years old), and younger patients with suspected concomitant labral pathology (**Fig. 2**). Because the labrum is not well evaluated with US, these younger patients were recommended to directly proceed to MR imaging. Otherwise, older patients should initially be evaluated with radiographs, followed by US for continued concern for cuff pathology. These patients would only move on to MR imaging following an US if their examination was considered "equivocal." Additionally, if there were findings on the radiographs that would prompt a concordant diagnosis (eg, calcific tendinosis), this would obviate further diagnostic imaging.

Shoulder Pain After Rotator Cuff Repair

In patients with a history of a rotator cuff repair, initial radiographs are indicated for evaluation of joint and hardware alignment, and for any osteoarthritis that could be contributing to pain. If the initial radiograph did not clearly demonstrate secondary evidence of a recurrent rotator cuff tear then US is recommended as the next imaging step. As before, MR imaging was only recommended if the US was equivocal (**Fig. 3**).

Shoulder Pain After Joint Arthroplasty

For patients with pain after an arthroplasty, a radiograph is recommended as the first step to evaluate for obvious hardware complications. Otherwise, US is recommended for evaluation of the rotator cuff, with MR imaging recommended only if the US was equivocal (**Fig. 4**).

CONTRAINDICATIONS

The contraindications for MR imaging have been well-documented[21] and largely relate to the safety of placing a patient in a high-field-strength magnetic bore with varying field gradients related to hardware, implanted devices, or thermal injury from metallic objects within these fields. Additionally, some patients are unable to tolerate an examination because of their size, problems with claustrophobia and anxiety, or inability to hold still

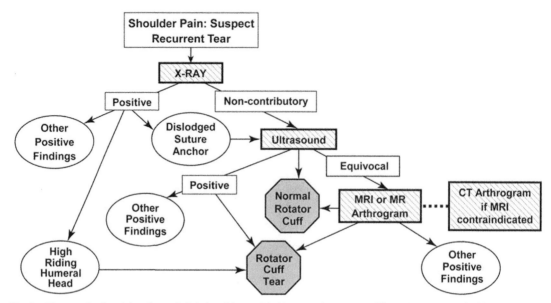

Fig. 3. Diagnostic algorithm for painful shoulders with history of rotator cuff repair suspected of having recurrent abnormality. CT, computed tomography. (*From* Nazarian LN, Jacobson JA, Benson CB, et al. Imaging algorithms for evaluating suspected rotator cuff disease: Society of Radiologists in Ultrasound consensus conference statement. Radiology 2013;267(2):593; with permission.)

for the duration of certain sequences. Although routine MR imaging examinations of the extremities do not require gadolinium-based imaging contrast agents, the use of gadolinium contrast for MR arthrograms or more specialized MR imaging examinations may also limit the number of eligible patients to receive this medication safely.

However, US has no absolute contraindications aside from the clinical stability of a patient to be able to sit through an examination.[17] Obese patients with more subcutaneous fat attenuate more of the sound waves, thus losing more acoustic

signal from deeper structures, which can limit the diagnostic performance of the examination (**Fig. 5**). Although these images may be suboptimal, US still provides an option for patients who would otherwise not be able to obtain MR imaging.

In addition, US is a portable modality that can easily be transported around a hospital, clinic, or even between different sites. For example, the utility of US in sports has increased substantially because it is quickly performed, and is easily portable to fit the needs of athletes and teams on the sidelines.[22]

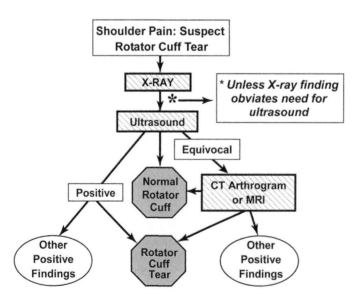

Fig. 4. Diagnostic algorithm for painful shoulders suspected of having rotator cuff pathology after arthroplasty. CT, computed tomography. (*From* Nazarian LN, Jacobson JA, Benson CB, et al. Imaging algorithms for evaluating suspected rotator cuff disease: Society of Radiologists in Ultrasound consensus conference statement. Radiology 2013;267(2):593; with permission.)

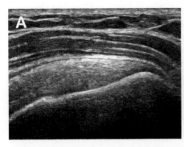
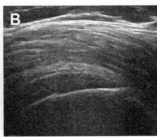

Fig. 5. Patient selection: body habitus. Long-axis US images of the supraspinatus tendon in a (*A*) thinner patient and (*B*) obese patient shows differences in imaging quality because of reduced penetration of the acoustic beam through thicker soft tissues. A lower transducer frequency is often required, resulting in lower spatial resolution.

TECHNIQUE CONSIDERATIONS
MR Imaging

Most institutions have a standard multiplanar, multisequence imaging protocol specifically for evaluation of the rotator cuff, labrum, and articular cartilage.[23] Because of continued advancements in sequence optimization and efficiency, the standard MR imaging protocol takes approximately 15 to 20 minutes to perform, in addition to 10 to 15 minutes of extra time for setup and repeated sequences. Some institutions have even begun to consider using rapid protocols that take up to 5 minutes, which have initially shown equivalent accuracy and interreader agreement to conventional MR imaging shoulder protocols.[24]

Ultrasound

US, however, is much more operator-dependent in terms of obtaining high-quality images that lead to accurate interpretation of pathology. Institutions with high-volume musculoskeletal (MSK) US examinations generally have dedicated MSK sonographers with special training in imaging joints and extremities. In recent times, specialty training of sonographers in MSK imaging has become more popular as MSK US has shown increased use.[25] Much like MR imaging, US evaluation of the shoulder follows a standard protocol of required images and planes to carefully evaluate all components of the joint.[9] In the hands of a skilled MSK sonographer, the standard shoulder US examination should take approximately 15 to 20 minutes to perform, and requires the patient to adopt several shoulder positions, which accentuates anatomy to locations that are superficial and more-easily imaged.

After the initial examination, the sonographer reviews the images with the interpreting radiologist, and more images are obtained if there are further questions or clarifications. The radiologist also has an opportunity to scan themselves should they wish to clarify findings in real time. With MR imaging, this postexamination review is not often performed. Also if there are quality issues with

the sequences obtained (eg, artifacts), the patient may have to be brought back to repeat portions of the examination.

Patients report better satisfaction scores with US in comparison with MR imaging because of the pain and discomfort encountered during the examination, and perceived length of the examination.[26] More patients report that they were willing to have the examination performed again with US, as opposed to those who had MR imaging.[26]

Standard Ultrasound Shoulder Examination

The standard US examination is performed with the patient sitting upright on a chair or swivel stool. When unable to sit upright, patients can also be examined laying down with a foam cushion placed under the patient's side as to allow the ipsilateral arm to be mobilized for evaluation of the rotator cuff. A linear, high-frequency transducer is generally used because most structures are superficially located.[27] This allows for exquisite detail of the tendon and muscle, to a greater degree than could be seen on MR imaging.[28]

Multiple shoulder positions have been well-described for optimal evaluation of each rotator cuff tendon, such as the Crass or modified Crass positions.[29] Although many patients are able to adopt these positions easily, some may have difficulty because of severe pain or frail state. Even with these limitations, a satisfactorily diagnostic examination can usually still be performed to accommodate patient discomfort, such as lying the patient supine on a stretcher and partially rolling the patient away from the sonographer to bring the rotator cuff anteriorly. In addition to these standard positions, additional maneuvers are also dynamically performed and recorded to assess for physiologic pathology that would only be evaluated during active movement, such as impingement assessment.[9]

ROTATOR CUFF TEARS

The workhorse of MR imaging and US evaluation of the shoulder involves imaging of the rotator

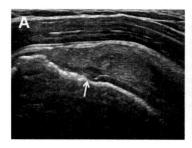
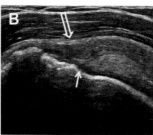

Fig. 6. Full-thickness rotator cuff tear with compression in a 71-year-old woman. Long-axis US images of the supraspinatus tendon (*A*) without and (*B*) with transducer compression shows dipping of the overlying deltoid muscle (*open arrow*) causing the full-thickness tear to become more apparent (*solid arrows*).

cuff tendons for tears or tendinopathy. Both modalities offer excellent visualization of the tendon size, integrity, and architecture. In addition to evaluation of the tendon itself, secondary evidence and predisposing features of larger or chronic tears, such as muscle atrophy, is visualized. Osseous features of subacromial impingement can also be easily evaluated. In combination, both of these elements can affect therapeutic options.

The multiplanar imaging of MR imaging offers a three-dimensional evaluation of all rotator cuff tendons from their myotendinous junction to the insertion on the greater and lesser tuberosity. The oblique course of the distal rotator cuff tendons, specifically the superior cuff, may lead to magic angle artifact when the tendon passes at a 55-degree angle to B_0 with respect to the magnetic field in structures with highly organized structures in parallel orientation, such as tendon fibers. This is specifically problematic in short-TE sequences, such as T1-weighted and proton-density-weighted acquisitions.[30,31]

US evaluation of the rotator cuff requires the patient to adopt multiple shoulder positions to accentuate each tendon, as previously described.[9,29] The parallel and highly organized nature of these tendons can lead to a well-known artifact known as anisotropy, where the tendon appears falsely hypoechoic when the transducer is not positioned perpendicular to the tendon of interest.[27,28,32,33] Fortunately, this artifact is well-known and is actively corrected, by "toggling" the transducer during the examination to reduce the risk of a false-positive diagnosis of tendinosis or tendon tear.

US also allows for dynamic compression of a suspected rotator cuff tear in real-time scanning. When a tear is present, the soft tissue (usually bursa) filling the torn tendon gap is compressed showing a characteristic dip in the deltoid and bursa in the tear defect (**Fig. 6**).

As a secondary sign on radiographs and US, cortical irregularities of the greater tuberosity footprint have been shown to be an indicator of an underlying partial- or full-thickness rotator cuff tear.[34] Sonographically, these are shown by a loss of the normal smooth contour of the underlying cortical surface, prompting careful investigation of the rotator cuff tendons (**Fig. 7**).

Sequela of chronic rotator cuff tears can also be easily seen on US and MR imaging including fatty infiltration of the muscle bellies.[35] Orthopedic surgeons often require evaluation of rotator cuff integrity and muscle composition for surgical management. Initially, fatty infiltration of the rotator cuff musculature was described and categorized using computed tomography evaluation,[36] although this has been extrapolated to MR imaging and US with similar efficacy, specifically when evaluating the supraspinatus muscle (**Fig. 8**).[37]

Because most degenerative tears are now thought to involve the junction of the posterior supraspinatus and anterior infraspinatus tendons, the superficial location of these muscles allows for easy visualization of the tendons. The integrity of these tendons seems to be a reliable surrogate for overall rotator cuff health, thus predicting postoperative outcomes for patients undergoing rotator cuff repair and joint replacement surgery.[38–40] When evaluating the rotator cuff muscles using US, capturing the cross-section of the supraspinatus and infraspinatus in one image is recommended using the extended field of view capability.[41] This allows for immediate comparison between the supraspinatus and infraspinatus muscle bellies for fatty infiltration and muscle atrophy. Contralateral comparison may also be necessary in case the supraspinatus and infraspinatus demonstrate fatty atrophy.

Comparison of Ultrasound and MR Imaging Evaluation of the Rotator Cuff

Multiple studies have been performed demonstrating the accuracy of rotator cuff US in comparison with MR imaging using arthroscopy as the gold standard.[42] US and MR imaging remain highly accurate in the diagnosis of full-thickness rotator

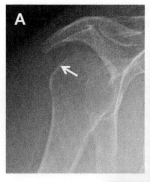 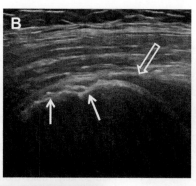

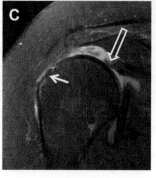

Fig. 7. Humeral head irregularity related to rotator cuff tendinopathy in an 81-year-old woman. (*A*) An anteroposterior oblique radiograph, (*B*) long-axis US view of the supraspinatus tendon, and (*C*) coronal T2 fat-saturated view of the shoulder on the same patient demonstrate irregularity of the humeral head cortex (*solid arrows*) related to a chronic, full-thickness supraspinatus rotator cuff tear (*open arrow*).

cuff tears. US also shows good diagnostic accuracy in the detection of partial-thickness tears, similar to MR imaging (**Figs. 9** and **10**).[28,43,44] MR arthrography maintains a slightly higher diagnostic accuracy of full- and partial-thickness tears in comparison with conventional MR imaging and US but is invasive.[45] As previously discussed, MR imaging and US also show equivalent accuracy in the evaluation of rotator cuff musculature for atrophy and fatty infiltration.[37]

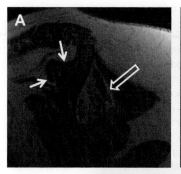 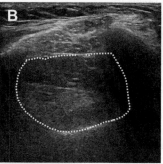

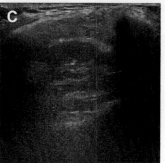

Fig. 8. Fatty infiltration and atrophy in a 66-year-old man. (*A*) Sagittal T1 MR imaging sequence demonstrates mild fatty atrophy of the supraspinatus muscle (*solid arrows*). (*B*) Long-axis ultrasound images of the left abnormal and (*C*) right normal supraspinatus muscles demonstrates mild fatty replacement and more echogenic appearance of the left supraspinatus muscle (surrounded by *dashed line*) related to a full-thickness tendon tear, in comparison with the normal right side. Note moderate atrophy of the infraspinatus muscle and on the MR imaging (*open arrow*).

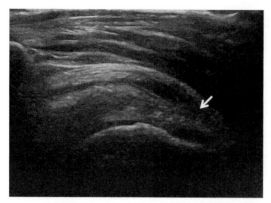

Fig. 9. Partial rotator cuff tear in a 69-year-old woman. Long-axis US image of the infraspinatus tendon shows irregularity and tearing along the bursal surface of the tendon, compatible with a low-grade partial-thickness tear of the bursal sided fibers (*arrow*).

BICEPS TENDON PATHOLOGY

The long and short heads of the biceps brachii tendon are unique because they are one of the few muscle-tendon units in the body that spans multiple consecutive articulations (shoulder and elbow).[46] Much like the rotator cuff, the tendon is subject to degeneration and tearing. Clinicians are often tasked with determining if a biceps tear is present within the proximal portion near the shoulder or distally near its insertion at the elbow.

The intra-articular portion of the long head biceps tendon (LHBT) is a complex structure extending from the biceps anchor to the pulley region composed of multiple components, including ligamentous, synovial, and labral. Although the extra-articular portion of the LHBT can easily be seen with US in select patients, thorough evaluation of the full tendon, including the intra-articular portions, is best performed with MR imaging, often using MR arthrography.[47]

US has shown excellent accuracy at evaluating normal tendons and full-thickness tears of the LHBT, but is less reliable in the diagnosis of partial-thickness tendon tears and nontear pathology (**Fig. 11**).[48] Evaluation of the proximal LHBT is

difficult on MR imaging because of the oblique positioning of the tendon on nearly all sequences rendering it vulnerable to magic-angle artifact on shorter and intermediate-TE sequences.[31]

SUBACROMIAL-SUBDELTOID BURSITIS

The subacromial-subdeltoid bursa is the largest bursa in the body, and can demonstrate distention with fluid, bursal wall thickening, and hyperemia in the setting of suspected symptomatic bursitis. Additionally, fluid distending the bursa can also communicate with the glenohumeral joint space in the setting of a full-thickness rotator cuff tear.[49] Bursal fluid is easily assessed on US by evaluating over the greater tuberosity, and along the anterior and posterior humeral head.[9] MR imaging clearly shows fluid within the bursa, specifically on fluid-sensitive, fat-saturated sequences (**Fig. 12**).[50]

OSTEOARTHRITIS

Degenerative joint disease involving the glenohumeral and acromioclavicular articulations is a common and debilitating cause of symptoms in the aging population. Although the glenohumeral cartilage is well-evaluated on MR imaging, the diagnosis is generally established by radiographs alone.[51] Secondary signs of osteoarthritis can also be seen on US, such as marginal osteophytes, intra-articular bodies, and joint effusion, but should not be the primary modality.

DYNAMIC ASSESSMENT

US provides a clear advantage for its real-time capability to assess for impingement, tendon subluxation, and dislocation during dynamic maneuvers. Although multiple investigational studies have begun to show the utility of dynamic MR imaging sequences (eg, cardiac MR imaging), standard imaging protocols continue to use only static sequences.[52] Although not dynamic, some static MR imaging sequences are performed with unique positional maneuvers to accentuate various pathologies.[53]

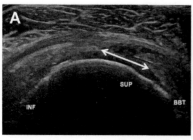
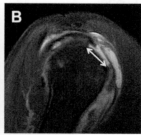

Fig. 10. Full-thickness rotator cuff tear in a 55-year-old woman. (*A*) Short-axis US of the superior cuff and (*B*) sagittal T2 fat-saturated image of the cuff demonstrate a similar appearance of a full-thickness tear involving the anterior and midsupraspinatus tendon (*arrows*). BBT, long head biceps tendon; INF, infraspinatus; SUP, supraspinatus.

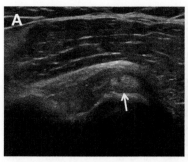
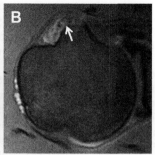

Fig. 11. Biceps tendon partial tear with medial subluxation in a 58-year-old man. (*A*) Short-axis US image of the proximal extra-articular biceps tendon, and (*B*) axial proton-density fat-saturated MR imaging image of the same patient demonstrates high-grade partial tearing and medial subluxation of the long head biceps tendon (*arrows*).

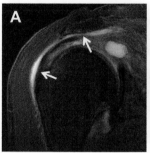
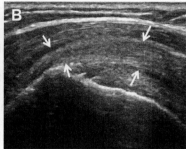

Fig. 12. Subacromial-subdeltoid bursitis in a 49-year-old woman. (*A*) Coronal T2 fat-saturated MR imaging sequence, and (*B*) long-axis US image of the supraspinatus tendon demonstrates bursal wall thickening and distention with fluid (*arrows*) in the setting of imaging and clinical bursitis.

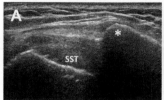
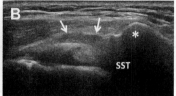

Fig. 13. Subacromial impingement in a 60-year-old woman. Longitudinal ultrasound images at the lateral margin of the acromion (*asterisk*) in (*A*) neutral and (*B*) abducted positions demonstrate bunching of bursal soft tissues in the abducted position (*arrows*), compatible with soft tissue impingement. SST, supraspinatus tendon.

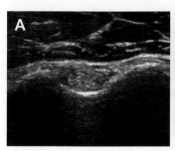
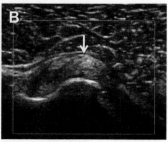

Fig. 14. Normal biceps position with subluxation. (*A*) Short-axis US images of the proximal extra-articular long head biceps tendon demonstrates normal positioning of the tendon in the bicipital groove. (*B*) In a different patient, a 63-year-old woman, external rotation of the arm during dynamic evaluation demonstrates medial subluxation of the tendon (*arrow*) caused by a partial-thickness subscapularis tendon tear.

Subacromial Impingement

Dynamic imaging with US can assess for subacromial impingement.[54] The US probe is placed long axis to the supraspinatus tendon just lateral to the acromial margin. With arm abduction and thumb pointing down, US can show bunching of the fluid-filled or thickened bursa (soft tissue impingement), the superior cuff, and/or superior elevation of the humeral head (osseous impingement) preventing further abduction (**Fig. 13**).[54] Additionally, the operator is able to directly ask the patient regarding associated pain during the maneuver, because not all impingement is shown to be symptomatic.[55]

Long Head Biceps Tendon Subluxation/Dislocation

As the humeral head undergoes internal and external rotation, the extra-articular LHBT can subluxate or even dislocate medially from the bicipital groove, usually with a concomitant injury to the adjacent subscapularis tendon as it continues from the lesser to the greater tuberosities as the transverse ligament.[56] This is visualized using dynamic US while the patient internally and externally rotates their arm with the elbow flexed at 90° (**Fig. 14**).[57] The static axial MR imaging sequence is generally performed in external rotation, and may result in a false-negative evaluation for LHBT stability.[58,59]

THE POSTOPERATIVE SHOULDER

Both MR imaging and US are used for imaging the postoperative shoulder, either after glenohumeral arthroplasty or a rotator cuff tendon repair. The metal from the joint prosthesis or rotator cuff suture anchor can result in susceptibility artifact on MR imaging, which can reduce diagnostic accuracy. Studies have shown high accuracy rates for the use of US in the rotator cuff repair population, approaching those of nonoperative shoulder,[60] and high accuracy for the evaluation of rotator cuff tears after joint arthroplasty.[61]

COST CONSIDERATIONS

As the health care system faces increased financial and resource burden, it is important to consider the costs of ordering various diagnostic studies. Although the exact cost of a service varies widely with different facility types, insurance providers, and reimbursement schedules, MR imaging consistently costs more than US, which often results in increased cost to the patient.[25] According to a 2016 single-state fee schedule, a routine MR imaging shoulder can cost USD $1400 to $2000.[62] The national average of the Medicare Physician Fee Schedule for shoulder MR imaging can cost up to USD $380, in comparison with a complete shoulder US costing approximately USD $120.[63,64]

However, US is time intensive and operator dependent, which are clear disadvantages compared with MR imaging. Radiologists often find it easier and quicker to read several MR imaging examinations than to perform just one diagnostic US over the same amount of time. MSK imaging is projected to account for $3.6 billion by 2020, with MR imaging accounting for greater than 55% of this cost.[65] With appropriate use of US instead of MR imaging, this could account for a substantial savings of an already strained health care system.[66] Although time intensive and at a lower cost, US may help provide value by adding to the complement of MSK imaging tools in a busy radiology clinical practice. Specifically, when patients are thought to have a full-thickness rotator cuff (supraspinatus) tear, both methods are thought to be cost-effective options for diagnosis.[67] An imaging center or organization must choose the most appropriate study based on their resource availability and clinical workflow.

INTERVENTION

MR imaging examinations provide static views of the patient's anatomy, which is generally interpreted after the completion of the examination. US, however, allows for the real-time interpretation of the examination, and if desired, a therapeutic intervention can also be performed at the same time after simple preparation in a matter of minutes. The following are examples of the most

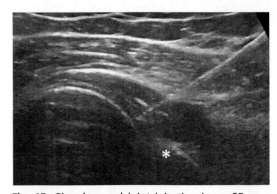

Fig. 15. Glenohumeral joint injection in an 85-year-old woman. US-guided injection of anesthetic and steroid via a posterior approach with a 22-gauge, 3.5-inch needle in plane with the transducer, into the posterior glenohumeral joint space. Note the posterior labrum is avoided (*asterisk*).

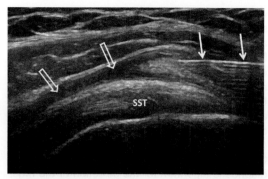

Fig. 16. Subacromial-subdeltoid bursal injection in a 41-year-old woman. US guidance over the anterolateral shoulder shows a 22-gauge, 1.5-inch needle (*solid arrows*) distending the subacromial-subdeltoid bursa (*open arrows*) with steroid and local anesthetic. SST, supraspinatus tendon.

commonly performed US-guided interventions in our clinic.

Glenohumeral Joint Injection

In the setting of osteoarthritis, labral tear, adhesive capsulitis, or rotator cuff tendinopathy, clinicians may order a therapeutic injection of steroid and anesthetic into the glenohumeral joint space.

Although this is often performed under fluoroscopic guidance, it can easily be performed under sonographic guidance, and has been shown to be a cost-effective treatment method in certain populations, such as those with adhesive capsulitis.[68] Generally, this is best performed by a posterior approach placing the needle tip at the posteromedial humeral head along the posterior joint space (**Fig. 15**).[69] The injected solution is easily seen flowing into the posterior joint recess. In patients with contrast allergies, this is an equally effective alternative that requires no contrast agent to confirm intra-articular location.

Bursal Injection

Subacromial-subdeltoid bursitis is a common entity that is treated by an injection of steroid and anesthetic directly into the bursa. Although some clinicians choose to perform a blind injection technique in their offices, US-guided injection has shown superior accuracy and better symptomatic improvement in patients with shoulder pain.[70] Visualization of injected solution appropriately placed into the bursa also allows the clinician to exclude an incorrectly positioned injection should symptomatic relief not meet expectations (**Fig. 16**).[70]

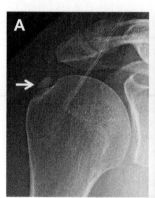
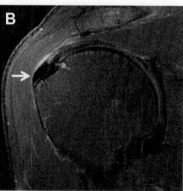
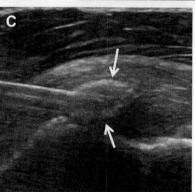

Fig. 17. Calcific lavage in a 67-year-old man. (*A*) Grashey radiograph and (*B*) coronal T2 fat-saturated MR imaging sequence show a focus of calcium hydroxyapatite deposition within the supraspinatus tendon at the footprint (*arrows*). (*C*) US shows 18-gauge, 3.5-inch needle placement within the deposit during percutaneous lavage.

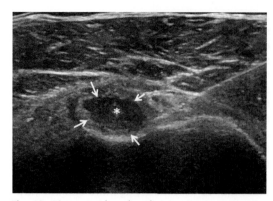

Fig. 18. Biceps tendon sheath injection in a 37-year-old woman. A 22-gauge, 1.5-inch needle is placed within the lateral and deep aspect of the bicipital groove, and distends the biceps tendon sheath (*arrows*) surrounding the long head biceps tendon (*asterisk*) with steroid and anesthetic.

Calcific Tendinitis Lavage

The diagnosis of calcific tendinitis is easily evaluated with MR imaging and US, demonstrating the size, location, and symptomatic nature of suspected calcium hydroxyapatite deposits usually first identified on radiographs.[71] If lavage is desired, this is easily performed under US-guidance.[72] During the procedure, a larger-gauge needle is placed into the center of the hydroxyapatite deposit, and the operator pulse-injects a solution of saline and anesthetic to break up and eventually aspirate the focus, which is watched on dynamic US (**Fig. 17**). Subsequently, a solution containing a steroid and anesthetic is placed into the overlying subacromial-subdeltoid bursa to hasten pain relief and prevent bursitis.[72–74]

Biceps Tendon Sheath Injection

In the setting of symptomatic biceps tendinopathy or tenosynovitis, clinicians may request for steroids and anesthetic to be injected directly into the LHBT sheath under US-guidance (**Fig. 18**). Of note, the biceps tendon sheath is an intra-articular, extrasynovial extension of the joint space that regularly communicates with the remainder of the glenohumeral joint space. However, studies have shown that most of the injected solution remains locally within the sheath when smaller volumes are injected.[47,75]

SUMMARY

For the evaluation of shoulder pain, radiographs, US, and MR imaging demonstrate well-described indications and benefits. US and MR imaging can often demonstrate similar diagnostic capabilities

with respect to the rotator cuff and surrounding soft tissues, with key differences related to their acquisition, technique, and limitations. Although MR imaging is a ubiquitous resource to many clinicians, US is limited to trained sonographers and radiologists who have experience in interpreting these studies. Advantages of US include dynamic assessments and interventional techniques for immediate pain relief.

The 2011 Society of Radiologists in Ultrasound Consensus Conference Statement[19] provides a diagnostic algorithm for the selection of the most appropriate imaging study in the setting of shoulder pain.

DISCLOSURE

D.C. Gimarc: none. K.S. Lee: grants from NBA/GE, Mitek; research support from SuperSonic Imagine; and royalties from Elsevier.

REFERENCES

1. Parsons S, Breen A, Foster NE, et al. Prevalence and comparative troublesomeness by age of musculoskeletal pain in different body locations. Fam Pract 2007;24(4):308–16.
2. Vecchio P, Kavanagh R, Hazleman BL, et al. Shoulder pain in a community-based rheumatology clinic. Rheumatology 1995;34(5):440–2.
3. Costa ML, Achten J, Parsons NR, et al. UK DRAFFT - A randomised controlled trial of percutaneous fixation with kirschner wires versus volar locking-plate fixation in the treatment of adult patients with a dorsally displaced fracture of the distal radius. BMC Musculoskelet Disord 2011;12:201.
4. Mitchell C, Adebajo A, Hay E, et al. Shoulder pain: diagnosis and management in primary care. BMJ 2005;331(7525):1124–8.
5. Tuite MJ, Small KM. Imaging evaluation of nonacute shoulder pain. Am J Roentgenol 2017;209(3):525–33.
6. Veeger HEJ, Van Der Helm FCT. Shoulder function: the perfect compromise between mobility and stability. J Biomech 2007;40:2119–29.
7. Ludewig PM, Reynolds JF. The association of scapular kinematics and glenohumeral joint pathologies. J Orthop Sports Phys Ther 2009;39(2):90–104.
8. Flores DV, Mejía Gómez C, Estrada-Castrillón M, et al. MR imaging of muscle trauma: anatomy, biomechanics, pathophysiology, and imaging appearance. Radiographics 2017;38(1):124–48.
9. Lee MH, Sheehan SE, Orwin JF, et al. Comprehensive shoulder US examination: a standardized approach with multimodality correlation for common shoulder disease. Radiographics 2016;36(6):1606–27.

10. Krzyżanowski W, Tarczyńska M. The use of ultrasound in the assessment of the glenoid labrum of the glenohumeral joint. Part II: examples of labral pathologies. J Ultrason 2012;12(50):329–41.

11. Waldt S, Burkart A, Lange P, et al. Diagnostic performance of MR arthrography in the assessment of lesions of the shoulder. Am J Roentgenol 2004; 182(April 2002):1271–8.

12. Magee T. 3-T MRI of the shoulder: is MR arthrography necessary? Am J Roentgenol 2009;192(1):86–92.

13. Saupe N, Pfirrmann CWA, Schmid MR, et al. Association between rotator cuff abnormalities and reduced acromiohumeral distance. Am J Roentgenol 2006;187(2):376–82.

14. Mayer V. Ultrasonography of the rotator cuff. J Ultrasound Med 1985;4(11):608.

15. Zappia M, Aliprandi A, Pozza S, et al. How is shoulder ultrasound done in Italy? A survey of clinical practice. Skeletal Radiol 2016;45(12):1629–34.

16. Ziskin MC. Fundamental physics of ultrasound and its propagation in tissue. Radiographics 1993;13(3): 705–9.

17. Nazarian LN. The top 10 reasons musculoskeletal sonography is an important complementary or alternative technique to MRI. Am J Roentgenol 2008; 190(6):1621–6.

18. Fessell DP, Jacobson JA, Craig J, et al. Using sonography to reveal and aspirate joint effusions. Am J Roentgenol 2000;174(5):1353–62.

19. Nazarian LN, Jacobson JA, Benson CB, et al. Imaging algorithms for evaluating suspected rotator cuff disease: Society of Radiologists in Ultrasound consensus conference statement. Radiology 2013; 267(2):589–95.

20. American College of Radiology. ACR appropriateness criteria: shoulder pain-traumatic and atraumatic. Reston (VA): American College of Radiology; 2019.

21. Dill T. Contraindications to magnetic resonance imaging. Heart 2008;94(7):943–8.

22. Dave RB, Stevens KJ, Shivaram GM, et al. Ultrasound-guided musculoskeletal interventions in American football: 18 years of experience. Am J Roentgenol 2014;203(6):W674–83.

23. University of Wisconsin - Madison; Department of Radiology. Upper extremity: MRI protocols.

24. Ciavarra GA, Beltran LS, Obuchowski NA, et al. Comparison of a fast 5-minute shoulder MRI protocol with a standard shoulder MRI protocol: a multiinstitutional multireader study. Am J Roentgenol 2017; 208(4):W146–54.

25. Tuite MJ. Musculoskeletal ultrasound: its impact on your MR practice. Am J Roentgenol 2009;193(3):605–6.

26. Middleton WD, Payne WT, Teefey SA, et al. Sonography and MRI of the shoulder: comparison of patient satisfaction. Am J Roentgenol 2004;183(5):1449–52.

27. Jacobson JA. Shoulder US: anatomy, technique, and scanning pitfalls. Radiology 2011;260(1):6–16.

28. Jacobson JA. Musculoskeletal ultrasound: focused impact on MRI. Am J Roentgenol 2009;193(3):619–27.

29. Jacobson JA. Fundamentals of musculoskeletal ultrasound. 3rd edition. Philadelphia: Elsevier; 2017.

30. Hayes CW, Parellada JA. The magic angle effect in musculoskeletal MR imaging. Top Magn Reson Imaging 1996;8(1):51–6.

31. Motamedi D, Everist BM, Mahanty SR, et al. Pitfalls in shoulder MRI. Part 2: biceps tendon, bursae and cysts, incidental and postsurgical findings, and artifacts. Am J Roentgenol 2014;203(3):508–15.

32. Yablon CM, Bedi A, Morag Y, et al. Ultrasonography of the shoulder with arthroscopic correlation. Clin Sports Med 2013;32(3):391–408.

33. Rutten MJCM, Jager GJ, Blickman JG. US of the rotator cuff: pitfalls, limitations, and artifacts. Radiographics 2007;26(2):589–604.

34. Wohlwend JR, Van Holsbeeck M, Craig J, et al. The association between irregular greater tuberosities and rotator cuff tears: a sonographic study. Am J Roentgenol 1998;171(1):229–33.

35. Chaudhury S, Dines JS, Delos D, et al. Role of fatty infiltration in the pathophysiology and outcomes of rotator cuff tears. Arthritis Care Res 2012;64(1):76–82.

36. Goutallier D, Postel JM, Bernageau J, et al. Fatty muscle degeneration in cuff ruptures. Pre- and postoperative evaluation by CT scan. Clin Orthop Relat Res 1994;304:78–83.

37. Khoury V, Cardinal É, Brassard P. Atrophy and fatty infiltration of the supraspinatus muscle: sonography versus MRI. Am J Roentgenol 2008;190(4):1105–11.

38. Kim HM, Dahiya N, Teefey SA, et al. Location and initiation of degenerative rotator cuff tears: an analysis of three hundred and sixty shoulders. J Bone Joint Surg Am 2010;92(5):1088–96.

39. Mochizuki T, Sugaya H, Uomizu M, et al. Humeral insertion of the supraspinatus and infraspinatus. J Bone Joint Surg Am 2008;90(5):962–9.

40. Lapner PLC, Jiang L, Zhang T, et al. Rotator cuff fatty infiltration and atrophy are associated with functional outcomes in anatomic shoulder arthroplasty clinical orthopaedics and related research. Clin Orthop Relat Res 2015;473:674–82.

41. Kavanagh EC, Koulouris G, Parker L, et al. Does extended-field-of-view sonography improve interrater reliability for the detection of rotator cuff muscle atrophy? Am J Roentgenol 2008;190(1):27–31.

42. Teefey SA, Hasan SA, Middleton WD, et al. Ultrasonography of the rotator cuff. A comparison of ultrasonographic and arthroscopic findings in one hundred consecutive cases. J Bone Jt Surg 2000; 82(4):498–504.

43. van Holsbeeck MT, Kolowich PA, Eyler WR, et al. US depiction of partial-thickness tear of the rotator cuff. Radiology 1995;197(2):443–6.

44. Fotiadou AN, Vlychou M, Papadopoulos P, et al. Ultrasonography of symptomatic rotator cuff tears

compared with MR imaging and surgery. Eur J Radiol 2008;68(1):174–9.

45. De Jesus JO, Parker L, Frangos AJ, et al. Accuracy of MRI, MR arthrography, and ultrasound in the diagnosis of rotator cuff tears: a meta-analysis. Am J Roentgenol 2009;192(6):1701–7.

46. Landin D, Thompson M, Jackson MR. Actions of the biceps brachii at the shoulder: a review. J Clin Med Res 2017;9(8):667–70.

47. Nakata W, Katou S, Fujita A, et al. Biceps pulley: normal anatomy and associated lesions at MR arthrography. Radiographics 2011;31:791–810.

48. Skendzel JG, Jacobson JA, Carpenter JE, et al. Long head of biceps brachii tendon evaluation: accuracy of preoperative ultrasound. Am J Roentgenol 2011;197(4):942–8.

49. Van Holsbeeck M, Strouse PJ. Pictorial essay sonography of the shoulder: evaluation of the subacromial-subdeltoid bursa. Am J Roentgenol 1993;160:561–4.

50. Monu JU V, Pruett S, Vanarthos WJ, et al. Isolated subacromial bursal fluid on MRI of the shoulder in symptomatic patients: correlation with arthroscopic findings. Skeletal Radiol 1994;23(7):529–33.

51. Millett PJ, Gobezie R, Boykin RE. Shoulder osteoarthritis: diagnosis and management. Am Fam Physician 2008;78(5):605–11.

52. Pierrart J, Lefèvre-Colau M-M, Skalli W, et al. New dynamic three-dimensional MRI technique for shoulder kinematic analysis. J Magn Reson Imaging 2014;39:729–34.

53. Beltran LS, Adler R, Stone T, et al. MRI and ultrasound imaging of the shoulder using positional maneuvers. Am J Roentgenol 2015;205(3):W244–54.

54. Bureau NJ, Beauchamp M, Cardinal E, et al. Dynamic sonography evaluation of shoulder impingement syndrome. Am J Roentgenol 2006;187(1):216–20.

55. Harrison AK, Flatow EL. Subacromial impingement syndrome. J Am Acad Orthop Surg 2011;19(11):701–8.

56. Gleason PD, Beall DP, Sanders TG, et al. The transverse humeral ligament. Am J Sports Med 2006;34(1):72–7.

57. Armstrong A, Teefey SA, Wu T, et al. The efficacy of ultrasound in the diagnosis of long head of the biceps tendon pathology. J Shoulder Elbow Surg 2006;15(1):7–11.

58. Khil EK, Cha JG, Yi JS, et al. Detour sign in the diagnosis of subluxation of the long head of the biceps tendon with arthroscopic correlation. Br J Radiol 2017;90(1070):20160375.

59. Dubrow S, Shishani Y, Streit J, et al. Diagnostic accuracy in detecting tears in the proximal biceps tendon using standard nonenhancing shoulder MRI. Open Access J Sports Med 2014;5:81–7.

60. Prickett WD, Teefey SA, Galatz LM, et al. Accuracy of ultrasound imaging of the rotator cuff in shoulders that are painful postoperatively. J Bone Joint Surg Am 2003;85-A(6):1084–9.

61. Sofka CM, Adler RS. Sonographic evaluation of shoulder arthroplasty. Am J Roentgenol 2003;180(4):1117–20.

62. Westermann RW, Schick C, Graves CM, et al. What does a shoulder MRI cost the consumer? Clin Orthop Relat Res 2017;475(3):580–4.

63. Hirahara AM, Panero AJ. A guide to ultrasound of the shoulder, part 1: coding and reimbursement. Am J Orthop (Belle Mead NJ) 2016;45(3):176–82.

64. Centers for Medicare & Medicaid Services. CY 2019 physician fee schedule. Available at: CMS.gov. Accessed August 7, 2019.

65. Parker L, Nazarian LN, Carrino JA, et al. Musculoskeletal imaging: Medicare use, costs, and potential for cost substitution. J Am Coll Radiol 2008;5(3):182–8.

66. Singh H, Debakey ME, Sittig DF. Reducing unnecessary shoulder MRI examinations within a capitated health care system: a potential role for shoulder ultrasound. J Am Coll Radiol 2016;13(7):780–7.

67. Gyftopoulos S, Guja KE, Subhas N, et al. Cost-effectiveness of magnetic resonance imaging versus ultrasound for the detection of symptomatic full-thickness supraspinatus tendon tears. J Shoulder Elbow Surg 2017;26(12):2067–77.

68. Gyftopoulos S, Abballe V, Virk MS, et al. Comparison between image-guided and landmark-based glenohumeral joint injections for the treatment of adhesive capsulitis: a cost-effectiveness study. Am J Roentgenol 2018;210(6):1279–87.

69. Chen CPC, Lew HL, Hsu C-C. Ultrasound-guided glenohumeral joint injection using the posterior approach. Am J Phys Med Rehabil 2015;94(12):e117–8.

70. Wu T, Song HX, Dong Y, et al. Ultrasound-guided versus blind subacromial-subdeltoid bursa injection in adults with shoulder pain: a systematic review and meta-analysis. Semin Arthritis Rheum 2015;45(3):374–8.

71. Hayes CW, Conway WF. Calcium hydroxyapatite deposition disease. Radiographics 2013;10(6):1031–48.

72. Lee KS, Rosas HG. Musculoskeletal ultrasound: how to treat calcific tendinitis of the rotator cuff by ultrasound-guided single-needle lavage technique. Am J Roentgenol 2010;195(3):W213.

73. Vignesh KN, McDowal A, Simunovic N, et al. Efficacy of ultrasound-guided percutaneous needle treatment of calcific tendinitis. Am J Roentgenol 2015;204(1):148–52.

74. Burke CJ, Adler RS. Ultrasound-guided percutaneous tendon treatments. Am J Roentgenol 2016;207(3):495–506.

75. Nwaka O, Miller T, Slaughter A, et al. Volume and movement affecting flow of injectate between the biceps tendon sheath and glenohumeral joint: a cadaveric study. AJR Am J Roentgenol 2016;206:373–7.

Printed and bound by CPI Group (UK) Ltd, Croydon, CR0 4YY

08/05/2025

01864694-0018